MW00585761

IMAGING IN PARKINSON'S DISEASE

IMAGING IN PARKINSON'S DISEASE

EDITED BY

David Eidelberg, MD

DIRECTOR, CENTER FOR NEUROSCIENCES

THE FEINSTEIN INSTITUTE FOR MEDICAL RESEARCH

NORTH SHORE-LIJ HEALTH SYSTEM

MANHASSET, NY

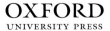

OXFORD
UNIVERSITY PRESS

Oxford University Press, Inc., publishes works that further Oxford University's objective of excellence
in research, scholarship, and education.

Oxford   New York
Auckland   Cape Town   Dar es Salaam   Hong Kong   Karachi
Kuala Lumpur   Madrid   Melbourne   Mexico City   Nairobi
New Delhi   Shanghai   Taipei   Toronto

With offices in
Argentina   Austria   Brazil   Chile   Czech Republic   France   Greece
Guatemala   Hungary   Italy   Japan   Poland   Portugal   Singapore
South Korea   Switzerland   Thailand   Turkey   Ukraine   Vietnam

Copyright © 2012 by Oxford University Press, Inc.

Published by Oxford University Press, Inc.
198 Madison Avenue, New York, New York 10016
www.oup.com

Oxford is a registered trademark of Oxford University Press

ISBN-13 978-0-19-539348-4

Cataloging-in-Publication data is on file with the Library of Congress

This material is not intended to be, and should not be considered, a substitute for medical or other professional advice.
Treatment for the conditions described in this material is highly dependent on the individual circumstances. And, while this
material is designed to offer accurate information with respect to the subject matter covered and to be current as of the time it
was written, research and knowledge about medical and health issues is constantly evolving and dose schedules for medications
are being revised continually, with new side effects recognized and accounted for regularly. Readers must therefore always
check the product information and clinical procedures with the most up-to-date published product information and data
sheets provided by the manufacturers and the most recent codes of conduct and safety regulation. The publisher and the
authors make no representations or warranties to readers, express or implied, as to the accuracy or completeness of this material.
Without limiting the foregoing, the publisher and the authors make no representations or warranties as to the accuracy or
efficacy of the drug dosages mentioned in the material. The authors and the publisher do not accept, and expressly disclaim,
any responsibility for any liability, loss or risk that may be claimed or incurred as a consequence of the use and/or application
of any of the contents of this material.

9 8 7 6 5 4 3 2 1
Printed in China
on acid-free paper

This book is dedicated in memory of my father, Professor Shlomo Eidelberg (1918-2010), who taught me how to think critically and love life at the same time.

Upon Israel and its rabbis and their students	עַל יִשְׂרָאֵל וְעַל רַבָּנָן וְעַל תַּלְמִידֵיהוֹן
and upon all their student's students	וְעַל כָּל תַּלְמִידֵי תַלְמִידֵיהוֹן.
and upon all those who engage in the Torah	וְעַל כָּל מָאן דְּעָסְקִין בְּאוֹרַיְתָא.
here and in all other places,	דִּי בְאַתְרָא הָדֵין וְדִי בְּכָל אֲתַר וַאֲתַר.
May they and you have much peace	יְהֵא לְהוֹן וּלְכוֹן שְׁלָמָא רַבָּא
grace and kindness and mercy and long life	חִנָּא וְחִסְדָּא וְרַחֲמֵי וְחַיֵּי אֲרִיכֵי
and plentiful nourishment and salvation	וּמְזוֹנֵי רְוִיחֵי וּפוּרְקָנָא
from before their Father in Heaven;	מִן קֳדָם אֲבוּהוֹן דְּבִשְׁמַיָּא
and say, Amen.	וְאִמְרוּ אָמֵן

(From the Kaddish D'Rabbanan, circa 200 CE)

PREFACE

In recent years, a series of advances in brain imaging technology have dramatically expanded the frontiers of human investigation in the neurosciences. Quantitative radiotracer imaging with positron emission tomography (PET) and single photon emission tomography (SPECT), once an exotic and methodologically demanding approach, has become commonplace and is now used routinely in patient-oriented research. Moreover, highly innovative magnetic resonance (MR) techniques have been (and continue to be) developed to provide unique information concerning structure-function relationships in the brain under normal and pathological conditions. In this regard, rigorous imaging techniques to assess changes in regional brain function in individual subjects have been successfully used in the study of the natural history of brain diseases and their response to treatment. Of note, these applications have generally focused on the mapping of local activation responses recorded during task performance or pharmacologic activation. Lately, however, resting state measurements of regional cerebral blood flow and metabolism – as well as fluctuations in brain oxygen level-dependent (BOLD) signal – have gained currency as providing a potentially simple means of quantifying disease progression and the therapeutic response.

The utility of these new imaging techniques has been further enhanced by parallel developments in computational methodology. The implementation of fast and unbiased software routines for voxel-by-voxel whole brain searches, as well as for the measurement of neural activity in pre-specified anatomical regions using probabilistic atlases, has impacted greatly on the accuracy and efficiency of imaging-based hypothesis testing. Additionally, mass-univariate methods have enabled hypothesis-generating analyses of scans from disease and control populations, as well as the comparison of imaging abnormalities involving human subjects with analogous findings from experimental disease models. Moreover, in recent years, complementary multivariate methods have been developed to identify disease-related changes at the system level. This is highly relevant to the study of degenerative diseases such as Parkinson's disease, in which neural dysfunction occurs not only at the known sites of pathology, but also in interconnected spatially removed brain regions. In addition to providing the ability to characterize topographically distinct large-scale brain networks associated with brain disease, multivariate approaches are well-suited for forward application, i.e. the prospective measurement of the activity of known networks in individual subjects and scans. Such voxel-wise computations, unthinkable a decade ago, permit the screening of new patient cohorts for a pre-defined disease topography, or the study of preclinical subjects such as those found to be genetically at risk. Prospective single case network computations are also crucial for the evaluation of subjects undergoing repeat scanning as part of natural history or experimental intervention studies. In effect, network analysis reduces the complex information embedded in a subject's brain image to one or more system-related quantitative measurements that capture the disease process at discrete time points or under different treatment conditions. Overall, these technical developments have set the stage for the remarkable advances achieved using imaging for the investigation of Parkinson's disease and related disorders.

In addition to contributing substantively to the current understanding of the anatomical and functional changes that underlie Parkinson's disease, imaging has had a profound impact on the clinical investigation of this disorder. As emphasized repeatedly in this volume, modern imaging tools have had a transformative role in the following key areas: differential diagnosis, assessment of disease progression, and evaluation of novel therapies.

Differential Diagnosis: Neurodegenerative disorders that manifest by signs and symptoms of parkinsonism constitute a group of frequently diagnosed conditions in neurological clinics. Current practice relies on clinical assessment and follow-up for the diagnosis and treatment of these disorders. However, postmortem studies indicate that diagnosis is only 75-80% accurate for patients believed clinically to have classical idiopathic Parkinson's disease. Differentiating between parkinsonian disorders on clinical grounds alone has proven unsatisfactory, particularly early after symptom onset. In approximately one-third of patients, the initial diagnosis changes by the fifth year of symptoms.

Indeed, reasonable diagnostic accuracy is achieved only after long-term serial assessment by a trained movement disorders specialist. As discussed in detail in Chapters 7 and 18, accurate early diagnosis is important for both prognosis and the formulation of an appropriate treatment strategy. Thus, the characterization of robust disease-specific biomarkers can improve the accuracy of differential diagnosis in patients with recent-onset symptoms as well as those with unclear clinical presentations.

Disease Progression: In addition to aiding in differential diagnosis, imaging biomarkers can be identified that are sensitive to the pathological processes that underlie disease progression. In Parkinson's disease, such biomarkers can be used in conjunction with clinical assessment to evaluate the efficacy of potential disease-modifying interventions. Despite similar underlying pathology, the various phenotypic subtypes of Parkinson's disease, such as the tremor predominant and the akinetic-rigid forms can progress at different rates. Even within clinical subtypes, progression in individual patients can vary depending on demographic factors such as age of onset. In clinical trials of new therapeutic agents, these differences can make the quantitative assessment of progression rate quite challenging if based solely upon standardized clinical ratings. Nonetheless, imaging-based progression biomarkers can provide a complementary and accurate means of gauging disease progression in natural history studies, neuroprotective trials, and potentially also as part of follow-up clinical assessment.

Therapeutics Assessment: Lastly, the past decade has seen major advances in the development of experimental therapies for Parkinson's disease and other neurodegenerative disorders. Clinical trials of novel interventions for these conditions have increasingly incorporated quantitative imaging outcome measures, notably the use of PET indices of striatal dopaminergic function, to assess cell-based therapies such as neural transplantation procedures (Chapter 16). More recently, metabolic network measurements have been used to evaluate the outcome of early phase gene therapy trials in advanced Parkinson's disease patients (see Chapter 17). The objective nature of these imaging assessments and their enhanced statistical power can serve to expedite the evaluation of new antiparkinsonian therapies. Moreover, image-based diagnostic algorithms (Chapter 7 and 18) can be used *a priori* to identify subjects with clinically similar "look-a-like' conditions who are likely not to response to the treatment in question.

Given these exciting developments in imaging applications for the study of Parkinson's disease, we believe this compilation to be a timely addition to the growing body of literature on this topic. The current need for such a volume was expressed uniformly by movement disorders experts, clinical investigators, and basic scientists when canvassed informally before the start of this project. Interestingly, the specific reasoning varied depending on the individual's research orientation, which led to a fascinating Rashomon effect. With very few exceptions, the basic science investigators believed that a book was necessary because of the recent proliferation of patient studies with too few well-articulated scientific hypotheses. By contrast, the clinical specialists and patient-oriented researchers stated that there have not been enough human studies to make sense of the many experimental hypotheses that have circulated in recent years. Which perception is correct? We'll leave that to the reader to decide.

TABLE OF CONTENTS

ACKNOWLEDGMENT

I thank the contributors who dedicated countless hours to this project merely for their "love of the game." Their enthusiasm and dedication are made clear by the consistently thoughtful and comprehensive overviews of the rather challenging topics that appear in this volume. I am deeply appreciative of the support offered by my colleagues at The Feinstein Institute for Medical Research, and especially Dr. Kevin J. Tracey, who encouraged the project despite its substantial time requirements. The members of the Center for Neurosciences at Feinstein were spectacular in their willingness to help. In particular, Drs. Vijay Dhawan and Chris C. Tang provided many valuable comments and suggestions on a variety of methodological issues. I am very grateful to Ms. Toni Fitzpatrick for her tireless editorial assistance, without which this work would certainly not have happened. Her professionalism at all phases of the project was truly inspirational. Finally, words cannot describe the seemingly endless patience and support offered by my editor Mr. Craig Panner (and assistant editors Mr. David D'Adonna and Ms. Kathryn Winder) at Oxford University Press. The team made producing this book an enjoyable and worthwhile experience.

On a personal note, I owe a profound debt of gratitude to my wife Hela and daughter Isabela who lived through this project. I can only hope that this work proves worthy of their unquestioning dedication and commitment.

David Eidelberg
Manhasset, NY
April 2011

CONTRIBUTORS

Angelo Antonini, M.D., Ph.D.
Azienda Ospedaliera
Istituti Clinici Di Perfezionamento
Parkinson Institute Milan
Department of Neuroscience
Milan, Italy

Anna L. Bartels
Department of Neurology
Groningen University Hospital
Groningen, The Netherlands

Daniela Berg, M.D.
Institute for Medical Genetics
Tübingen, Germany

Ferdinand Binkofski, Ph.D.
Department of Neurology
University Hospital Schleswig-Holstein
Lübeck, Germany

Nicolaas I. Bohnen, M.D., Ph.D.
Functional Neuroimaging
Cognitive and Mobility Laboratory
Departments of Radiology and Neurology
The University of Michigan
Ann Arbor, MI

David J. Brooks, M.D.
Division of Neuroscience and MRC Clinical
    Sciences Centre
Faculty of Medicine
Hammersmith Hospital
Imperial College London
London, UK

Maren Carbon, M.D.
Center for Neurosciences
The Feinstein Institute for Medical Research
North Shore-LIJ Health System
Manhasset, NY

Alain Dagher, Ph.D.
McConnell Brain Imaging Centre
Montreal Neurological Institute and Hospital
McGill University
Montreal, Quebec
Canada

Vijay Dhawan, Ph.D.
Center for Neurosciences
The Feinstein Institute for Medical Research
North Shore-LIJ Health System
Manhasset, NY

David Eidelberg, M.D.
Center for Neurosciences
The Feinstein Institute for Medical Research
North Shore-LIJ Health System
Manhasset, NY

Andrew Feigin, M.D.
Center for Neurosciences
The Feinstein Institute for Medical Research
North Shore-LIJ Health System
Manhasset, NY

Kirk A. Frey, M.D., Ph.D.
Departments of Neurology and Radiology
Director, Positron Emission Tomography (PET)
    Neuropharmacology Section
Co-Director, Movement Disorders Clinic
Division Chief, Nuclear Medicine
The University of Michigan
Ann Arbor, MI

Biju Gopalakrishnan, M.B.B.S, M.D., D.M.
University Hospital
Faculty of Medicine/UBC Site
Vancouver, British Columbia
Canada

Shigeki Hirano, M.D.
Department of Neurology,
    Chiba University School of Medicine
Chiba, Japan
Molecular Neuroimaging Group,
    Molecular Imaging Center,
        National Institute of Radiological Sciences
Chiba, Japan

Ioannis U. Isaias, M.D.
Parkinson Institute
Milan, Italy

Klaus L. Leenders, M.D., Ph.D.
Department of Neurology
Groningen University Hospital
Groningen, The Netherlands

Yilong Ma, Ph.D.
Center for Neurosciences
The Feinstein Institute for Medical Research
North Shore-LIJ Health System
Manhasset, NY

Paul J. Mattis, Ph.D.
Center for Neurosciences
The Feinstein Institute for Medical Research
North Shore-LIJ Health System
Manhasset, NY

Martin Niethammer, M.D., Ph.D.
Center for Neurosciences
The Feinstein Institute for Medical Research
North Shore-LIJ Health System
Manhasset, NY

Shichun Peng, Ph.D.
Center for Neurosciences
The Feinstein Institute for Medical Research
North Shore-LIJ Health System
Manhasset, NY

Paola Piccini, M.D.
MRC Clinical Sciences Centre and Division of
    Neurosciences
Imperial College London
Hammersmith Hospital
London, UK

Werner Poewe, M.D.
Chairman Department of Neurology
Medical University Innsbruck
Innsbruck, Austria

Mario Politis
MRC Clinical Sciences Centre and Division of
    Neurosciences
Imperial College London
Hammersmith Hospital
London, UK

Kathleen L. Poston, M.D.
Department of Neurology and Neurological Sciences
Stanford University
Stanford, CA

L.K. Prashanth , M.B.B.S., D.M.(Neurology)
Movement Disorders Center
Toronto Western Hospital
Toronto

Kathrin Reetz, M.D.
Department of Neurology
University Hospital Schleswig-Holstein
Campus Lübeck,
Lübeck, Germany

Christoph Scherfler, M.D.
Department of Neurology
Innsbruck Medical University
Innsbruck, Austria

A. Jon Stoessl, M.D.
University Hospital
Faculty of Medicine/UBC Site
Vancouver, British Columbia
Canada

Antonio P. Strafella, M.D., Ph.D.
Toronto Western Hospital
Toronto, Ontario
Canada

Chris C. Tang, M.D.
Center for Neurosciences
The Feinstein Institute for Medical Research
North Shore-LIJ Health System
Manhasset, NY

IMAGING IN PARKINSON'S DISEASE

1

DOPAMINERGIC IMAGING IN PARKINSON'S DISEASE: PET

Biju Gopalakrishnan and A. Jon Stoessl

INTRODUCTION

Parkinson's disease (PD) is characterized pathologically by the loss of dopamine (DA) neurons in the substantia nigra (SN) pars compacta. The neuronal loss is usually asymmetric and, when it reaches around 50%, patients develop clinical signs consisting mainly of a combination of resting tremor, rigidity, and bradykinesia (Fearnley and Lees 1991). Later, dementia, autonomic dysfunction, and bulbar dysfunction also develop in a variable proportion of patients. Positron emission tomography (PET) is a functional imaging technique utilized in PD largely to assess the integrity of the nigrostriatal system.

FUNDAMENTALS OF PET

PET imaging is particularly useful for imaging the distribution and metabolism of small molecules in vivo. The molecule of interest is labeled with a positron-emitting radionuclide; the molecular probe is then injected into the subject and its distribution can be imaged in a quantitative fashion, based upon the detection of pairs of photons (511 KeV) traveling in opposite directions that result from the annihilation of a positron with an electron. Any isotope that decays by releasing positrons can be used for PET imaging. Those most commonly used include ^{11}C, ^{13}N, ^{15}O, and ^{18}F (Williams 2008).

DOPAMINE SYNTHESIS AND FUNCTION

Dopamine is synthesized in the terminals of the dopaminergic neurons. The first step is the conversion of tyrosine to L-3,4-dihydroxyphenylalanine (L-dopa) by the enzyme tyrosine hydroxylase. L-dopa is then decarboxylated by L-aromatic amino acid decarboxylase (L-AADC) to dopamine. Dopamine is then taken up into presynaptic vesicles

via the vesicular monoamine transporter type 2 (VMAT2). This dopamine is released into the synaptic cleft following depolarization by an action potential.

The action of dopamine is terminated in one of three ways: (1) catechol-O-methyltransferase (COMT) mediated conversion; (2) monoamine oxidase (MAO) mediated catabolism; or (3) reuptake into the presynaptic terminal by the plasmalemmal dopamine transporter (DAT). Dopamine that has been taken back up into the nerve terminal can then be used again or can be metabolized by intracellular MAO to 3,4-dihydroxyphenylacetic acid (DOPAC). DOPAC is converted to homovanillic acid (HVA) by COMT.

Dopamine is thought to have multiple functions in the human brain. It modulates motor activity through the direct and indirect basal-ganglia-thalamocortical loops, implicated in the motor dysfunction of PD. Dopamine is also considered important in human thought processing and decision-making ability, as evidenced by its role in impulse control disorders, addiction, and related issues, via its activity in the mesolimbic and mesocortical pathways. Many psychiatric disorders including schizophrenia are linked to alterations in dopamine function. In PD, dopamine and its metabolites are decreased, as are DAT and VMAT2 density.

PET TRACERS

Positron emission tomography (PET) is a radiotracer-based method that helps in assessing the in vivo function of the dopaminergic and other systems in PD. PET can also be used to assess the progression of dopamine deficiency in vivo.

The usual methods for assessing presynaptic dopamine function by PET are: (1) [^{18}F]fluoro-L-dopa (FD), used to study the uptake of levodopa and its decarboxylation to dopamine (fluorodopamine; FDA) and the subsequent storage of FDA in synaptic vesicles; (2) a variety of [^{18}F]

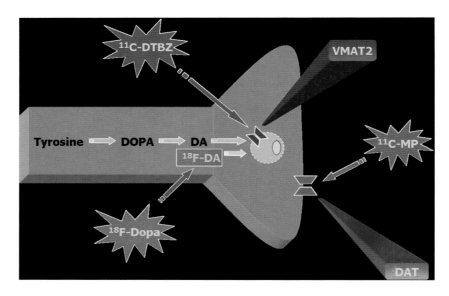

Figure 1 6-[18F]fluoro-L-dopa (18FD) uptake represents the striatal uptake of levodopa, AADC (aromatic amino acid decarboxylase) activity, and presynaptic vesicular storage; 11C-dihydrotetrabenazine (DTBZ) labels the vesicular monoamine transporter type 2 (VMAT2), which is responsible for pumping monoamines including dopamine from the cytosol into presynaptic vesicles, and in the striatum, is predominantly associated with dopaminergic terminals; 11C-d-*threo*-methylphenidate (MP) labels the plasmalemmal dopamine transporter (DAT), which mediates the reuptake of dopamine (DA) from the synaptic cleft into the dopaminergic terminal. 18F-DA = [18F]fluoro-dopamine; L-DOPA = L-3,4-dihydroxyphenylalanine; TH = tyrosine hydroxylase. (Nandhagopal et al. 2008b)

and [11C] labeled antagonists can be used to assess DAT density; and (3) [11C]dihydrotetrabenazine (DTBZ) is used to measure the VMAT2 density.

For assessing postsynaptic dopamine receptor binding sites at D_1 receptors [11C]SCH 23390 and at D_2 receptors [11C]raclopride or [18F]fallypride are used (Au et al. 2005).

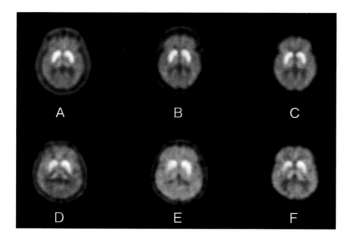

Figure 2 Striatal uptake of presynaptic dopaminergic PET tracers in a healthy subject and in Parkinson's disease (PD). Upper panel (A–C): Striatal uptake of presynaptic dopaminergic PET tracers in a healthy subject. Lower panel (D–F): In PD, reduced tracer uptake is asymmetric and is more pronounced in putamen than in caudate. FD = 6-[18F] fluoro-L-dopa; DTBZ = [11C]-dihydrotetrabenazine; MP = [11C]- d-threo-methylphenidate. (Nandhagopal et al. 2008b)

PET IMAGING IN PD

Patients are scanned in a tomograph following the administration of a radiotracer chosen to optimally target the purpose of the study. Single- or multiple-tracer studies can be performed. In most centers, the predominant use of PET is for research purposes, although PET and other functional imaging techniques may on occasion be helpful for diagnosis.

PRESYNAPTIC FUNCTION

In idiopathic Parkinson's disease, markers of VMAT2, DAT, and FD all show an asymmetric reduction of radioactivity, with a rostrocaudal gradient, such that the caudate nucleus is relatively preserved while there is a progressive reduction of uptake from anterior to posterior putamen. DAT binding may be the most sensitive marker of early disease. Reduced DAT binding is in part due to the loss of dopaminergic nerve terminals, but may also reflect downregulation of the DAT in early disease, in an effort to preserve synaptic DA levels. FD uptake tends to be less affected than DTBZ or DAT binding in early disease. This may in part reflect a compensatory upregulation of decarboxlase activity in surviving dopaminergic nerve terminals, as well as expression of decarboxylase in non-dopaminergic neurons (Brown et al. 1999; Lee et al. 2000; Moore et al. 2003).

F-DOPA

The usual technique for PET measurement of FD uptake is to acquire radioactivity counts over the first 90–120 minutes following tracer injection and to then assess either the striatum-to-background ratio or an influx constant (K_i). The latter is determined by relating radioactivity in the region of interest (striatum) to the integrated input function, derived from either metabolite-corrected arterial plasma or from a reference tissue region such as the occipital cortex. FD uptake determined over 90–120 minutes predominantly reflects decarboxylation to FDA and storage in synaptic vesicles, and the analysis is based on an assumption of unidirectional transport (Martin et al. 1989). However, if longer scanning times are used, FDA egresses from the nerve terminal and is then subject to metabolism (Holden et al. 1997). This can be used to advantage to estimate DA turnover, which is increased early in PD and continues to increase with disease progression (Sossi et al. 2002).

The pattern of presynaptic dopaminergic FD uptake in the parkinsonian brain is in striking contrast to the normal brain. Reduction in FD uptake is greater in the putamen compared to the caudate. Patients with bilateral disease show corresponding asymmetric reductions in FD uptake in both striata. Patients with unilateral disease show reductions predominantly in the contralateral striatum, but the clinically unaffected striatum is also involved. Reductions of FD uptake correlate with bradykinesia and rigidity (Vingerhoets et al. 1997), but not with severity of tremor (Doder et al. 2003).

DOPAMINE TRANSPORTER (DAT)

DAT is a 620-amino acid protein with 12 α-helical hydrophobic transmembrane domains, two to four extracellular glycosylation sites, and up to five intracellular phosphorylation sites. It is found exclusively in DA axons and dendrites. DAT levels correlate with striatal DA concentrations. DAT binding is accordingly considered a potential marker of DA nerve terminal density. DAT ligands used in PET include several tropane (cocaine-like) analogs such as [^{11}C]-2-h-carbomethoxy-3-h-[4-fluorophenyl] tropane (CFT), [^{18}F]CFT, [^{11}C]RTI-32, and [^{11}C]altropane, as well as the non-tropane [^{11}C]d-threo-methylphenidate [MP]. DAT binding correlates with the clinical severity of PD (Seibyl et al. 1995). The potential disadvantage of DAT is that its regulation in response to compensatory changes and pharmacological therapy may render it less suitable as a marker of disease progression,

although this is almost certainly true of FD as well as and to a lesser extent for VMAT2. DAT binding is affected by normal ageing (De Keyser, Ebinger, and Vauquelin 1990; Volkow et al. 1996), and its interpretation therefore requires the appropriate correction.

VESICULAR MONOAMINE TRANSPORTER TYPE 2 (VMAT2)

VMAT2 is a 515-amino acid protein responsible for the uptake of cytoplasmic monoamines into synaptic vesicles. Tetrabenazine binds to VMAT2 and blocks the uptake of monoamines into the vesicles. [^{11}C]dihydrotetrabenazine (DTBZ) has been used in humans to study the integrity of striatal monoaminergic nerve terminal density. VMAT2 is thought to not be regulated by conditions affecting dopamine metabolism, and its expression is not subject to pharmacological regulation (Vander Borght et al. 1995; Wilson and Kish 1996). However, the effects of aging on DTBZ binding are still not clear. Furthermore, DTBZ binding is in fact subject to competition from intravesicular DA (Fuente-Fernandez et al. 2003). Thus, marked depletion of vesicular DA can lead to false elevations in VMAT2 binding, which may be reversed following replenishment with exogenous L-dopa (Fuente-Fernandez et al. 2009). One important disadvantage of VMAT is that it is not specific for DA; however, the majority of binding in the striatum is to dopaminergic neurons.

ASSESSMENT OF POSTSYNAPTIC DA FUNCTION

D_1 and D_2 receptors can also be evaluated using PET with selective radiotracers. [^{18}F]fallypride, [^{11}C]FLB-457, and [^{11}C]epidepride have a high affinity and can therefore be used to assess extrastriatal D_2 receptors. [^{11}C]raclopride (RAC) has a lower affinity and is therefore used to assess striatal DA receptor availability. RAC competes with endogenous DA for in vivo binding to D_2 receptors, and changes in binding, especially in response to interventions, can be used to estimate changes in synaptic DA concentration (Laruelle 2000; Seeman, Guan, and Niznik 1989). Tracer binding is also dictated by age and, to some extent, the stage of PD and DA replacement therapy (DRT). Increased binding is seen in the more affected putamen in early (untreated) PD, but in advanced PD and with chronic DRT, normalization of binding in the putamen and decreased binding in the caudate are seen (Antonini et al. 1997). D_1 binding assessed using [^{11}C]SCH 23390 PET is normal in PD but may be decreased in multiple system atrophy (Shinotoh et al. 1993).

EARLY PD AND DISEASE PROGRESSION

The symptoms of PD typically appear when patients have lost about 80% of striatal dopamine content, or about 50% of nigral dopamine neurons. Presymptomatic stages can be detected using PET to assess DAT binding. Thus, PET imaging of asymptomatic carriers of LRRK2 mutations showed normal FD uptake and abnormal DAT binding, with an intermediate degree of reduction in VMAT2 binding (Adams et al. 2005; Nandhagopal et al. 2008a). Even though the detection of PD at a preclinical stage may be of limited clinical relevance at this time owing to the lack of established neuroprotective therapies, the ability to detect such changes may be of potential benefit in the future as such therapies become available. Detection of preclinical abnormalities may also be of benefit in reassigning phenotype in individuals who come from families with inherited PD. In situations where it has not yet been identified, this may assist in the identification of the causative mutation.

The progression of PD can be assessed using PET, and several studies have demonstrated the previously noted anteroposterior gradient in the striatum and, in the early stages, greater involvement of the putamen contralateral to the affected limb. Longitudinal studies have also shown that the anteroposterior gradient of dopamine denervation is maintained throughout the course of the illness. However, the asymmetry tends to disappear over time (Nandhagopal et al. 2009). Preservation of the anteroposterior gradient is compatible with the view that those factors responsible for disease initiation (which result in differential involvement of DA fibers projecting to the posterior putamen) are likely different from those contributing to disease progression (which affect all striatal subregions to an equal degree). FD PET techniques in various studies have shown similar rates of disease progression, with a mean annual reduction of approximately 5%–10% in the putamen (Morrish et al. 1998; Nurmi et al. 2001).

Dyskinesia arises as a drug-induced complication that emerges over the course of the disease. As time progresses, dopaminergic nerve terminals are lost and with that, the capacity to store dopamine. However, in some patients, dyskinesias can appear early and may not correlate with DA terminal density as evaluated with FD uptake. By performing longer (4-hour) scans with FD, it is possible to demonstrate that younger PD patients have a higher dopamine

turnover, thereby potentially contributing to larger swings in synaptic dopamine levels (Sossi et al. 2006). Dopamine turnover is also inversely correlated to DAT expression—thus the greater the degree of DAT downregulation (beyond the degree of DAT reduction explained by nerve terminal loss), the greater the dopamine turnover (Sossi et al. 2007), and the increased probability of levodopa-induced dyskinesias (Troiano et al. 2009). This is further elaborated in the following section and in Chapter 14.

STUDIES OF DOPAMINE RELEASE

As [^{11}C]raclopride is subject to competition from dopamine, changes in its binding can be used to infer alterations in DA release in response to a variety of interventions. This can be used to study the motor complications of levodopa therapy. In patients with a stable response to levodopa, a short lived change (<4 hours) in [^{11}C]raclopride binding following oral levodopa is associated with the later development of motor fluctuations, whereas subjects with prolonged (4 hours or more) changes in binding maintain a stable response to medication for at least three years (Fuente-Fernandez et al. 2001). Similarly, changes in [^{11}C]raclopride binding potential are of relatively greater magnitude and less sustained in patients with levodopa-induced dyskinesias (Fuente-Fernandez et al. 2004). These findings are entirely compatible with increased DA turnover demonstrated on prolonged FD scans. Taking these observations together, one must conclude that, irrespective of any changes downstream to DA receptors (which may occur secondarily), presynaptic alterations in the central pharmacokinetics of levodopa/dopamine play an important role in the development of these complications.

In addition to the demonstration of sensitized levodopa-induced DA release in the dorsal striatum of dyskinetic PD patients, [^{11}C]raclopride PET has also been used to demonstrate enhanced levodopa-induced DA release in the ventral striatum of patients with the dopamine disequilibrium syndrome (Evans et al. 2006) and in response to a gambling task in patients with dopamine agonist-associated pathological gambling (Steeves et al. 2009).

The sensitized responses in the ventral striatum are in keeping with the known role of dopamine in signaling reward or reward expectation in this structure, and similar changes can be seen during the performance of tasks associated with monetary reward (Koepp et al. 1998).

In keeping with the importance of dopamine release for signaling reward expectation, [^{11}C]raclopride PET has also been used to demonstrate that the placebo effect in PD can be attributed to the release of dopamine in the striatum. In the original study, patients were scanned in open baseline condition and on four occasions following injection of the drug—either apomorphine (a dopamine agonist; 3/4 injections) or placebo (1/4 injections). There was a substantial release of dopamine following injection of the placebo (approximately 17% decrease in [^{11}C]raclopride binding, corresponding to a change of 200% or more in extracellular dopamine concentration and comparable to the response to amphetamine in healthy subjects with an intact dopamine system) (Fuente-Fernandez et al. 2001). In that study, dopamine release in the motor areas of the striatum (putamen and dorsal caudate) was greater in those patients who reported subjective improvement in their symptoms following the placebo injection. As improvement in clinical symptoms can be seen as a very powerful reward to patients with disability, the finding led to the suggestion that activation of mesolimbic dopamine pathways might be a necessary underpinning of placebo responses in conditions other than Parkinson's (Fuente-Fernandez, Schulzer, and Stoessl 2004; Lidstone et al. 2005). This appears to be the case for pain and depression. More recently, we have used [^{11}C]raclopride PET to assess the relationship between the strength of expectation (i.e., the probability of receiving active medication) and placebo-induced dopamine release. Interestingly, we found that placebo-induced dopamine release was seen when the expected probability of receiving active medication was 75%, but not at higher or lower probabilities (Lidstone et al. 2010).

Dopamine release, as shown by reduced [^{11}C]raclopride binding, has also been demonstrated in healthy controls and PD patients during pre-learned sequential motor tasks (Goerendt et al. 2003), during the performance of a set-shift task (Monchi, Ko, and Strafella 2006), and during performance of a spatial working memory task (Sawamoto et al. 2008).

PET FOR DIAGNOSIS OF PD

PET or other functional imaging techniques such as SPECT should reliably detect evidence of dopaminergic dysfunction by the time symptoms appear and may therefore be helpful for differentiating between essential tremor and PD. However, the more challenging diagnostic problem is the differentiation between typical PD and atypical forms of parkinsonism such as multiple system atrophy (MSA) or progressive supranuclear palsy (PSP). The demonstration of dopamine dysfunction without the rostrocaudal gradient typical of PD (i.e., without relative sparing of the anterior striatum) may be suggestive of one of these diagnoses, as may the concurrent demonstration of reduced dopamine D$_2$ receptor binding. However, this is not entirely reliable, as a pattern of presynaptic dysfunction virtually identical to that of PD may be seen in MSA (Antonini et al. 1997). Scans of glucose metabolism may actually provide greater capacity to differentiate between PD and atypical syndromes (Eckert et al. 2005), as may the demonstration of cardiac sympathetic denervation (typical of PD, not seen in MSA where sympathetic dysfunction is preganglionic) (Braune et al. 1999). These applications are discussed elsewhere in this volume.

PET AND NON-MOTOR SYMPTOMS OF PD

It is now increasingly appreciated that non-motor complications of PD significantly affect the quality of life of patients as well as caregivers. The important non-motor complications are cognitive decline, autonomic dysfunction, psychiatric problems, pain, and sleep disturbances (Barone et al. 2009). Some of the observations made with PET in PD patients include the following:

(1) Preferential decrease in occipital glucose metabolism (Minoshima et al. 2001), widespread decreases in cholinesterase activity (Bohnen et al. 2003), and variably increased amyloid deposition (Edison 2008; Gomperts 2008; Maetzler 2009) in cases of PD with dementia; cognitive abilities are associated with dopaminergic integrity of the caudate nucleus (Rinne 2000)

(2) Reduced dopamine/noradrenaline transporter binding in the ventral striatum, thalamus, and locus coeruleus (Remy 2005) and increased serotonin transporter binding in depressed PD patients (Boileau et al. 2008)

(3) Increased dopamine release in the ventral striatum in response to exogenous levodopa administration (Evans et al. 2006) or gambling (Steeves et al. 2009) in patients with impulse control disorders

(4) DA denervation in the posterior putamen in cases of isolated REM sleep behavior disorder (RBD) (Albin et al. 2000) and inverse relationship of REM sleep duration to lateral and dorsal mesopontine FD uptake in early PD (Hilker et al. 2003)

(5) Increased blood flow activation in the insula, prefrontal, and anterior cingulate cortex in PD patients with pain elicited by cold water immersion, a response that was reduced following levodopa (Brefel-Courbon et al. 2005)

(6) Reduced cardiac uptake of 6-[¹⁸F]fluorodopamine (Goldstein et al. 2002) or [¹¹C]hydroxyephedrine in PD patients with autonomic dysfunction (Berding et al. 2003).

PET IN PD DUE TO GENETIC MUTATIONS

PET studies of PD due to LRRK2 mutation reveal asymmetric reduction of all markers of presynaptic dopaminergic function, with a rostral-caudal gradient, identical to the pattern seen in sporadic PD (Adams et al. 2005). Asymptomatic mutation carriers display abnormal DAT binding with the later development of reduced VMAT2 binding. Development of symptoms was associated with the emergence of abnormal FD uptake (Adams et al. 2005; Nandhagopal et al. 2008a).

PET studies in parkin mutation patients have demonstrated significant reductions of FD uptake in the caudate, putamen, ventral striatum, locus coeruleus, midbrain raphe, and pallidum. Comparison of parkin with IPD patients showed that the hypothalamus was more involved in IPD while the midbrain raphe was more involved in parkin-related disease (Pavese et al. 2010). In both PINK1 and parkin, asymptomatic heterozygotes have been reported to show monoaminergic dysfunction (Khan et al. 2002a; Khan et al. 2002b), but the significance is not clear.

SCANS WITHOUT EVIDENCE OF DOPAMINERGIC DEFICIT (SWEDDs)

There is a subgroup of patients described in the very early stage of suspected PD in whom dopaminergic imaging was normal. While the basis for this observation is still not fully resolved, follow-up studies suggest that there is no progression, that the response to dopaminergic medication is questionable (Marshall et al. 2006), that dopamine innervation remains intact, and that glucose metabolic patterns remain normal (Eckert et al. 2007). Recent evidence suggests that a number of these patients may have dystonic tremor rather than PD (Schneider et al. 2007; Schwingenschuh et al. 2010).

LIMITATIONS

Radiotracer methods have numerous potential limitations. PET is currently available in only a few centers; its clinical use (especially for assessment of specific neurochemical functions) is limited, and it is used mainly for research. There is some exposure to radioactivity during the scans that, while quite low, may be of concern, especially when imaging children or women of reproductive age, especially when multitracer studies are being contemplated. Image acquisition for PET often requires prolonged periods of scanning and may be difficult for Parkinson patients to tolerate. Both the temporal and spatial resolution of PET is limited compared to those of fMRI. The interpretation of PET imaging is also complex, and it should be remembered that one is simply measuring radioactivity and that the biological meaning must be interpreted based on biological models and assumptions.

CONCLUSION

PET scanning of DA terminals helps to assess the function of the dopaminergic system in PD and is also able to detect preclinical dysfunction and progression. However, the methods have limitations and results must be interpreted with caution. The last few years have seen substantial improvements in spatial resolution as well as the capacity to concurrently perform PET and other higher-resolution anatomical or functional imaging. PET has the enormous advantage of allowing the investigator to probe a variety of molecular processes.

REFERENCES

Adams, J. R., H. van Netten, M. Schulzer, E. Mak, J. McKenzie, A. Strongosky, V. Sossi, T. J. Ruth, C. S. Lee, M. Farrer, T. Gasser, R. J. Uitti, D. B. Calne, Z. K. Wszolek, A. J. Stoessl. 2005. PET in LRRK2 mutations: Comparison to sporadic Parkinson's disease, evidence for presymptomatic compensation. *Brain* 128, no. 12: 2777–2785.

Albin, R. L., R. A. Koeppe, R. D. Chervin, F. B. Consens, K. Wernette, K. A. Frey, and M. S. Aldrich. 2000. Decreased striatal dopaminergic innervation in REM sleep behavior disorder. *Neurology* 55, no. 9:1410–1412.

Antonini, A., K. L. Leenders, P. Vontobel, R. P. Maguire, J. Missimer, M. Psylla, and I. Gunther. 1997. Complementary PET studies of striatal neuronal function in the differential diagnosis between multiple system atrophy and Parkinson's disease. *Brain* 120, no. 12: 2187–2195.

Antonini, A., J. Schwarz, W. H. Oertel, O. Pogarell, and K. L. Leenders. 1997. Long-term changes of striatal dopamine D2 receptors in patients with Parkinson's disease: A study with positron emission tomography and [11C] raclopride. *Mov Disord* 12, no. 1:33–38.

Au, W. L., J. R. Adams, A. R. Troiano, and A. J. Stoessl. 2005. Parkinson's disease: In vivo assessment of disease progression using positron emission tomography. *Brain Res Mol Brain Res* 134, no. 1:24–33.

Barone, P., A. Antonini, C. Colosimo, R. Marconi, L. Morgante, T. P. Avarello, E. Bottacchi, A. Cannas, G. Ceravolo, R. Ceravolo, G. Cicarelli, R. M. Gaglio, R. M. Giglia, F. Iemolo, M. Manfredi, G. Meco, A. Nicoletti, M. Pederzoli, A. Petrone, A. Pisani, F. E. Pontieri, R. Quatrale, S. Ramat, R. Scala, G. Volpe, S. Zappulla, A. R. Bentivoglio, F. Stocchi, G. Trianni, and P. D. Dotto. 2009. The PRIAMO study: A multicenter assessment of nonmotor symptoms and their impact on quality of life in Parkinson's disease. *Mov Disord* 24, no. 11:1641–1649.

Berding, G., C. H. Schrader, T. Peschel, J. van den Hoff, H. Kolbe, G. J. Meyer, R. Dengler, and W. H. Knapp. 2003. [N-methyl 11C] meta-Hydroxyephedrine positron emission tomography in Parkinson's disease and multiple system atrophy. *Eur J Nucl Med Mol Imaging* 30, no. 1:127–131.

Bohnen, N. I., D. I. Kaufer, L. S. Ivanco, B. Lopresti, R. A. Koeppe, J. G. Davis, C. A. Mathis, R. Y. Moore, and S. T. DeKosky. 2003. Cortical cholinergic function is more severely affected in parkinsonian dementia than in Alzheimer disease: An in vivo positron emission tomographic study. *Arch Neurol* 60, no. 12:1745–1748.

Boileau, I., J. J. Warsh, M. Guttman, J. A. Saint-Cyr, T. McCluskey, P. Rusjan, S. Houle, A. A. Wilson, J. H. Meyer, and S. J. Kish. 2008. Elevated serotonin transporter binding in depressed patients with Parkinson's disease: A preliminary PET study with [11C]DASB. *Mov Disord*. 23, no. 12:1776–1780.

Braune, S., M. Reinhardt, R. Schnitzer, A. Riedel, and C. H. Lucking. 1999. Cardiac uptake of [123I]MIBG separates Parkinson's disease from multiple system atrophy. *Neurology* 53, no. 5:1020–1025.

Brefel-Courbon, C., P. Payoux, C. Thalamas, F. Ory, I. Quelven, F. Chollet, J. L. Montastruc, and O. Rascol. 2005. Effect of levodopa on pain threshold in Parkinson's disease: A clinical and positron emission tomography study. *Mov Disord* 20, no. 12:1557–1563.

Brown, W. D., M. D. Taylor, A. D. Roberts, T. R. Oakes, M. J. Schueller, J. E. Holden, L. M. Malischke, O. T. DeJesus, and R. J. Nickles. 1999. FluoroDOPA PET shows the nondopaminergic as well as dopaminergic destinations of levodopa. *Neurology* 53, no. 6:1212–1218.

De Keyser, J., G. Ebinger, and G. Vauquelin. 1990. Age-related changes in the human nigrostriatal dopaminergic system. *Ann Neurol* 27, no. 2:157–161.

Doder, M., E. A. Rabiner, N. Turjanski, A. J. Lees, and D. J. Brooks. 2003. Tremor in Parkinson's disease and serotonergic dysfunction: An 11C-WAY 100635 PET study. *Neurology* 60, no. 4:601–605.

Eckert, T., A. Barnes, V. Dhawan, S. Frucht, M. F. Gordon, A. S. Feigin, and D. Eidelberg. 2005. FDG PET in the differential diagnosis of parkinsonian disorders. *Neuroimage* 26, no. 3:912–921.

Eckert, T., A. Feigin, D. E. Lewis, V. Dhawan, S. Frucht, and D. Eidelberg. 2007. Regional metabolic changes in parkinsonian patients with normal dopaminergic imaging. *Mov Disord* 22, no. 2:167–173.

Edison P., C. C. Rowe, J. O. Rinne, S. Ng, I. Ahmed, N. Kemppainen, V. L. Villemagne, G. O'Keefe, K. Någren, K. R. Chaudhury, C. L. Masters, and D. J. Brooks. 2008. Amyloid load in Parkinson's disease dementia and Lewy body dementia measured with [11C]PIB positron emission tomography. *J Neurol Neurosurg Psychiatry* 79 (12):1331–8.

Evans, A. H., N. Pavese, A. D. Lawrence, Y. F. Tai, S. Appel, M. Doder, D. J. Brooks, A. J. Lees, and P. Piccini. 2006. Compulsive drug use linked to sensitized ventral striatal dopamine transmission. *Ann Neurol* 59, no. 5:852–858.

Fearnley, J. M. and A. J. Lees. 1991. Ageing and Parkinson's disease: Substantia nigra regional selectivity. *Brain* 114 (5):2283–2301.

Fuente-Fernandez, R., J. Q. Lu, V. Sossi, S. Jivan, M. Schulzer, J. E. Holden, C. S. Lee, T. J. Ruth, D. B. Calne, and A. J. Stoessl. 2001. Biochemical variations in the synaptic level of dopamine precede motor fluctuations in Parkinson's disease: PET evidence of increased dopamine turnover. *Ann Neurol* 49, no. 3:298–303.

Fuente-Fernandez, R., T. J. Ruth, V. Sossi, M. Schulzer, D. B. Calne, and A. J. Stoessl. 2001. Expectation and dopamine release: Mechanism of the placebo effect in Parkinson's disease. *Science* 293, no. 5532: 1164–1166.

Fuente-Fernandez, R., S. Furtado, M. Guttman et al. 2003. VMAT2 binding is elevated in dopa-responsive dystonia: Visualizing empty vesicles by PET. *Synapse* no. 49:20–28.

Fuente-Fernandez, R., M. Schulzer, and A. J. Stoessl. 2004. Placebo mechanisms and reward circuitry: Clues from Parkinson's disease. *Biol Psychiatry* 56, no. 2:67–71.

Fuente-Fernandez, R., V. Sossi, Z. Huang, S. Furtado, J. Q. Lu, D. B. Calne, T. J. Ruth, and A. J. Stoessl. 2004. Levodopa-induced changes in synaptic dopamine levels increase with progression of Parkinson's disease: Implications for dyskinesias. *Brain* 127, no. 12:2747–2754.

Fuente-Fernandez, R., V. Sossi, S. McCormick, M. Schulzer, T. J. Ruth, and A. J. Stoessl. 2009. Visualizing vesicular dopamine dynamics in Parkinson's disease. *Synapse* 63, no. 8:713–716.

Goerendt, I. K., C. Messa, A. D. Lawrence, P. M. Grasby, P. Piccini, and D. J. Brooks. 2003. Dopamine release during sequential finger movements in health and Parkinson's disease: A PET study. *Brain* 126, no. 2:312–325.

Goldstein, D. S., C. S. Holmes, R. Dendi, S. R. Bruce, and S. T. Li. 2002. Orthostatic hypotension from sympathetic denervation in Parkinson's disease. *Neurology* 58, no. 8:1247–1255.

Gomperts, S. N., D. M. Rentz, E. Moran, J. A. Becker, J. J. Locascio, W. E. Klunk, C. A. Mathis et al. 2008. Imaging amyloid deposition in Lewy body diseases. *Neurology* 71, no. 12:903–10.

Hilker, R., N. Razai, M. Ghaemi, S. Weisenbach, J. Rudolf, B. Szelies, and W. D. Heiss. 2003. [18F]fluorodopa uptake in the upper brainstem measured with positron emission tomography correlates with decreased REM sleep duration in early Parkinson's disease. *Clin Neurol Neurosurg* 105, no. 4:262–269.

Holden, J. E., D. Doudet, C. J. Endres, G. L. Chan, K. S. Morrison, F. J. Vingerhoets, B. J. Snow, B. D. Pate, V. Sossi, K. R. Buckley, and T. J. Ruth. 1997. Graphical analysis of 6-fluoro-L-dopa trapping: Effect of inhibition of catechol-O-methyltransferase. *J Nucl Med* 38, no. 10:1568–1574.

Khan, N. L., D. J. Brooks, N. Pavese, M. G. Sweeney, N. W. Wood, A. J. Lees, and P. Piccini. 2002a. Progression of nigrostriatal dysfunction in a parkin kindred: An [18F]dopa PET and clinical study. *Brain* 125, no. 10:2248–2256.

Khan, N. L., E. M. Valente, A. R. Bentivoglio, N. W. Wood, A. Albanese, D. J. Brooks, and P. Piccini. 2002b. Clinical and subclinical dopaminergic dysfunction in PARK6-linked parkinsonism: An 18F-dopa PET study. *Ann Neurol* 52, no. 6:849–853.

Koepp, M. J., R. N. Gunn, A. D. Lawrence, V. J. Cunningham, A. Dagher, T. Jones, D. J. Brooks, C. J. Bench, and P. M. Grasby. 1998. Evidence for striatal dopamine release during a video game. *Nature* 393, no. 6682:266–268.

Laruelle, M. 2000. Imaging synaptic neurotransmission with in vivo binding competition techniques: A critical review. *J Cereb Blood Flow Metab* 20, no. 3:423–451.

Lee, C. S., A. Samii, V. Sossi, T. J. Ruth, M. Schulzer, J. E. Holden, J. Wudel, P. K. Pal, R. Fuente-Fernandez, D. B. Calne, and A. J. Stoessl. 2000. In vivo positron emission tomographic evidence for compensatory changes in presynaptic dopaminergic nerve terminals in Parkinson's disease. *Ann Neurol* 47, no. 4:493–503.

Lidstone, S., R. de la Fuente-Fernandez, and A. J. Stoessl. 2005. The placebo response as a reward mechanism. *Sem Pain Med*, no. 3:37–42.

Lidstone, S. C., M. Schulzer, K. Dinelle, E. Mak, V. Sossi, T. J. Ruth, R. de la Fuente-Fernandez, A. G. Phillips, and A. J. Stoessl. 2010. Great expectations: Placebos mimic the effect of active medication in Parkinson's disease. *Arch Gen Psychiatry* 67:857–865.

Marshall, V. L., J. Patterson, D. M. Hadley, K. A. Grosset, and D. G. Grosset. 2006. Two-year follow-up in 150 consecutive cases with normal dopamine transporter imaging. *Nucl Med Commun* 27, no. 12:933–937.

Martin, W. R., M. R. Palmer, C. S. Patlak, and D. B. Calne. 1989. Nigrostriatal function in humans studied with positron emission tomography. *Ann Neurol* 26, no. 4:535–542.

Maetzler, W., I. Liepelt, M. Reimold, G. Reischl, C. Solbach, C. Becker, C. Schulte, et al. 2009. Cortical PIB binding in Lewy body disease is associated with Alzheimer-like characteristics. *Neurobiol Dis* 34, no. 1:107–12.

Minoshima, S., N. L. Foster, A. A. Sima, K. A. Frey, R. L. Albin, and D. E. Kuhl. 2001. Alzheimer's disease versus dementia with Lewy bodies: Cerebral metabolic distinction with autopsy confirmation. *Ann Neurol* 50, no. 3:358–365.

Monchi, O., J. H. Ko, and A. P. Strafella. 2006. Striatal dopamine release during performance of executive functions: A [(11)C] raclopride PET study. *Neuroimage* 33, no. 3:907–912.

Moore, R. Y., A. L. Whone, S. McGowan, and D. J. Brooks. 2003. Monoamine neuron innervation of the normal human brain: An 18F-DOPA PET study. *Brain Res* 982, no. 2:137–145.

Morrish, P. K., J. S. Rakshi, D. L. Bailey, G. V. Sawle, and D. J. Brooks. 1998. Measuring the rate of progression and estimating the preclinical period of Parkinson's disease with [18F]dopa PET. *J Neurol Neurosurg Psychiatry* 64, no. 3:314–319.

Nandhagopal, R., L. Kuramoto, M. Schulzer, E. Mak, J. Cragg, C. S. Lee, J. McKenzie, S. McCormick, A. Samii, A. Troiano, T. J. Ruth, V. Sossi, R. Fuente-Fernandez, D. B. Calne, and A. J. Stoessl. 2009. Longitudinal progression of sporadic Parkinson's disease: A multitracer positron emission tomography study. *Brain* 132, no. 11: 2970–2979.

Nandhagopal, R., E. Mak, M. Schulzer, J. McKenzie, S. McCormick, V. Sossi, T. J. Ruth, A. Strongosky, M. J. Farrer, Z. K. Wszolek, and A. J. Stoessl. 2008a. Progression of dopaminergic dysfunction in a LRRK2 kindred: A multitracer PET study. *Neurology* 71, no. 22:1790–1795.

Nandhagopal, R., M. J. McKeown, and A. J. Stoessl. 2008b. Functional imaging in Parkinson disease. *Neurology* 70, no. 16 Pt 2:1478–1488.

Nurmi, E., H. M. Ruottinen, J. Bergman, M. Haaparanta, O. Solin, P. Sonninen, and J. O. Rinne. 2001. Rate of progression in Parkinson's disease: A 6-[18F]fluoro-L-dopa PET study. *Mov Disord* 16, no. 4:608–615.

Pavese, N., R. Y. Moore, C. Scherfler, N. L. Khan, G. Hotton, N. P. Quinn, K. P. Bhatia, N. W. Wood, D. J. Brooks, A. J. Lees, and P. Piccini. 2010. In vivo assessment of brain monoamine systems in parkin gene carriers: A PET study. *Exp Neurol* 222, no. 1: 120–124.

Remy, P., M. Doder, A. Lees, N. Turjanski, and D. Brooks. 2005. Depression in Parkinson's disease: Loss of dopamine and noradrenaline innervation in the limbic system. *Brain* 128, no. 6:1314–1322.

Rinne, J. O., R. Portin, H. Ruottinen, E. Nurmi, J. Bergman, M. Haaparanta, and O. Solin. 2000. Cognitive impairment and the brain dopaminergic system in Parkinson disease: [18F]fluorodopa positron emission tomographic study. *Arch Neurol* 57, no. 4: 470–475.

Sawamoto, N., P. Piccini, G. Hotton, N. Pavese, K. Thielemans, and D. J. Brooks. 2008. Cognitive deficits and striato-frontal dopamine release in Parkinson's disease. *Brain* 131, no. 5:1294–1302.

Schneider, S. A., M. J. Edwards, P. Mir, C. Cordivari, J. Hooker, J. Dickson, N. Quinn, and K. P. Bhatia. 2007. Patients with adult-onset dystonic tremor resembling parkinsonian tremor have scans without evidence of dopaminergic deficit (SWEDDs). *Mov Disord* 22, no. 15:2210–5.

Schwingenschuh, P., D. Ruge, M. J. Edwards, C. Terranova, P. Katschnig, F. Carrillo, L. Silveira-Moriyama, et al. 2010. Distinguishing SWEDDs patients with asymmetric resting tremor from Parkinson's disease: A clinical and electrophysiological study. *Mov Disord* 2010 [Epub ahead of print].

Seeman, P., H. C. Guan, and H. B. Niznik. 1989. Endogenous dopamine lowers the dopamine D2 receptor density as measured by [3H] raclopride: Implications for positron emission tomography of the human brain. *Synapse* 3, no. 1:96–97.

Seibyl, J. P., K. L. Marek, D. Quinlan, K. Sheff, S. Zoghbi, Y. Zea-Ponce, R. M. Baldwin, B. Fussell, E. O. Smith, D. S. Charney, C. van Dyck, P. B. Hoffer and R. B. Innis. 1995. Decreased single-photon emission computed tomographic [123I]beta-CIT striatal uptake correlates with symptom severity in Parkinson's disease. *Ann Neurol* 38, no. 4:589–598.

Shinotoh, H., O. Inoue, K. Hirayama, A. Aotsuka, M. Asahina, T. Suhara, T. Yamazaki, and Y. Tateno. 1993. Dopamine D1 receptors in Parkinson's disease and striatonigral degeneration: A positron emission tomography study. *J Neurol Neurosurg Psychiatry* 56, no. 5:467–472.

Silveira-Moriyama, L., P. Schwingenschuh, A. O'Donnell, S. A. Schneider, P. Mir, F. Carrillo, C. Terranova, A. Petrie, D. G. Grosset, N. P. Quinn, K. P. Bhatia, and A. J. Lees. 2009. Olfaction in patients with suspected parkinsonism and scans without evidence of dopaminergic deficit (SWEDDs). *J Neurol Neurosurg Psychiatry* 80, no. 7:744–748.

Sossi, V., R. Fuente-Fernandez, J. E. Holden, D. J. Doudet, J. McKenzie, A. J. Stoessl, and T. J. Ruth. 2002. Increase in dopamine turnover occurs early in Parkinson's disease: Evidence from a new modeling approach to PET 18 F-fluorodopa data. *J Cereb Blood Flow Metab* 22, no. 2:232–239.

Sossi, V., R. Fuente-Fernandez, M. Schulzer, J. Adams, and J. Stoessl. 2006. Age-related differences in levodopa dynamics in Parkinson's: Implications for motor complications. *Brain* 129, no. 4:1050–1058.

Sossi, V., R. Fuente-Fernandez, M. Schulzer, A. R. Troiano, T. J. Ruth, and A. J. Stoessl. 2007. Dopamine transporter relation to dopamine turnover in Parkinson's disease: A positron emission tomography study. *Ann Neurol* 62, no. 5:468–474.

Steeves, T. D., J. Miyasaki, M. Zurowski, A. E. Lang, G. Pellecchia, T. Van Eimeren, P. Rusjan, S. Houle, and A. P. Strafella. 2009. Increased striatal dopamine release in Parkinsonian patients with pathological gambling: A [11C] raclopride PET study. *Brain* 132, no. 5:1376–1385.

Troiano, A. R., R. Fuente-Fernandez, V. Sossi, M. Schulzer, E. Mak, T. J. Ruth, and A. J. Stoessl. 2009. PET demonstrates reduced dopamine transporter expression in PD with dyskinesias. *Neurology* 72, no. 14:1211–1216.

Vander, Borght T., M. Kilbourn, T. Desmond, D. Kuhl, and K. Frey. 1995. The vesicular monoamine transporter is not regulated by dopaminergic drug treatments. *Eur J Pharmacol* 294, no. 2–3:577–583.

Vingerhoets, F. J., M. Schulzer, D. B. Calne, and B. J. Snow. 1997. Which clinical sign of Parkinson's disease best reflects the nigrostriatal lesion? *Ann Neurol* 41, no. 1:58–64.

Volkow, N. D., Y. S. Ding, J. S. Fowler, G. J. Wang, J. Logan, S. J. Gatley, R. Hitzemann, G. Smith, S. D. Fields, and R. Gur. 1996. Dopamine transporters decrease with age. *J Nucl Med* 37, no. 4:554–559.

Williams, L. E. 2008. Anniversary paper: Nuclear medicine: Fifty years and still counting. *Med Phys*, no. 35(7):3020–9.

Wilson, J. M., and S. J. Kish. 1996. The vesicular monoamine transporter, in contrast to the dopamine transporter, is not altered by chronic cocaine self-administration in the rat. *J Neurosci* 16, no. 10:3507–3510.

2

DOPAMINERGIC IMAGING IN PARKINSON'S DISEASE: SPECT

Christoph Scherfler and Werner Poewe

INTRODUCTION

While a clinical diagnosis of idiopathic Parkinson's disease (PD) can be made with high degrees of accuracy in cases with full expression of classical motor features, diagnostic uncertainty is common in early disease with subtle or ambiguous signs. Diagnostic error rates by neurologists not specialized in movement disorders can be as high as 25% (Hughes et al. 2001; Hughes et al. 2002; Rajput et al. 1991). The major sources of error are related to the differentiation of PD from atypical degenerative parkinsonian disorders like multiple system atrophy (MSA) or progressive supranuclear palsy (PSP) and to the classification of isolated rest or dystonic tremor, drug-induced, psychogenic, or vascular parkinsonism (Deuschl 1999). In recent years, a number of ancillary tests have been developed with the aim to enhance the accuracy of a clinical diagnosis of PD and other forms of parkinsonism. These include testing for dopaminergic responsiveness using levodopa or apomorphine, tests of autonomic or smell function and a variety of neuroimaging procedures, based on MR or positron emission tomography (PET) and single photon emission computed tomography (SPECT). This chapter will review methodological aspects of dopamine transporter (DAT) SPECT imaging and its clinical ability in the differential diagnosis of parkinsonian syndromes as well as its potential as a tool to monitor disease progression. Lastly, the potential of DAT-SPECT to identify subjects at risk for PD will be discussed.

METHODOLOGICAL PRINCIPLES OF MEASURING DAT BINDING USING SPECT

The DAT is a sodium chloride–dependent protein on the presynaptic dopaminergic nerve terminals mediating the reuptake of free dopamine from the intrasynaptic cleft. Recent studies revealed that DAT expression is a markedly regulated rather than a static factor in dopamine signaling (Melikian and Buckley 1999). Amphetamine can decrease DAT membrane expression (Kahlig et al. 2004), while insulin via phosphatidylinositol 3-kinase and akt kinase increases membrane trafficking of the DAT (Garcia et al. 2005). Other kinases, such as protein kinase C or mitogene-activated protein kinase 1, also alter DAT function (Khoshbouei et al. 2004; Lin et al. 2003). Several SPECT radioligands for DAT are available, including [123I]2β-carboxymethoxy-3β-(4-iodophenyl) tropane ([123I]2β-CIT) and [123I]N-w-fluoropropyl-2β-carbomethoxy-3β-(4-iodophenyl) nortropane ([123I]FP-CIT). These SPECT radiotracers are commercially available and frequently used in clinical routine and research endeavors. Both tracers were reported to have high binding potentials to DAT and to a lower extent to the serotonin transporters, which are poorly expressed in the striatum. Other [123I]-labeled DAT radioligands used in some imaging centers include [123I]-2β-carbomethoxy-3β-(4-fluorophenyl)-N-(1-iodoprop-1-en-3-yl)nortropane ([123I]-Altropane), [123I]-N-(3-iodopropen-2-yl)-2β-carbomethoxy-3β-(4-chlorophenyl) tropane ([123I]-IPT), and [123I]-labeled N-(3-iodoprop-(2E)-enyl)-2β-carboxymethoxy-3β-(4-methylphenyl)nortropane ([123I]-PE2I). Among other SPECT radioligands, [99mTc]-TRODAT-1 ([99mTc]-[2-[[2-[[[3-(4-chlorophenyl)-8-methyl-8-azabicyclo[3.2 0.1]oct-2-yl]methyl](2-mercaptoethyl)amino]ethyl]amino]ethanethiolato(3-)-N2,N2',S2,S2']oxo-[1R-(exo-exo)]]) is the only available technetium labeled radioligand and has drawn attention because of its potential for routine clinical use (Varrone and Halldin 2010). Detailed guidelines for DAT-SPECT are available (EANM procedure guidelines, EJNM 2010). Pre-injection thyroid block (e.g., perchlorate 1 g, orally) following slow intravenous bolus injection over several seconds of a dose of 185 MBq has been recommended by the European Association of Nuclear Medicine and the manufacturer of FP-CIT. Optimal image acquisition at ligand-to-receptor equilibrium was determined at 18 to

24 hours after injection of [^{123}I]β-CIT, and 3 to 6 hours after injection of [^{123}I]FP-CIT. Signal acquisition is then achieved by multiple detectors system with appropriate collimators (LEHR, LEUHR, or medium energy) and scanning times that allow for higher than 3 million total counts. Subsequently filtered backprojection or iterative algorithms enable 3D image reconstruction comprising the entire brain volume. Following low-pass filtering, images undergo attenuation correction to minimize signal altera-tions from variably deep brain structures such as the stria-tum. For diagnostic purposes, a visual assessment of DAT binding using high-quality images (Acton et al. 2006) and a semiquantitative analysis using regions of interest (ROI) compared to absent (or low) background DAT expression (e.g., occipital cortex, cerebellum) is commonly performed in the routine clinical setting. ROI size should be at least twice the full width at half maximum of the scanner's spa-tial resolution, and shape should be standardized (e.g., using templates) (Schwarz et al. 2004) and based on morphologi-cal information (e.g., from MRI) if available. Routine clini-cal assessment of DAT-SPECT has so far focused primarily on the striatum as the brain area with the highest DAT uptake, whereas estimation of DAT density in brain regions with somewhat lower but still detectable signal encounters difficulties due to the lack of anatomical detail provided by DAT-SPECT. Novel evaluation procedures based on the fully automated voxel-by-voxel assignment of the individ-ual's image to a brain template have recently provided additional information on DAT distribution (Koch et al. 2005; Scherfler et al. 2005; Seppi et al. 2006; Scherfler and Nocker 2009).

Regulatory effects by levodopa or dopamine agonists on DAT expression or affinity have remained controversial, although the majority of studies addressing this issue have failed to provide clear evidence for such effects. Hence, in clinical routine, dopaminergic therapy does not need to be discontinued. On the contrary, CNS stimulants and sero-tonin reuptake inhibitors are known to have a significant influence on radioligand binding and therefore need to be stopped prior to the scan (Table 1).

PARKINSON'S DISEASE

In PD, motor symptoms develop when approximately 60%–70% of dopamine neurons have been lost. Several studies have shown that DAT ligand uptake is severely reduced in the early stage of PD when compared with age-matched healthy subjects, indicating a potential role of

DAT-SPECT in PD diagnosis of patients presenting with mild symptoms (Marek et al. 1996; Chouker et al. 2001; Pirker et al. 2002; Staffen et al. 2000). However, sensitivity of DAT-SPECT imaging to detect nigrostriatal presynaptic abnormalities in patients with clinically probable PD is less than 100%. When studying 38 patients with a clinical diag-nosis of probable PD according to step 1 of the UK PD Brain Bank Criteria, Benamer and colleagues found visu-ally normal FP-CIT-SPECT results in 5 patients (13%) presenting with unilateral rest tremor and variable degrees of bradykinesia (Benamer et al. 2003). This figure corre-sponds to the results from clinical trials using [^{123}I]β-CIT SPECT and [^{18}F]dopa PET as surrogate markers for dis-ease progression reporting that a proportion of 5.7% to 14.7% diagnosed as early PD have normal scans (Whone et al. 2003; Parkinson Study Group 2002; Parkinson Study Group 2004).

For such individuals, the term "SWEDD" (subject without evidence of dopaminergic deficit) has recently come into use (Parkinson Study Group 2002; Parkinson Study Group 2004). Possible explanations for such discrep-ancies between clinical diagnosis and imaging findings are that reductions of striatal DAT availability in early PD would be below the detection threshold or that the cases were clinically misdiagnosed. There is strong experimen-tal and clinical evidence that DAT availability measured with SPECT mirrors the decline in levels of striatal dop-amine (Uhl et al. 1994; Bezard et al. 2001; Scherfler et al. 2002) and, given that 80% of striatal dopamine and 50% of nigral dopamine cells are lost when symptoms first appear, it is improbable that DAT imaging would be normal in initial early disease. In addition, abnormal DAT imaging has been found in preclinical or subclinical phases of PD (Berendse et al. 2001; Sommer et al. 2004; Stiasny-Kolster et al. 2005, Iranzo et al. 2010), including bilateral deficits in patients with unilateral symptoms (Tissingh et al. 1998). Follow-up investigations of the 11% of patients with ini-tially normal [^{18}F]dopa PET scans in the REAL-PET study showed that these scans remained normal at 2 years. Follow-up in patients with normal DAT-SPECT in the ELLDOPA study reported normal scans in all who were rescanned (numbers falling from 19 at 9 months to 10 at 4 years). Blinded video evaluation by five movement disor-der experts of UPDRS "off-state" examinations showed that 3 or more evaluators doubted the diagnosis of PD in most of these cases. In conclusion, these observations sug-gest that patients with normal striatal DAT availability and clinical signs of parkinsonism or tremor disorders are unlikely to have early degeneration of the nigrostriatal

TABLE 1: RELEVANT DRUG INTERACTION WITH DOPAMINE TRANSPORTER SINGLE PHOTON EMISSION COMPUTED TOMOGRAPHY (DAT-SPECT)

Minor* effect on DAT-SPECT	To be stopped prior to DAT-SPECT	Significant† effect on DAT-SPECT	To be stopped prior to DAT-SPECT
Citalopram	8 days	Cocaine	2 days
Fluoxetine	45 days	Amfetamine	7 days
Paroxetine	5 days	Methylamfetamine	3 days
Venlafaxine	3 days	Methylphenidate	1 days
Duloxetine	3 days	Methylphenidate	2 days
Escitalopram	8 days	Dexamfetamine	7 days
Fluvoxamine	5 days	Mazindol	3 days
Sertraline	6 days	Phentermine	14 days
Imipramine	5 days	Modafinil	3 days
Clomipramine	21 days	Bupropion or amfebutamone	8 days
Pimozide	28 days	Benzatropine	5 days
Ziprasidone	2 days		
Memantine	5 days		
Amantadine	6 days		
Budipine	6 days		
Ephedrine, epinephrine	6–10 h		
Phenylephrine			
Pseudoephedrine			
Xylometazoline			

* May have a small effect on uptake (at most 15%). This is acceptable for routine DAT-SPECT but not for research.

† All of these drugs are likely to alter (usually decrease) radioligand uptake by at least 20% and often substantially more, and therefore have to be stopped prior to routine DAT-SPECT.

dopaminergic pathway. In those cases, alternative diagnoses need to be considered.

NON-PARKINSON'S DISEASE TREMOR

Distribution, frequency, severity, age of onset, evolution, and additional clinical signs all help with the clinical classification of tremor entities. Diagnostic uncertainties may arise when additional clinical signs are apparent that overlap with another diagnostic entity. Such discrepancies are encountered when a rest tremor component is found in patients whose clinical features would otherwise be compatible with classical essential tremor. In addition, a number of studies have suggested that patients with essential tremor

(ET) are at risk of developing PD later in life (Benito-Leon et al. 2009). Indeed, some patients with PD have a history of longstanding asymmetrical postural tremor preceding the onset of parkinsonism by years or even decades, and DAT imaging was found abnormal in some patients with a clinical phenotype of ET (Chaudhuri et al. 2005; Parkinson Study Group 2000). Vice versa, patients with essential tremor may be mistaken for PD as reported in 12.4% of 402 patients erroneously treated with anti-parkinson therapy (Meara et al. 1999). Other sources of error might occur in patients with dystonic tremor and, when presenting with additional rest tremor, increased limb tone, or impaired arm swing, all features that may suggest PD (Schrag et al. 2000; Schneider et al. 2007). Diagnostic difficulties may also be encountered in patients with autosomal-recessive parkinsonism (PARK 2, 6, and 7), where cases with bilateral hand tremor without any associated features of parkinsonism have been described (Pellecchia et al. 2007).

On the other hand, patients fulfilling essential tremor criteria without overlapping clinical features or other confounders invariably have normal presynaptic DAT imaging (Asenbaum et al. 1998; Benamer et al. 2000a). Comparing ET to early PD (Hoehn & Yahr stage 1) showed no evidence of subclinical dopaminergic disruption in essential tremor. Also, patients with adult-onset dystonic tremor were reported to have normal striatal DAT availability (Scheider et al. 2007). Hence, it can be concluded that abnormal striatal DAT-SPECT findings rule out a diagnosis of essential and dystonic tremor.

ATYPICAL PARKINSONIAN DISORDERS

Particularly in early disease stages, the differentiation of PD from atypical parkinsonian disorders like MSA or PSP can raise considerable difficulties. Poor levodopa responsiveness and more rapid clinical deterioration are typical for these atypical parkinsonian disorders, which involve pre- and postsynaptic dopaminergic degeneration. Although marked asymmetry in reductions of putamenal DAT finding is more typical for PD as compared to other degenerative parkinsonian disorders, SPECT imaging using DAT ligands usually does not help to differentiate between those entities (Pirker et al. 2000, Figure 1).

However, a recent study using statistical parametric mapping (SPM) found reduced midbrain [123I]β-CIT uptake in patients with the Parkinson variant of multiple system atrophy (MSA-P), and based on this technique the authors were able to correctly classify 95% of MSA-P and PD patients (Scherfler et al. 2005). Using the same technique in a group of patients with fully developed PSP revealed severe DAT-SPECT signal decline in the caudate and midbrain, which was different in its distribution when compared to MSA-P and PD (Seppi et al. 2006; Göbel et al. 2010 revised). Whether this finding is able to discriminate patients with subtle or ambiguous signs needs to be investigated.

PET and DAT-SPECT studies have also shown that even clinically pure forms of MSA-C have some decrease in DAT binding but less compared with MSA-P or PD (Rinne et al. 1995). This finding could be of some diagnostic impact in the differential diagnosis of MSA-C to idiopathic late-onset cerebellar ataxia. Striatal DAT loss in CBD is in the same range as it is in PD and other forms of atypical parkinsonism although it is much more asymmetrical and less pronounced than seen in MSA and PSP (Pirker et al. 2000; Klaffke et al. 2006).

PSYCHOGENIC PARKINSONISM

Psychogenic parkinsonism (PsyP) can be difficult to differentiate from PD and other parkinsonian disorders. Clinical pointers of PsyP are sudden onset and static course of motor symptoms, deliberate slowness, active resistance to limb movements, and variability of tremor and limb rigidity with distraction or during activation of movements in opposite limbs and bizarre gait disorders (Lang et al. 1995). Despite such clinical hints, it can be difficult to rule out organic parkinsonism on clinical grounds alone. Psychogenic movement disorders can coexist with an underlying organic disease and may respond to placebo, complicating the interpretation of a positive levodopa challenge test (Factor et al. 1995; Lang et al. 1995). However, early and accurate diagnosis is important to offer an adequate prognosis, to provide an adequate treatment, and to avoid unnecessary diagnostic procedures. Studies using DAT-SPECT in patients with PsyP are limited to case control studies but have consistently found striatal

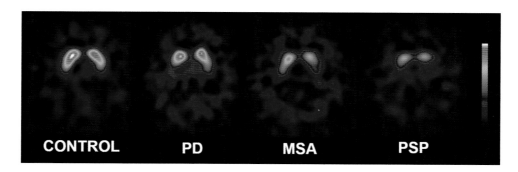

Figure 1 Striatal dopamine transporter availability in a healthy subject and patients with Parkinson's disease, multiple system atrophy, and progressive supranuclear palsy.

DAT availability in the range of normal controls (Booij 2001; Gaig et al. 2006; Jennings et al. 2004). These observations suggest that DAT-SPECT is useful in the differentiation of psychogenic from degenerative parkinsonism.

VASCULAR PARKINSONISM

The clinical presentations of vascular parkinsonism overlap with degenerative forms and hence cause difficulties for the clinician even if CT or MRI brain scans are available. Vascular lesions are a common incidental finding in pathologically confirmed PD, and a large proportion of patients with late onset PD have some white-matter changes on CT/MRI scans, complicating the untangling of true vascular from degenerative parkinsonism. Recently, Zijlmans et al. were able to delineate the clinical and pathophysiological features of 17 cases of VP based on careful post-mortem neuropathological diagnosis and proposed criteria for the clinical diagnosis of vascular parkinsonism, including i) bradykinesia, ii) cerebrovascular disease visualized by CT or MRI, and iii) a temporal relationship between the location of vascular lesions and the appearance of parkinsonian symptoms or the presence of extensive subcortical white-matter lesions and bilateral symptoms at onset (Zijlmans et al. 2004). Proposed diagnostic criteria suggest exclusion of other causes of parkinsonism as space occupying lesions, pharmacological and toxic effects, head trauma, or encephalitis. Presynaptic dopaminergic circuitry is generally preserved in VP, although a slight reduction in lateral substantia nigra is probably due to trans-neuronal degeneration (Zijlmans et al. 2004), and moderate cell nerve loss in substantia nigra in cases with massive unilateral basal ganglia infarction has been reported (Forno 1983). Studies assessing the utility of DAT-SPECT in the differentiation of vascular from degenerative parkinsonism have yielded inconsistent results. Gerschlager et al. found that the whole striatal DAT binding and the putamen/caudate ratio were normal or only mildly reduced in patients with VP (Gerschlager et al. 2002). Other authors reported reduced striatal DAT binding in vascular parkinsonism, with values ranging in between levels of normal and cases with PD (Tzen et al. 2001). Similarly, in 20 patients with parkinsonism with cerebrovascular disease and without pre-existing PD (Lorberboym et al. 2004), striatal DAT binding was diminished in more than half (Zijlmans et al. 2007). Variable striatal DAT availability ranging from normal to pathological values in VP and overlapping in part with those observed in PD makes it difficult to separate those two entities even with the use of in vivo striatal DAT markers.

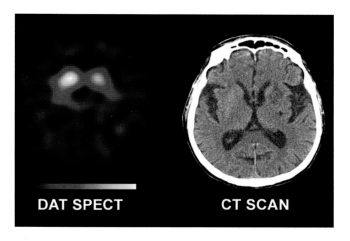

Figure 2 Case vignette: 78-year-old patient with acute hemiparesis following left striatocapsular infarct. The patient developed left-sided hemiparkinsonism seven months after stroke.

The true value is in cases with clinical parkinsonism and vascular lesions on MRI or CT in whom DAT-SPECT is normal. These would then be classified as vascular parkinsonism using the criteria by Zijlmans et al. A proportion of those fulfilling these criteria may, however, also have abnormal tracer binding, which would not be incompatible with a diagnosis of vascular parkinsonism (Figure 2).

DAT-SPECT IN DRUG-INDUCED PARKINSONISM

Drug-induced parkinsonism (DIP) is caused predominantly by neuroleptics interfering with the postsynaptic D2 receptors and calcium-channel blockers as well as tetrabenazine, which exerts additional presynaptic effects. DIP cannot be reliably distinguished from neurodegenerative parkinsonism on clinical grounds alone. Although commonly associated with symmetric symptoms, several authors reported the occurrence of unilateral parkinsonian features in about one-third of patients (Arblaster et al. 1993; Lavalaye et al. 2001). The affinity of neuroleptics to the DAT and its influence toward changes of DAT density is negligible, making DAT-SPECT a valuable tool to separate DIP from degenerative parkinsonism (Reader et al. 1998).

However, the interpretation of the causal relationship between drug-exposure and clinical parkinsonism is complicated by the possibility that patients with incipient or preclinical idiopathic PD may be unmasked by the exposure to dopamine-blocking drugs. In a study including 19 patients with DIP, striatal DAT availability was reduced in nine participants and remained unchanged within a follow-up period of two years (Tinazzi et al. 2009).

Interestingly, the UPDRS motor score worsened solely in patients with abnormal DAT-SPECT, corroborating the concept of antidopaminergic drugs unmasking PD. It can be concluded that DAT-SPECT is likely to be normal in DIP unless presymptomatic degenerative parkinsonism is present and hence is important to guide appropriate therapeutic management.

DEMENTIA WITH LEWY BODIES

Diffuse Lewy Body Disease (DLB) and PD are characterized by striatal DAT loss, making DAT-SPECT not helpful in the differential diagnosis. Together with vascular dementia, DLB is one of the commonest forms of dementia after Alzheimer's disease (AD). Operationalized clinical diagnostic criteria have been agreed for all of these syndromes, but even in specialist research settings, they have limited accuracy when compared with postmortem findings. Distinguishing AD from DLB is of clinical relevance in terms of prognosis and appropriate treatment. Patients with AD do not show severe nigrostriatal degeneration (Piggot et al. 1999).

The usefulness of DAT imaging in distinguishing DLB from AD was confirmed in a study that compared in-life diagnosis, DAT imaging, and neuropathology in 20 demented patients (Walker et al. 2007). Amongst the eight pathological confirmed DLB patients, of which four showed coexisting AD and cerebrovascular pathology, all but one patient presented with reduced striatal DAT-SPECT signal. More importantly, all seven individuals with in-life diagnosis of DLB but with normal striatal DAT had their diagnosis reversed to other forms of dementias at the time of autopsy, indicating that DAT imaging substantially enhances the accuracy of diagnosing DLB by comparison with clinical criteria alone. Abnormal DAT imaging was therefore also included as a suggestive feature in the DLB consensus criteria in 2005 (McKeith et al. 2005).

SCREENING OF AT-RISK INDIVIDUALS FOR DEVELOPING PARKINSON'S DISEASE

Although the interval between the onset of nigral dopaminergic degeneration and the onset of clinical symptoms of PD is unknown, postmortem examination of nigral cell loss in a series of PD brains suggested a preclinical window of around six years (Fearnley and Lees 1991). Imaging studies estimate the onset of nigrostriatal degeneration to be less than seven years before clinical symptom onset, assuming

a linear relationship between disease duration and putaminal [18 F]dopa uptake (Morrish et al. 1998). These time intervals are in accord with calculations based on sequential DAT imaging (Marek et al. 2001). Further evidence arises from examining striatal dopamine terminals in early, strictly hemiparkinsonian patients (Marek et al. 1996), in whom bilateral striatal loss occurs before bilateral clinical signs. In asymptomatic but hyposmic first-degree relatives of PD patients, an increased rate of decline in DAT-SPECT binding was found in 12.5%, who developed PD within five years, indicating again that DAT-SPECT might be able to detect presymptomatic PD (Ponsen et al. 2010). At present, however, there is no agreed-upon and clearly defined at-risk population to be investigated with DAT-SPECT, raising the issue of cost versus effectiveness for this procedure as a primary screening tool. Further, to the identification of hyposmia as a potential marker to identify subjects at risk of developing PD, the visualization of hyperechogenic signals in the region of the SN by transcranial ultrasound and a diagnosis of the idiopathic REM sleep behavior disorder (RBD), both suggested to be present before the onset of symptoms (Sommer et al. 2004, Unger et al. 2008), could narrow the candidates subjected to DAT-SPECT. However, before applying DAT-SPECT as a secondary or confirmatory screening tool for subjects at risk of developing PD, the following practical limitations need to be solved. First, it is unknown when, how often, and at what intervals these individuals would have to be scanned to detect their preclinical window. Second, it is unknown if abnormal DAT-SPECT results in asymptomatic persons would predict invariably the onset of clinical disease at a later time. Finally, and most importantly, there is currently no treatment or intervention that would prevent or significantly delay the onset of clinically overt disease in asymptomatic patients with neuroimaging evidence of nigrostriatal terminal dysfunction.

A BIOMARKER FOR DISEASE PROGRESSION

Criteria for an appropriate biomarker to study disease progression in PD include 1) objective and reproducible measurement in early PD patients, 2) sensitivity to deterioration of the nigrostriatal dopaminergic system, 3) correlation with global disability over time, and 4) absence of confounding effects of symptomatic therapy. DAT-SPECT retesting for [123 I]β-CIT and [123 I]FP-CIT in seven and 10 early PD patients respectively scanned 7–21 days apart gave test/retest reliability of mean striatal DAT availability ranging from 5% to 16% (SD 13%) (Seibyl et al. 1997;

Booij et al. 1998). Striatal DAT availability measured with SPECT relates to the amount of rat nigral dopaminergic neurons (Scherfler et al. 2002), reflects striatal dopamine levels in MPTP-treated monkeys (Bezard et al. 2001), and is reduced in PD brains (Uhl et al. 1994), fulfilling the sensitivity criterion for the process of nigral degeneration. In longitudinal studies assessing PD progression, the annual rate of reduction of striatal DAT uptake is between 6% and 13% in PD patients versus 0% to 2.5% in healthy controls and is significantly correlated with clinical stages measured by the Hoehn and Yahr rating scale (Staffen et al. 2000; Chouker et al. 2001; Pirker et al. 2002; Benamer et al. 2000b; Figure 3) and the severity of bradykinesia and rigidity but not tremor (Seibyl et al. 1995; Asenbaum et al. 1997). The percent of change from baseline of striatal DAT-SPECT has been used as an index for disease progression in clinical trials with levodopa, selegiline, and pramipexole (Parkinson Study Group 2004; Innis et al. 1999 Parkinson Study Group 2002). No significant alterations of striatal DAT binding in PD patients treated with selegiline or pramipexole were found compared to levodopa in the short term (4 to 10 weeks) (Innis et al. 1999). In contrast, after 46 months of treatment, there was a significant one-third reduction in relative rates of decline of striatal $[^{123}I]\beta$-CIT uptake in the pramipexole versus levodopa treated patients (Parkinson Study Group 2002). Since there may be different effects of dopamine agonists and levodopa on the regulation of DAT expression, and differences in radiotracer affinity and receptor occupancy cannot be completely excluded, there are major difficulties in the interpretation of the clinical relevance of such findings (Ahlskog 2003; Wooten 2003). Before serial SPECT assessments of striatal DAT binding can be accepted as a valid biomarker

for progression of nigrostriatal pathology in PD, these issues need to be clarified in appropriate studies.

USE OF DAT-SPECT IN ROUTINE CLINICAL PRACTICE

A majority of patients with PD or ET can be diagnosed clinically. The principal role of DAT-SPECT comes in when clinical signs are inconclusive or vague and a diagnosis of early PD cannot be made with confidence. However, to avoid overuse of DAT-SPECT, the judicious selection of patients presenting with subtle or ambiguous signs, insufficient for a confident diagnosis on the basis of clinical criteria, requires assessment by clinicians with movement disorder expertise. The accuracy of DAT-SPECT to identify neurodegenerative parkinsonism in patients with inconclusive clinical symptoms at their initial neurological visit has been evaluated in three studies (Catafau et al. 2004, Tolosa et al. 2007; Marshall et al. 2009; Jennings et al. 2004). Sensitivity varies in two studies between 78% and 92%, specificity between 96% and 100% for DAT-SPECT to correctly classify neurodegenerative PD, compared with the judgment of an expert movement disorder clinician or consensus video-rating six months and 36 months after the initial visit. A third study was conducted to investigate the impact of DAT-SPECT on the diagnosis and changes in therapeutic management in patients with inconclusive parkinsonism, and reported that results from DAT-SPECT imaging were not consistent with the initial diagnosis in 36% of cases with neurodegenerative parkinsonism and 54% of cases with nonpresynaptic parkinsonism (Catafau et al. 2004). The mismatch of the clinical assessment and DAT-SPECT results led to a change of diagnosis in 52% of patients. In all three studies the diagnostic accuracy and reliability of DAT-SPECT have invariably been evaluated against the clinical examination. However, to determine most accurately the discriminant power of DAT-SPECT separating neurodegenerative from other causes of parkinsonism, correlations of imaging with results from autopsy are needed.

CONCLUSION

We conclude that DAT-SPECT can provide valuable additional information in patients presenting with inconclusive parkinsonian symptoms, particularly early in the disease where correct treatment decisions have far-reaching implications not only in control of symptoms but also in cost-efficiency for national health care systems (Dodel et al. 2003). Additional potential roles of DAT-SPECT that have not yet

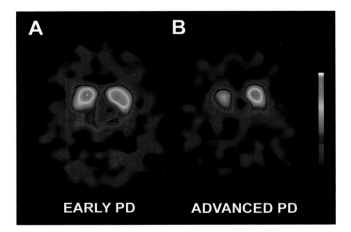

Figure 3 Decline of striatal dopamine transporter availability in early (1 year; A) and advanced (10 years; B) Parkinson's disease.

been validated include (i) use as a secondary screen for persons at risk for developing PD as was reported for first-degree relatives, gene mutation carriers, hyposmic individuals, and subjects with RBD, and (ii) its use in the longitudinal monitoring of the striatal dopaminergic dysfunction in treated PD patients as a measure for disease progression.

REFERENCES

Acton, P. D., A. Newberg, K. Ploessl, and P. D. Mozley. 2006. Comparison of region-of-interest analysis and human observers in the diagnosis of Parkinson's disease using [99mTc]Trodat-1 and SPECT. *Phys Med Biol* 51:757–585.

Ahlskog, J. E. 2003. Slowing Parkinson's disease progression: Recent dopamine agonist trials. *Neurology* 60:381–389.

Arblaster, L. A., M. Lakie, W. J. Mutch, and M. Semple. 1993. A study of the early signs of drug induced parkinsonism. *J Neurol Neurosurg Psychiatry* 56:301–303.

Asenbaum, S., T. Brucke, W. Pirker, I. Podreka, P. Angelberger, S. Wenger et al. 1997. Imaging of dopamine transporters with iodine-123-beta-CIT and SPECT in Parkinson's disease. *J Nucl Med* 38:1–6.

Asenbaum, S., W. Pirker, P. Angelberger, G. Bencsits, M. Pruckmayer, and T. Brucke. 1998. [123I]beta-CIT and SPECT in essential tremor and Parkinson's disease. *J Neural Transm* 105:1213–1228.

Benamer, H. T., W. H. Oertel, J. Patterson et al. 2003. Prospective study of presynaptic dopaminergic imaging in patients with mild parkinsonism and tremor disorders: Part 1. Baseline and 3-month observations. *Mov Disord* 18:977–984.

Benamer, H. T. S., J. Patterson, D. G. Grosset et al. 2000a. Accurate differentiation of parkinsonism and essential tremor using visual assessment of [123I]FP-CIT SPECT imaging: The [123I]FP-CIT SPECT study group. *Mov Disord* 15:503–510.

Benamer, H. T. S., J. Patterson, D. J. Wyper, D. M. Hadley, G. J. A. Macphee, and D. G. Grosset. 2000b. Correlation of Parkinson's disease severity and duration with FP-CIT SPECT striatal uptake. *Mov Disord* 15:692–698.

Benito-León, J., E. D. Louis, F. Bermejo-Pareja, Neurological Disorders in Central Spain Study Group. 2009. Risk of incident Parkinson's disease and parkinsonism in essential tremor: A population based study. *J Neurol Neurosurg Psychiatry* 80: 423–5.

Berendse, H. W., J. Booij, C. M. J. E. Francot, P. L. M. Bermans, R. Hijman, J. C. Stoof et al. 2001. Subclinical dopaminergic dysfunction in asymptomatic Parkinson's disease patients' relatives with decreased sense of smell. *Ann Neurol* 50:34–41.

Bezard, E., S. Dovero, C. Prunier, P. Ravenscroft, S. Chalon, D. Guilloteau et al. 2001. Relationship between the appearance of symptoms and the level of nigrostriatal degeneration in a progressive 1-methyl-4phenyl-1,2,3,6-tetrahydropyridine-lesioned macaque model of Parkinson's disease. *J Neurosci* 21:6853–6861.

Booij, J., J. B. Habraken, P. Bergmans, G. Tissingh, A. Winogrodzka, E. C. Wolters et al. 1998. Imaging of dopamine transporters with iodine-123-FP-CIT SPECT in healthy controls and patients with Parkinson's disease. *J Nucl Med* 39:1879–1884.

Booij, J., J. D. Speelman, H. W. Horstink, and E. C. Wolters. 2001. The clinical benefit of imaging striatal dopamine transporters with [123I] FP-CIT SPECT in differentiating patients with presynaptic parkinsonism from those with other forms of parkinsonism. *Eur J Nucl Med* 28:266–272.

Catafau, A. M., and E. Tolosa. 2004. Impact of dopamine transporter SPECT using 123I-Ioflupane on diagnosis and management of patients with clinically uncertain Parkinsonian syndromes. *Mov Disord* 19:1175–1182.

Chaudhuri, K. R., M. Buxton-Thomas, V. Dhawan et al. 2005. Long duration asymmetrical postural tremor is likely to predict development of Parkinson's disease and not essential tremor: Clinical follow up study of 13 cases. *J Neurol Neurosurg Psychiatry* 76:115–17.

Chouker, M., K. Tatsch, R. Linke, O. Pogarell, K. Hahn, and J. Schwarz. 2001. Striatal dopamine transporter binding in early to moderately advanced Parkinson's disease: Monitoring of disease progression over 2 years. *Nucl Med Commun* 22:721–725.

Deuschl, G. 1999. Differential diagnosis of tremor. *J Neural Transm Suppl* 56:211–220.

Dodel, R. C., H. Hoffken, J. C. Moller, B. Bornschein, T. Klockgether, T. Behr et al. 2003. Dopamine transporter imaging and SPECT in diagnostic work-up of Parkinson's disease: A decision-analytic approach. *Mov Dis* 18 Suppl 7:52–62.

Darcourt, J., J. Booij, K. Tatsch, A. Varrone, T. Vander, Ö. L. Kapucu, K. Någren, F. Nobili, Z. Walker, and K. Van Laere. 2010. EANM procedure guidelines for brain neurotransmission SPECT using 123I-labelled dopamine transporter ligands, version 2. *Eur J Nucl Med Mol Imaging* 37:443–450.

Factor, S. A., G. D. Podskalny, and E. S. Molho. 1995. Psychogenic movement disorders: Frequency, clinical profile, and characteristics. *J Neurol Neurosurg Psychiatry* 59:406–12.

Fahn, S., D. Oakes, I. Shoulson, K. Kieburtz, A. Rudolph, A. Lang et al. 2004. Levodopa and the progression of Parkinson's disease. *N Engl J Med* 351:2498–2508.

Fearnley, J. M, and A. J. Lees. 1991. Ageing and Parkinson's disease: Substantia nigra regional selectivity. *Brain* 114:2283–2301.

Forno, L. 1983. Reaction of the substantia nigra to massive basal ganglia infarction. *Acta Neuropathol (Berl)* 62:96–102.

Gaig, C., M. J. Marti, E. Tolosa, F. Valldeoriola, P. Paredes, F. J. Lomena et al. 2006. [123I]-ioflupane SPECT in the diagnosis of suspected psychogenic Parkinsonism. *Mov Disord* 21:1994–1998.

Garcia, B. G., Y. Wei, J. A. Moron, R. Z. Lin, J. A. Javitch, and A. Galli. 2005. Akt is essential for insulin modulation of amphetamine-induced human dopamine transporter cell-surface redistribution. *Mol Pharmacol* 68:102–109.

Gerschlager, W., G. Bencsits, W. Pirker, B. R. Bloem, S. Asenbaum, D. Prayer et al. 2002. [123I]beta-CIT distinguishes vascular parkinsonism from Parkinson's disease. *Mov Disord* 17:518–523.

Goebel, G., K. Seppi, E. Donnemiller, B. Warwitz, G. K. Wenning, I. Virgolini, W. Poewe, and C. Scherfler. 2011. A novel computer-assisted image analysis of [123I]β-CIT SPECT images improves the diagnostic accuracy of parkinsonian disorders. *Eur J Nucl Med Mol Imaging* 38:702–710.

Hughes, A. J., Y. Ben-Shlomo, S. E. Daniel, and A. J. Lees. 1992/2001. What features improve the accuracy of clinical diagnosis in Parkinson's disease: A clinicopathologic study. *Neurology* (2001); 57(10 Suppl 3): S34–S38.

Hughes, A. J., S. E. Daniel, Y. Ben-Shlomo, and A. J. Lees. 2002. The accuracy of diagnosis of parkinsonian syndromes in a specialist movement disorder service. *Brain* 125: 861–870.

Innis, R. B., K. L. Marek, K. Sheff, S. Zoghbi, J. Castronuovo, A. Feigin et al. 1999. Effect of treatment with L-dopa/carbidopa or L-selegiline on striatal dopamine transporter SPECT imaging with [123I]beta-CIT. *Mov Disord* 14:436–442.

Innis, R. B., J. P. Seibyl, B. E. Scanley, M. Laruelle, A. Abi-Dargham, E. Wallace et al. 1993. Single photon emission computed tomographic imaging demonstrates loss of striatal dopamine transporters in Parkinson disease. *Proc Natl Acad Sci USA* 90:11965–11969.

Iranzo, A., F. Lomeña, H. Stockner, F. Valldeoriola, I. Vilaseca, M. Salamero, J. L. Molinuevo, M. Serradell, J. Duch, J. Pavía, J. Gallego, K. Seppi, B. Högl, E. Tolosa, W. Poewe, J. Santamaria; for the Sleep Innsbruck Barcelona (SINBAR) group. 2010. Decreased striatal dopamine transporters uptake and substantia nigra hyperechogenicity as risk markers of synucleinopathy in patients with idiopathic rapid-eye-movement sleep behaviour disorder: A prospective study. *Lancet Neurol* 9:1070–1077.

Jennings, D. L., J. P. Seibyl, D. Oakes, S. Eberly, J. Murphy, and K. Marek. 2004. [123I] beta-CIT and single-photon emission computed tomographic imaging vs clinical evaluation in Parkinsonian syndrome: Unmasking an early diagnosis. *Arch Neurol* 61:1224–1229.

Kägi, G., K. P. Bhatia, and E. Tolosa. 2010. The role of DAT-SPECT in movement disorders. *J Neurol Neurosurg Psychiatry* 81:5–12.

Kahlig, K. M., J. A. Javitch, and A. Galli. 2004. Amphetamine regulation of dopamine transport. Combined measurements of transporter currents and transporter imaging support the endocytosis of an active carrier. *J Biol Chem* 279:8966–8975.

Khoshbouei, H., N. Sen, B. Guptaroy, L. Johnson, D. Lund, M. E. Gnegy et al. 2004. N-terminal phosphorylation of the dopamine transporter is required for amphetamine-induced efflux. *PLoS Biol* 2:E78.

Klaffke, S., A. A. Kuhn, M. Plotkin et al. 2006. Dopamine transporters, D2 receptors, and glucose metabolism in corticobasal degeneration. *Mov Disord* 21:1724–7.

Koch, W., P. E. Radau, C. Hamann, and K. Tatsch. 2005. Clinical testing of an optimized software solution for an automated, observer-independent evaluation of dopamine transporter SPECT studies. *J Nucl Med* 46:1109–1118.

Lang, A. E., W. C. Koller, and S. Fahn. 1995. Psychogenic parkinsonism. *Arch Neurol* 52:802–10.

Lavalaye, J., D. H. Linszen, J. Booij, L. Reneman, B. P. Gersons et al. 2001. Dopamine transporter density in young patients with schizophrenia assessed with [123]FP-CIT SPECT. *Schizophr Res* 47:59–67.

Lin, Z., P. W. Zhang, X. Zhu, J. M. Melgari, R. Huff, R. L. Spieldoch et al. 2003. Phosphatidylinositol 3-kinase, protein kinase C, and MEK1/2 kinase regulation of dopamine transporters (DAT) require N-terminal DAT phosphoacceptor sites. *J Biol Chem* 278:20162–20170.

Lorberboym, M., R. Djaldetti, E. Melamed, M. Sadeh, and Y. Lampl. 2004. [123I]FP-CIT SPECT Imaging of dopamine transporters in patients with cerebrovascular disease and clinical diagnosis of vascular parkinsonism. *J Nucl Med* 45:1688–1693.

Marek, K., R. Innis, C. van Dyck, B. Fussell, M. Early, S. Eberly et al. 2001. [123I]beta-CIT SPECT imaging assessment of the rate of Parkinson's disease progression. *Neurology* 57:2089–2094.

Marek, K. L., J. P. Seibyl, S. S. Zoghbi et al. 1996a. [123I]-beta-CIT/SPECT imaging demonstrates bilateral loss of dopamine transporters in hemi-Parkinson's disease. *Neurology* 46:231–237.

Marshall, V. L., C. B. Reininger, M. Marquardt, J. Patterson, D. M. Hadley, W. H. Oertel, H. T. Benamer, P. Kemp, D. Burn, E. Tolosa, J. Kulisevsky, L. Cunha, D. Costa, J. Booij, K. Tatsch, K. R. Chaudhuri, G. Ulm, O. Pogarell, H. Höffken, A. Gerstner, and D. G. Grosset. 2009. Parkinson's disease is overdiagnosed clinically at baseline in diagnostically uncertain cases: A 3-year European multicenter study with repeat [123I]FP-CIT SPECT. *Mov Disord* 24(4):500–8.

McKeith, I. G., D. W. Dickson, J. Lowe et al. 2005. Diagnosis and management of dementia with Lewy bodies: Third report of the DLB consortium. *Neurology* 65:1863–72.

Meara, J., B. K. Bhowmick, and P. Hobson. 1999. Accuracy of diagnosis in patients with presumed Parkinson's disease. *Age Ageing.* 28:99–102.

Melikian, H. E., and K. M. Buckley. 1999. Membrane trafficking regulates the activity of the human dopamine transporter. *J Neurosci* 19:7699–7710.

Morrish, P. K., J. S. Rakshi, D. L. Bailey, G. V. Sawle, and D. J. Brooks. 1998. Measuring the rate of progression and estimating the preclinical period of Parkinson's disease with [18F]dopa PET. *J Neurol Neurosurg Psychiatry* 64:314–319.

Parkinson Study Group. 2000. A multicenter assessment of dopamine transporter imaging with DOPASCAN/SPECT in parkinsonism. *Neurology* 55:1540–7.

Parkinson Study Group. 2002. Dopamine transporter brain imaging to assess the effects of pramipexole vs levodopa on Parkinson disease progression. *JAMA* 287:1653–1661.

Pellecchia, M. T., A. Varrone, G. Annesi et al. 2007. Parkinsonism and essential tremor in a family with pseudo-dominant inheritance of PARK2: An FP-CIT SPECT study. *Mov Disord* 22:559–63.

Piggott, M. A., E. F. Marshall, N. Thomas et al. 1999. Striatal dopaminergic markers in dementia with Lewy bodies, Alzheimer's and Parkinson's diseases: Rostrocaudal distribution. *Brain* 122:1449–68.

Pirker, W., S. Asenbaum, G. Bencsits, D. Prayer, W. Gerschlager, L. Deecke et al. 2000. [123I]beta-CIT SPECT in multiple system atrophy, progressive supranuclear palsy, and cortical degeneration. *Mov Dis* 15:1158–1167.

Pirker, W., S. Djamshidian, S. Asenbaum, W. Gerschlager, G. Tribl, M. Hoffmann, and T. Brucke. 2002. Progression of dopaminergic degeneration in Parkinson's disease and atypical parkinsonism: A longitudinal beta-CIT SPECT study. *Mov Disord* 17:45–53.

Ponsen, M. M., D. Stoffers, ECh. Wolters, J. Booij, and H. W. Berendse. 2010. Olfactory testing combined with dopamine transporter imaging as a method to detect prodromal Parkinson's disease. *J Neurol Neurosurg Psychiatry* 81(4):396–9.

Rajput, A. H., B. Rozdilsky, and A. Rajput. 1991. Accuracy of clinical diagnosis in parkinsonism—a prospective study. *Can J Neurol Sci* 18:275–278.

Reader, T. A., A. R. Ase, N. Huang et al. 1998. Neuroleptics and dopamine transporters. *Neurochem Res* 23:73–80.

Rinne, J. O., D. J. Burn, C. J. Mathias et al. 1995. Positron emission tomography studies on the dopaminergic system and striatal opioid binding in the olivopontocerebellar atrophy variant of multiple system atrophy. *Ann Neurol* 37:568–73.

Scherfler, C., E. Donnemiller, M. Schocke, K. Dierkes, C. Decristoforo, M. Oberladstatter et al. 2002. Evaluation of striatal dopamine transporter function in rats by in vivo beta-[123I]CIT pinhole SPECT. *Neuroimage* 17:128–141.

Scherfler, C., and M. Nocker. 2009. Dopamine transporter SPECT: How to remove subjectivity? *Mov Disord.* 24 Suppl 2:S721–4.

Scherfler, C., K. Seppi, E. Donnemiller, G. Goebel, C. Brenneis, I. Virgolini et al. 2005. Voxel-wise analysis of [123I]beta-CIT SPECT differentiates the Parkinson variant of multiple system atrophy from idiopathic Parkinson's disease. *Brain* 128:1605–1612.

Schneider, S. A., M. J. Edwards, P. Mir, C. Cordivari, J. Hooker, J. Dickson, N. Quinn, and K. P. Bhatia. 2007. Patients with adult-onset dystonic tremor resembling parkinsonian tremor have scans without evidence of dopaminergic deficit (SWEDDs). *Mov Disord* 22 (15):2210–5.

Schrag, A., A. Munchau, K. P. Bhatia et al. 2000. Essential tremor: An overdiagnosed condition? *J Neurol* 247:955–9.

Schwarz, J., A. Storch, W. Koch, O. Pogarell, P. E. Radau, and K. Tatsch. 2004. Loss of dopamine transporter binding in Parkinson's disease follows a single exponential rather than linear decline. *J Nucl Med* 45:1694–1697.

Seibyl, J. P., K. Marek, K. Sheff, R. M. Baldwin, S. Zoghbi, Y. Zea-Ponce et al. 1997. Test/retest reproducibility of iodine-123-betaCIT SPECT brain measurement of dopamine transporters in Parkinson's patients. *J Nucl Med* 38:1453–1459.

Seibyl, J. P., K. L. Marek, D. Quinlan, K. Sheff, S. Zoghbi, Y. Zea-Ponce et al. 1995. Decreased single-photon emission computed tomographic [123I] beta-CIT striatal uptake correlates with symptom severity in Parkinson's disease. *Ann Neurol* 38:589–598.

Seppi, K., C. Scherfler, E. Donnemiller, I. Virgolini, M. F. H. Schocke, G. Goebel et al. 2006. Topography of dopamine transporter availability in progressive supranuclear palsy: A voxel wise [123I]beta CIT SPECT analysis. *Arch Neurol* 63:1154–1160.

Sommer, U., T. Hummel, K. Cormann, A. Mueller, J. Frasnelli, J. Kropp et al. 2004. Detection of presymptomatic Parkinson's disease: Combining smell tests, transcranial sonography, and SPECT. *Mov Disord* 19:1196–1202.

Staffen, W., A. Mair, J. Unterrainer, E. Trinka, and G. Ladurner. 2000. Measuring the progression of idiopathic Parkinson's disease with [123I]beta-CIT SPECT. *J Neural Transm* 107:543–552.

Stiasny-Kolster, K., Y. Doerr, J. C. Möller, H. Höffken, T. M. Behr, W. H. Oertel et al. 2005. Combination of "idiopathic" REM sleep behaviour disorder and olfactory dysfunction as possible indicator for alpha-synucleinopathy demonstrated by dopamine transporter FP-CIT-SPECT. *Brain* 128:126–137.

The Parkinson Study Group. 2004. Levodopa and the progression of Parkinson's disease. *N Engl J Med* 351:2498–2508.

Tinazzi, M., A. Antonini, T. Bovi, I. Pasquin, M. Steinmayr, G. Moretto, A. Fiaschi, and S. Ottaviani. 2009. Clinical and [123I]FP-CIT SPET imaging follow-up in patients with drug-induced parkinsonism. *J Neurol* 256:910–915.

Tissingh, G., P. Bergmans, J. Booij, A. Winogrodzka, E. A. van Royen, J. C. Stoof et al. 1998. Drug-naïve patients with Parkinson's disease in Hoehn and Yahr stages I and II show a bilateral decrease in striatal dopamine transporters as revealed by [123I]beta-CIT SPECT. *J Neurol* 245:14–20.

Tolosa, E., T. V. Borght, E. Moreno, DaTSCAN Clinically Uncertain Parkinsonian Syndromes Study Group. 2007. Accuracy of DaTSCAN (123I-Ioflupane) SPECT in diagnosis of patients with clinically uncertain parkinsonism: 2-year follow-up of an open-label study. *Mov Disord* 22 (16): 2346–51.

Tzen, K. Y., C. S. Lu, T. C. Yen, S. P. Wey, and G. Ting. 2001. Differential diagnosis of Parkinson's disease and vascular parkinsonism by [99mTc]-TRODAT-1. *J Nucl Med* 42:408–413.

Uhl, G. R., D. Walther, D. Mash, B. Faucheux, and F. Javoy-Agid. 1994. Dopamine transporter messenger RNA in Parkinson's disease and control substantia nigra neurons. *Ann Neurol* 35:494–498.

Unger, M. M., J. C. Möller, K. Stiasny-Kolster, K. Mankel, D. Berg, U. Walter, H. Hoeffken, G. Mayer, and W. H. Oertel. 2008. Assessment of idiopathic rapid-eye-movement sleep behavior disorder by transcranial sonography, olfactory function test, and FP-CIT-SPECT. *Mov Disord* 23 (4):596–9.

Varrone, A., and C. Halldin. 2010. Molecular imaging of the dopamine transporter. *J Nucl Med* 51:1331–1334.

Varrone, A., K. L. Marek, D. Jennings, R. B. Innis, and J. P. Seibyl. 2001. [123I]beta-CIT SPECT imaging demonstrates reduced density of striatal dopamine transporters in Parkinson's disease and multiple system atrophy. *Mov Disord* 16:1023–1032.

Walker, Z., E. Jaros, R. W. H. Walker et al. 2007. Dementia with Lewy bodies: A comparison of clinical diagnosis, FP-CIT single photon emission computed tomography imaging and autopsy. *J Neurol Neurosurg Psychiatry* 78:1176–81.

Whone, A. L., R. L. Watts, A. J. Stoessl et al. 2003. Slower progression of Parkinson's disease with ropinirole versus levodopa: The REAL PET study. *Ann Neurol* 54:93–101.

Wooten, G. F. 2003. Agonists vs. levodopa in PD: The thrilla of whitha. *Neurology* 60:360–362.

Zijlmans, J., A. Evans, F. Fontes, R. Katzenschlager, S. Gacinovic, A. J. Lees, and D. Costa. 2007. [123I] FP-CIT spect study in vascular parkinsonism and Parkinson's disease. *Mov Disord* 22 (9): 1278–85.

Zijlmans, J. C. M., S. E. Daniel, A. J. Hughes, T. Révész, and A. J. Lees. 2004. Clinicopathological investigation of vascular parkinsonism, including clinical criteria for diagnosis. *Mov Disord* 19:630–640.

3

CEREBRAL GLUCOSE METABOLISM AND BLOOD FLOW IN PARKINSON'S DISEASE

Yilong Ma, Shichun Peng, Vijay Dhawan, and David Eidelberg

INTRODUCTION

Functional brain imaging with positron emission tomography (PET) and single photon emission computed tomography (SPECT) has provided insights into the pathophysiology of Parkinson's disease (PD) and related movement disorders. The integrity of the presynaptic nigrostriatal dopaminergic system can be evaluated by measuring dopa decarboxylase activity using [18F]fluoro-dopa (FDOPA) PET or dopamine transporter (DAT) binding using cocaine derivative tracers such as [123I]βCIT, or [123I]FPCIT SPECT, or [18F]FPCIT PET (see Thobois et al. 2004;Dhawan and Eidelberg 2007). The postsynaptic dopamine system can be assayed with radioligands that bind specifically to D_1 or D_2 neuroreceptors. In addition, studies of brain metabolism and blood flow have contributed considerably to the understanding of the abnormal neuronal circuitry underlying the pathophysiology of PD. In particular, PET has been used to study regional neuronal activity in this disorder by quantifying rest-state regional cerebral glucose metabolism (rCMRglc) with [18F]fluoro-deoxyglucose (FDG) PET (Dhawan and Eidelberg 2007) and cerebral blood flow (rCBF) with O^{15}-labeled water ($H_2^{15}O$) PET. Perfusion tracers such as ^{99m}Tc-ethyl cysteinate dimer (ECD) (Feigin et al. 2002; Van Laere et al. 2004; Eckert et al. 2007a) and arterial spin labeling (ASL) MRI (Ma et al. 2010) methods have also been employed to study resting functional brain changes in PD. (The study of abnormal brain activation response in PD utilizing [15O]H_2O PET and functional magnetic resonance imaging (fMRI) is reviewed in Chapter 9).

Functional brain imaging has been particularly useful for assessing the downstream consequences of nigrostriatal dopamine loss in PD on the functional organization of the basal ganglia and the cortico-striato-pallido-thalamocortical (CSPTC) loops (DeLong and Wichmann 2007). Although the primary pathological abnormality in PD is confined to the substantia nigra, degeneration of nigrostriatal dopaminergic projections leads to widespread alterations in the functional activity of the motor network as a whole (Eidelberg 2009). On a basic level, the functional organization of the basal ganglia predicts that the loss of inhibitory dopaminergic input to the striatum is associated with enhanced inhibitory (GABAergic) output from the putamen to the external globus pallidus (GPe), leading to diminished inhibitory GPe output to the subthalamic nucleus (STN). PD is functionally defined by overactivity of the STN and its excitatory (glutamatergic) projections to the internal globus pallidus (GPi), which in turn leads to an increase in pallidothalamic inhibition and concomitant reductions in ventrolateral and intralaminar thalamic output to the motor cortex. These circuit changes are paralleled by corresponding alterations in local synaptic activity as measured by specific regional- and network-level abnormalities observed on scans of cerebral metabolism or blood flow (Eidelberg et al. 1994, 2009).

This chapter provides a review of recent functional brain imaging studies, mainly involving the regional mapping of changes in cerebral metabolism and blood flow in PD patients. Additionally, recent imaging data will be presented to illustrate the clinical applications of network-based techniques in delineating mechanisms of the treatment response to novel antiparkinsonian therapies.

FUNCTIONAL BRAIN IMAGING: UNIVARIATE ANALYSES

Resting state scans of cerebral metabolism and blood flow have been employed extensively to identify alterations in regional brain function in PD patients analogous to those discerned in experimental animal models of parkinsonism (Brownell et al. 2003; Guigoni et al. 2005; Peng et al. 2010). The bulk of this effort has been based on the use of statistical parametric mapping (SPM) to localize abnormal regional changes as well as clinical-imaging correlations in PD patients. Typically, in this univariate approach, functional brain images are spatially transformed into a standard anatomical space to allow for the use of voxel-by-voxel analytical methods.

CEREBRAL GLUCOSE METABOLISM

Because the regional rate of glucose metabolism reflects local synaptic activity, FDG PET has been generally used to study abnormal brain function in PD. A dual-tracer PET study with FDG and $[^{15}O]H_2O$ showed that regional energy metabolism is increased in the putamen and pallidum in early unmedicated PD patients (Powers et al. 2008). Increases in resting cerebellar metabolic activity have also been described in early-stage and advanced PD patients, which have been associated with akinetic rigidity (Ghaemi et al. 2002; Hilker et al. 2004), although parkinsonian tremor can also contribute to functional changes in this brain region (Mure et al. 2011). Reductions in cortical metabolic activity have also been observed in PD. A study reported occipital hypometabolism (greater in the hemisphere contralateral to the more severely affected body side) in PD (Bohnen et al. 1999) and also in patients with diffuse Lewy body disease (Minoshima 2001). Hypometabolism of frontal and occipital cortical regions has been reported in non-demented PD patients (Hosokai et al. 2009). These changes have been found to be more widespread with advancing PD (Hilker 2004; Huang 2007b), and are not correlated with reductions in global metabolic activity (Spetsieris 2011). In a recent study of de novo PD patients there was evidence of a significant negative relationship between Unified Parkinson's Disease Rating Scale (UPDRS) motor ratings and rCMRglc in premotor cortex (PMC) (Berti et al. 2010). A positive relationship was found between putamen DAT binding and measurements of regional metabolism in premotor and dorsolateral and anterior prefrontal regions, and in the orbitofrontal cortex. In a subsequent study (Tang et al. 2010a), putamen DAT binding exhibited an inverse relationship with metabolic activity measured in the same brain region, linking metabolic increases in the basal ganglia with nigrostriatal dopaminergic attrition. Taken together, these findings suggest a correlation between PD-related metabolic changes and motor deficits. Given that in PD both measures exhibit only modest correlations with nigrostriatal deficits, it is likely that the observed clinical and metabolic changes are not epiphenomena of disease-related dopaminergic dysfunction (Eckert 2007b).

Rest-state imaging has also been used to investigate metabolic correlates with cognitive impairment in PD. Recent studies reported extensive metabolic reductions in the posterior cortical regions (including the temporo-parieto-occipital junction, precuneus, and inferior temporal cortex) in PD patients with mild cognitive impairment (Huang et al. 2008; Hosokai et al. 2009). Significant correlations have been reported between these regional metabolic deficits and cognitive dysfunction in a combined cohort of PD patients with and without dementia (Liepelt et al. 2009). This is in agreement with the finding that intellectual impairment in PD correlates negatively with measurements of glucose metabolism in the posterior cortical association regions (Wu et al. 2000). These findings therefore suggest that posterior cortical dysfunction is a consistent imaging feature of cognitive impairment in PD patients.

CEREBRAL BLOOD FLOW

Prior to the routine use of fMRI in brain activation experiments, $H_2^{15}O$ PET was used for the quantification of changes in regional cerebral blood flow (rCBF) during task performance. This method is still used in activation studies when absolute quantification is needed, as when an intervention is found to influence baseline neural activity, or dissociate rCBF from regional glucose utilization (Hirano et al. 2008). This technique is also preferred when fMRI is not routinely doable as is the case with implanted deep brain stimulation (DBS) electrodes (Fukuda et al. 2001a; Hirano et al. 2008; Mure et al. 2011). That said, $H_2^{15}O$ PET has also been utilized to measure rCBF changes in PD patients scanned in the rest-state. Scans of cerebral blood flow and metabolism acquired in the same PD patients have yielded similar patterns of abnormal regional activity, consistent with the presence of tight coupling between these rest-state measures (Ma and Eidelberg 2007), at least in the absence of dopaminergic medication(Hirano et al. 2008). Moreover, CBF findings with $H_2^{15}O$ PET are comparable to those obtained using resting state SPECT perfusion imaging. In an early imaging study of mildly affected PD patients, rCBF was found to increase in the caudate and lenticular nuclei contralateral to the more affected body side (Miletich et al. 1994). Parametric maps of globally normalized rCBF were also compared in PD patients and age-matched healthy volunteers scanned with ECD SPECT (Imon et al. 1999). In patients with early-stage PD, rCBF was elevated in the putamen and hippocampus relative to controls. In patients with late-stage PD, rCBF increased in the putamen, globus pallidus, hippocampus, cerebellum/dentate nuclei, ventrolateral thalamus, and right insula and inferior temporal gyrus. Thus, rCBF findings in PD are consistent with the changes in the functional architecture of CSPTC loops observed with FDG PET.

In advanced PD patients (Hoehn & Yahr Stage III/IV) regional cerebral blood flow was found to decline in the supplementary motor area (SMA) and in the dorsolateral prefrontal cortex (DLPFC), as demonstrated by ^{99m}Tc-hexamethyl propylene amine oxime (HMPAO) SPECT (Kikuchi et al. 2001). Another study using N-isopropyl-p-[^{123}I]iodoamphetamine (IMP) SPECT showed reduced rCBF in the posterior parietal and occipital cortices in non-demented PD patients (Abe et al. 2003). In PD, a positive correlation has been reported between performance on a visual processing task and rCBF decreases in the visual association area, suggesting that the latter is a consistent feature of the disease, even in the absence of dementia. By contrast, in PD patients with dementia, more extensive rCBF reductions were noted involving frontal, parietal, and temporal association regions (Matsui et al. 2007; Firbank et al. 2003; Osaki et al. 2005). These findings may have utility in classifying PD patients with and without dementia on imaging grounds.

FUNCTIONAL BRAIN IMAGING: MULTIVARIATE ANALYSES

Local measurements of cerebral blood flow and glucose metabolism may not fully account for the complex nature of the neural systems that are involved in neurodegenerative processes and their response to treatment. The functional natural history of a progressive neurodegenerative disorder such as PD may be better represented at the systems level through an analysis of specific spatially distributed networks associated with the disease process. A variety of multivariate computational algorithms have been developed for the characterization of disease-related spatial covariance pattern (i.e., functional brain networks) in the resting state (Eidelberg 2009; Chen et al. 2009; Habeck and Stern 2010). These approaches are generally based on principal component analysis (PCA) to identify sets of linearly independent (orthogonal) covariance patterns in functional imaging data (Gwadry et al. 2001; Spetsieris and Eidelberg 2011).

METABOLIC NETWORK ANALYSIS

PD is one of the most extensively studied brain diseases from the standpoint of network analysis. In this disorder, the Scaled Subprofile Model (SSM) (Alexander and Moeller

1994; Habeck and Stern 2010; Spetsieris and Eidelberg 2011), a PCA-based computational algorithm has been used successfully to identify, validate, and prospectively quantify the activity of PD-related metabolic brain networks (Tang and Eidelberg 2010). The details of SSM/PCA for the analysis of PD imaging data have been provided elsewhere (Eidelberg 2009; Spetsieris and Eidelberg 2011). This approach uses PCA to identify regional covariance patterns in imaging datasets of combined samples of patients and controls. This analysis is blind to subject class designation and utilizes the variance across the entire population to define specific patterns associated with the disease. The resulting disease-related patterns reflect covarying increases or decreases in regional brain function in patients relative to the control population. The SSM/PCA approach also allows for prospective quantification of pattern expression in brain images of individual subjects on a single case basis. These network values (termed subject scores) can be correlated with independently obtained clinical or physiological disease descriptors. In contrast to the neurochemical dopaminergic markers described above, the subject scores have the attribute of increasing signal-to-noise with advancing disease. This property offers potentially greater sensitivity in the detection of longitudinal changes in network expression with disease progression (Huang et al. 2007b; Tang et al. 2010 a) or treatment (Asanuma et al. 2006). For these reasons, this network method has been found to be well suited for the study of the changes in functional brain organization that occur in PD and other neurodegenerative disorders (Eidelberg 2009; Habeck and Stern 2010).

SSM/PCA analysis of metabolic brain images from PD patients and healthy controls has consistently revealed an abnormal spatial covariance pattern in PD patients characterized by increased metabolism in the putamen/globus pallidus, thalamus, cerebellum, pons, and sensorimotor cortex (SMC), with reduced metabolism in the lateral frontal, paracentral, and parieto-occipital areas (Figure 1A). Subject scores for this PD-related covariance pattern (PDRP) were abnormally elevated in PD patients and correlated positively with clinical motor ratings (Figure 1B) and negatively with independent PET measurements of synaptic nigrostriatal dopaminergic functioning (Kaasinen et al. 2006; Huang et al. 2007b; Tang et al. 2010a). Indeed, the PDRP topography has been validated in seven independent cohorts of PD patients and healthy subjects scanned using different imaging techniques on a variety of tomographic platforms (Eckert et al. 2007; Eidelberg 2009). Prospectively computed PDRP values have been found to have excellent test–retest reproducibility in repeat FDG PET sessions separated by up to eight weeks

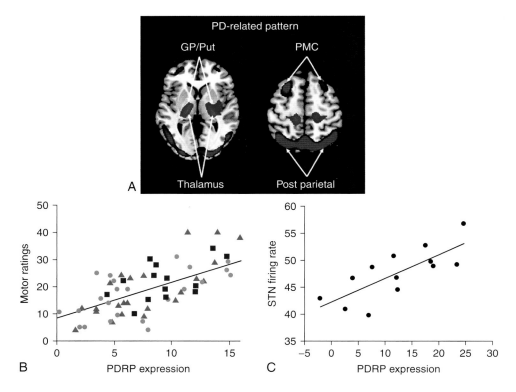

Figure 1 Parkinson's disease-related pattern: Validation and correlates. **A.** Parkinson's disease-related pattern (PDRP). This motor-related metabolic spatial covariance pattern is characterized by hypermetabolism in the thalamus, globus pallidus (GP), pons, and primary motor cortex, associated with relative metabolic reductions in the lateral premotor cortex (PMC) and posterior parietal areas (Ma et al. 2007). [In the representative slices, relative metabolic increases are displayed in red; relative metabolic decreases are displayed in blue. Slices were overlaid on a standard MRI brain template.] **B.** PDRP expression correlates with Unified Parkinson's Disease Rating Scale (UPDRS) motor scores from a combined group of three independent PD populations (n = 65; r = 0.68, p < 0.001) (Eidelberg et al. 1995; Lozza et al. 2004; Asanuma et al. 2006). These correlations were also significant within each of the individual patient cohorts (*circles*: n = 27, r = 0.66, p < 0.001; *squares*: n = 15, r = 0.65, p < 0.01; *triangles*: n = 23, r = 0.76, p < 0.001). **C.** PDRP expression correlates with intraoperative measurements of spontaneous subthalamic nucleus (STN) firing rate (n = 17, r = 0.76, p < 0.007) recorded in PD patients undergoing the implantation of deep brain stimulation (DBS) electrodes (Lin et al. 2008). The regression line includes corrections for individual differences in disease duration and motor ratings across the subjects. [*Reproduced with permission from Eidelberg 2009, 32:548-57.*]

(Ma et al. 2007). Interestingly, preoperative measurements of PDRP expression were found to correlate with individual differences in STN firing rate recorded during DBS surgery (Lin et al. 2008) (Figure 1C). Of note, distinct disease-specific spatial covariance patterns have also been characterized for atypical parkinsonian syndromes, such as multiple system atrophy (MSA) and progressive supranuclear palsy (PSP) (Eckert et al. 2008; Tang et al. 2010b). Recent studies indicate how these disease-related metabolic patterns can be used in concert with PDRP quantification to classify individual patients with parkinsonism at a time when the final clinical diagnosis is not yet known (Tang et al. 2010b). Accurate differentiation of typical and atypical forms of parkinsonism may be critical in determining suitable candidates for stereotaxic surgery and for enrollment in clinical trials of new therapies for PD.

Network analysis has also led to the identification of a specific metabolic network associated with cognitive dysfunction in PD. Using this approach to evaluate scan data from non-demented PD patients, Huang et al. (2007a) described a significant spatial covariance pattern that correlated with performance on tests of memory and executive functioning, but not with UPDRS motor scores. This PD-related cognitive pattern (PDCP) was characterized by metabolic reductions in frontal and parietal association areas with relative increases in the cerebellar vermis and dentate nuclei (Figure 2A). In prospective studies, PDCP values were found to predict memory performance, visuospatial function, and perceptual motor speed in three independent validation samples of PD patients with similar disease duration and severity (Figure 2B). As with PDRP expression, PDCP scores also exhibited excellent test–retest reliability (Huang et al. 2007a). Of relevance, PDCP

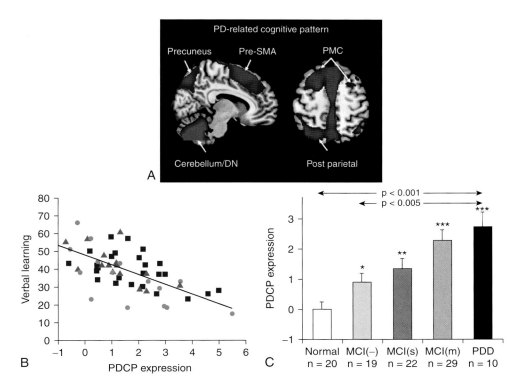

Figure 2 Parkinson's disease-related cognitive pattern: validation and correlates. **A.** Parkinson's disease-related cognitive pattern (PDCP). This cognition-related metabolic spatial covariance pattern is characterized by hypometabolism of dorsal premotor cortex (PMC), rostral supplementary motor area (preSMA), precuneus, and posterior parietal regions, associated with relative metabolic increases in the cerebellum (Huang et al. 2007a). [In the representative slices, relative metabolic increases are displayed in red; relative metabolic decreases are displayed in blue. Slices were overlaid on a standard MRI brain template.] **B.** PDCP expression correlates with performance on neuropsychological tests of memory and executive functioning in non-demented PD patients. For the California Verbal Learning Test: Sum 1 to 5 (CVLT sum), this correlation was significant for the entire cohort (n = 56, r = −0.67, p < 0.001), as well as for the original group used for pattern derivation (*circles*: n = 15, r = −0.71, p = 0.003) and in two prospective validation groups (*squares*: n = 25, r = −0.53, p = 0.007; *triangles*: n = 16, r = −0.80, p < 0.001) (Huang et al. 2007a). **C.** Bar graph of PDCP expression (mean ± SE) in PD patients with dementia (PDD), multiple domain mild cognitive impairment (MCI(m)), single domain mild cognitive impairment (MCI(s)), PD patients without mild cognitive impairment (MCI(−)), and in healthy control subjects. There was a significant difference in PDCP expression across the patient and control groups (F(4,70) = 8.87, p < 0.001; one-way ANOVA) and among the PD groups (F(3,56) = 4.84; p < 0.005), with higher expression in the PDD and MCI(m) cohorts compared to the MCI(−) cohort (p < 0.03; Tukey-Kramer HSD). For each PD group, PDCP expression was separately compared to healthy control values using Student *t*-tests. The asterisks denote significant increases in network activity relative to controls (*p < 0.05, **p < 0.005, ***p < 0.0001) in all PD categories including MCI(−). [*Reproduced with permission from Eidelberg 2009, 32:548–57.*]

scores were found to have a stepwise relationship with progressing levels of cognitive impairment (Figure 2C) independent of global metabolic rate (Huang et al. 2008; Spetsieris and Eidelberg 2011).

NETWORK ANALYSIS USING CEREBRAL BLOOD FLOW IMAGING

Spatial covariance analysis can be used to identify and prospectively assess PD-related brain networks in scans of cerebral blood flow acquired with PET, SPECT, or ASL MRI. SSM/PCA of resting ECD SPECT data from PD patients and healthy volunteer subjects revealed a significant disease-related pattern of similar topography to that identified with FDG PET (Feigin et al. 2002), with elevated

pattern expression in the PD patients relative to MSA and healthy cohorts. Interestingly, subject scores for the PET-derived PDRP computed in individual ECD SPECT scans were also found to discriminate PD patients from healthy controls and MSA patients with an overall diagnostic accuracy of 0.91 (Eckert et al. 2007). This indicates that the PDRP network identified from FDG PET data can be reliably applied to SPECT perfusion scans, a finding substantiated in a recent ASL MRI study (Ma et al. 2010). Of note, the PDRP topographies derived from images of cerebral metabolism and blood flow using SSM/PCA have been found to be similar to those identified using independent component analysis (ICA), a form of multivariate analysis in which each of the resulting components (patterns) is computed to contain unique information concerning the

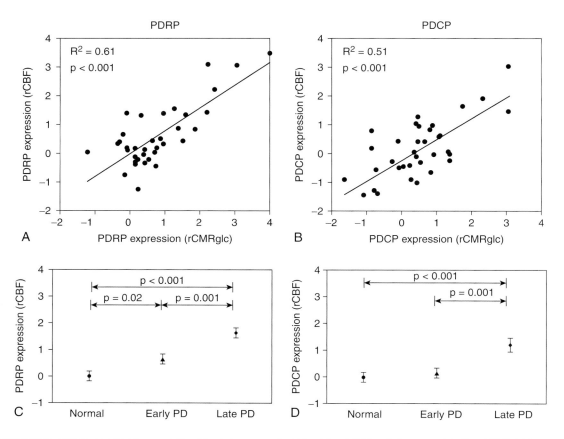

Figure 3 A/B: Regression analysis revealed linear relationships between cerebral blood flow (rCBF) and glucose metabolism (rCMRglc) in expressions of motor- (PDRP) and cognition-related (PDCP) brain networks in patients with Parkinson's disease (PD). The expression of each brain network was computed prospectively from resting state FDG and H_2O PET scans acquired concurrently in 36 PD patients (Ma et al. 2007). Subject scores were significantly correlated between rCBF and rCMRglc data in both PDRP (the fitted regression line: $y = 0.80 x - 0.03$) and PDCP ($y = 0.72 x - 0.26$). C/D: Discrimination of early and advanced PD by expressions of PDRP and PDCP brain networks. The expression of each brain network was computed prospectively with resting state H_2O PET scans in the same cohort of patients and age-matched normal controls (Ma and Eidelberg 2007). PDRP scores were abnormally elevated in early PD (n = 19) and significantly discriminated between early and late PD (n = 17) as well as control (n = 14) groups. PDCP scores remained normal in early PD but were elevated in late PD relative to controls, with comparable accuracy as PDRP (p < 0.001). Subject scores (mean ± SE) were obtained in individual case analysis conducted using an automated routine that was blind to diagnostic category.

sources of variability found in the data (i.e., the mutual information in any pair of components is minimized) (Bell and Sejnowski 1995). A SPECT study compared differences in rCBF between PD patients and controls after decomposing the images into disease-related and unrelated components (Hsu et al. 2007). The disease-related ICA pattern was found to resemble the PDRP in that the disease-related network was also characterized by perfusion increases in the putamen, globus pallidus, thalamus, brainstem, and anterior cerebellum, as well as covarying reductions in the parieto-temporo-occipital cortex, DLPFC, insula, and cingulate gyrus. The ICA approach appears to be especially promising as a means of data processing to remove extraneous image signals and for the detection of "blind sources" in the data (Jung et al. 2001).

Both the PDRP and PDCP have been validated as reliable measures of motor and cognitive dysfunction by

prospective computation of their respective network values in independent PD and control populations (Ma and Eidelberg 2007). PDRP/PDCP expression was significantly elevated in $H_2^{15}O$ and FDG PET scans of PD patients. For each network, there was a significant correlation between subject scores computed from $H_2^{15}O$ and FDG images in subjects scanned with both tracers (Figure 3A,B). Importantly, the PDRP (but not PDCP) scores computed in the CBF scans from these subjects separated early-stage PD from normal, whereas the expression of both networks discriminated more advanced PD patients from healthy subjects (Figure 3C,D). This is in line with the observation from a longitudinal FDG PET progression study (Huang et al. 2007b) that manifestation of motor symptoms precedes cognitive dysfunction in early PD. The test-retest reliability of PDRP/PDCP expression computed in scans of rCBF was also excellent, comparing favorably to the reproducibility of the network values computed in scans of glucose utilization (Ma et al. 2007; Huang 2007a). Further evidence for the comparability of network computations performed using perfusion imaging comes from a recent study in which CBF scans were generated non-invasively using ASL MRI (Ma et al. 2010). In aggregate, these findings support the utility of PDRP and PDCP computations in rCBF scans of PD patients. Pattern derivation and prospective individual case network quantitative assessments can be obtained from FDG PET data, and from rCBF data obtained using PET, SPECT, or ASL MRI. It is likely that network measurements will become available through the analysis of rest-state fMRI data (e.g., Wu et al. 2009).

FUNCTIONAL BRAIN IMAGING IN THE ASSESSMENT OF THERAPEUTIC INTERVENTIONS

Reliable in vivo biomarkers are in increasing use for the objective assessment of new therapeutic interventions for brain disease. Clinical rating instruments often have substantial variability that can limit their use, particularly in the evaluation of outcomes from early-phase trials. By contrast, resting state measures of cerebral function, at both the region and network levels, can provide an objective and accurate means of assessing the efficacy of new therapies. The advantages of such an approach are illustrated by several recent studies of established and experimental treatments for PD.

EFFECTS OF DOPAMINERGIC THERAPY ON BRAIN FUNCTION

Functional brain imaging has been applied to quantify regional changes associated with effective drug therapy for PD and related disorders. Levodopa (LD) treatment is associated with reduced regional glucose metabolism in the putamen, thalamus, cerebellum, and primary motor cortex in PD (Feigin et al. 2001; Asanuma et al. 2006). A significant decline in PDRP expression was also present, which correlated with improvement in UPDRS motor ratings (Figure 4). These findings are consistent with the idea that metabolic overactivity in PD can be reversed by dopaminergic treatment and that effective interventions are associated with PDRP network modulation. Interestingly, this network effect has been found to differ depending on whether PDRP expression was quantified in scans of cerebral metabolism or blood flow (Hirano et al. 2008).

Levodopa infusion was associated with PDRP reductions when computed in FDG PET scans—but with substantial elevations when quantified in $H_2^{15}O$ PET scans obtained in the same scanning sessions. At the regional level, treatment-mediated dissociation of blood flow and metabolism was localized to the putamen/globus pallidus, dorsal midbrain/pons, STN, and ventral thalamus. The elevations in rCBF may be attributed to a direct action of drug on the micro-vasculature in areas rich in dopa decarboxylase enzyme activity. Flow-metabolism dissociation appears to be a distinctive consequence of levodopa therapy that is exaggerated in patients with drug-induced dyskinesia.

STEREOTAXIC SURGICAL THERAPIES

Stereotaxic surgical procedures can provide effective symptomatic relief in patients with advanced disease through localized interventions at key components of the motor CSPTC loop and related functional-anatomic circuits. As opposed to ablative (lesioning) techniques, high-frequency DBS offers a reversible solution for PD patients. Moreover, DBS tuning parameters can be adjusted for optimal clinical benefit on an individual basis. Functional neuroimaging has contributed greatly to the current understanding of the mechanisms underlying the therapeutic effects of these procedures.

Pallidotomy and pallidal DBS

Preoperative metabolic imaging with FDG PET has been found to have use in the prediction of clinical outcome following internal pallidal interventions for advanced PD. Although individual differences in the size and location of pallidotomy targets had minimal influence on surgical outcome, preoperative measurements of lentiform nucleus (putamen and globus pallidus) metabolic activity proved to predict clinical benefit at six months following surgery (Eidelberg et al. 1996; Kazumata et al. 1997). Pallidal lesioning also resulted in a metabolic decline in the thalamus and an increase in primary and associative motor cortical regions in patients undergoing this procedure. This suggests that the clinical response to pallidal interventions is associated with the modulation of large-scale networks comprised of interconnected brain regions remote from the actual surgical target (Eidelberg et al. 1996, 1997).

Measurements of regional cerebral blood flow have also been used to study mechanisms of pallidal stimulation in PD. A $H_2^{15}O$ PET study showed an increase in rCBF in ipsilateral PMC during GPi stimulation for PD, with corresponding improvement in rigidity and bradykinesia

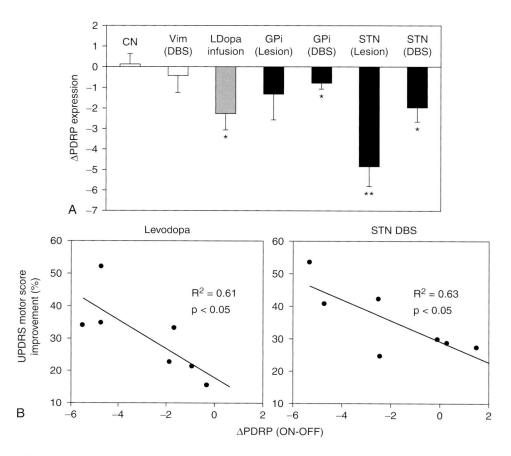

Figure 4 Network modulation and clinical correlation with antiparkinsonian interventions in patients assessed with FDG PET (Feigin et al. 2001; Asanuma et al. 2006). **A.** Bar graph illustrating relative changes in the expression of the PD-related metabolic covariance pattern (PDRP) during antiparkinsonian therapy with levodopa infusion (shaded bar) and ventral pallidotomy, pallidal and STN DBS, and subthalamotomy (filled bars). Reduction in PDRP activity was greater comparing lesion vs. DBS at the same target or comparing STN vs. GPi with either lesion or DBS. For the unilateral surgical interventions, PDRP reflects changes in network activity in the operated hemispheres. With levodopa infusion, the PDRP changes were averaged across hemispheres. [Asterisks represent p values relative to the untreated condition. *p < 0.01; **p < 0.005].
B. Correlations between clinical improvement in UPDRS motor ratings and treatment-mediated changes in PDRP activity. Clinical outcome in individual patients was significantly associated with the degree of PDRP suppression following levodopa administration (*left*) and STN stimulation (*right*).

ratings (Davis et al. 1997). In a subsequent ECD SPECT study, GPi DBS was associated with a reduction in CBF involving the ipsilateral thalamus and striatum (van Laere et al. 2000). There was a significant correlation between these changes and concurrent motor ratings in patients with clinical improvement. These findings are consistent with those reported with FDG PET in patients undergoing GPi stimulation (Fukuda et al. 2001b). Pallidal stimulation also resulted in a significant decline in PDRP expression ipsilateral to stimulation, which correlated with clinical improvement in motor ratings.

Thalamic DBS

DBS targeting the ventral intermediate (Vim) thalamic nucleus has been employed clinically for the control of parkinsonian tremor. Rest-state imaging with $H_2^{15}O$ PET

showed reduced rCBF in the SMA, cerebellum, and SMC during thalamic stimulation (Davis et al. 1997). Additionally, blood flow increased in the frontal and ipsilateral occipital regions. Similarly, in PD patients with severe tremor, Vim DBS led to rCBF reductions in the SMC and cerebellum, along with concurrent increases in the ventral thalamus (Fukuda et al. 2004). Stimulation-mediated rCBF changes in the SMC and SMA regions correlated with changes in tremor amplitude in these patients. After controlling for the effects of Vim DBS on tremor amplitude, voxel-based regression analysis disclosed a correlation between changes in tremor frequency and rCBF measured in the dentate nucleus and pons. These results suggest that Vim DBS improves PD tremor by modulating the activity of cerebello-thalamocortical pathways and that specific tremor characteristics may relate to regional brain activity in different nodes of this system. The metabolic topography of the brain networks mediating PD tremor has been recently investigated using a new within-subject supervised PCA algorithm (Mure et al. 2011; c.f., Habeck et al. 2005). This and related imaging studies of parkinsonian tremor are described in detail in Chapter 7.

Subthalamic lesioning and DBS

The subthalamic nucleus (STN) is perhaps the most common surgical target for DBS therapy to improve the akinetic-rigid manifestations of PD (Krack et al. 1998). Stimulation of this region is thought to be more effective than GPi because this intervention is directed more proximally in the motor pathway. Trost et al. (2006) reported reduced metabolism in the GPi and caudal midbrain but elevated posterior parietal metabolism following STN lesioning (subthalamotomy) and stimulation (DBS). PDRP expression was similarly reduced with both interventions. In another study, STN DBS and levodopa were each associated with significant metabolic reductions in the putamen/globus pallidus, SMC, and cerebellar vermis, as well as with increases in the precuneus (Asanuma et al. 2006). Comparable declines in PDRP activity were also observed with the two interventions (Figure 4A), which correlated with clinical improvement (Figure 4B). These results are in agreement with previous reports of metabolic network modulation following subthalamotomy, pallidotomy, and GPi stimulation (Trost et al. 2006; Fukuda et al. 2001b; Eidelberg et al. 1996; Wang et al. 2010). While the magnitude of the treatment-mediated changes in PDRP expression differed across the various surgical procedures (lesion vs. DBS) and targets (GPi vs. STN), therapies for PD appear to share PDRP network modulation as a distinctive metabolic outcome of intervention. Indeed, PDRP modulation is currently being explored as a biomarker of the response to STN adeno-associated virus (AAV)-borne glutamic acid decarboxylase (GAD) gene therapy, a potentially new surgical intervention for this disorder (Feigin et al. 2007).

The effects of STN stimulation for PD have been examined by measuring rest-state rCBF changes with SPECT. In a long-term follow-up study, Sestini et al. (2005) reported an increase in rCBF in the pre-SMA, PMC, and DLPFC regions five months following stimulation. At 42 months, rCBF remained increased in these regions, and additionally improved function was noted in the primary sensorimotor cortex, globus pallidus, ventral lateral thalamus, and cerebellum at this time point. Additionally, stimulation-mediated rCBF increases in the pre-SMA and PMC correlated with improvement in clinical ratings. Overall, STN stimulation leads to progressive CBF increases in the motor and associative cortical areas, and in the long-term, in critical subcortical elements of the CSPTC loops and related motor pathways.

In summary, functional imaging of cerebral blood flow and metabolism is a useful experimental method to assess the modulation of structure-functional relationships during the treatment of PD. High-frequency DBS offers a reversible amelioration of PD symptoms through alterations in functional brain circuitry at both the regional and network levels. Indeed, clinical improvement correlates consistently with changes in PDRP expression, involving the modulation of synaptic activity at key network nodes.

CONCLUSION

Functional brain imaging has been widely used to identify alterations of regional cerebral metabolism and blood flow in PD patients. These measurements provide unique information regarding the topography of the widespread network changes that take place during the progression of PD and with its treatment. Indeed, these circuit-level features of PD cannot typically be discerned with presynaptic dopaminergic markers or postsynaptic radioligands. Considerable attention has been dedicated to the development of novel analytical methods for the characterization and quantification of neural networks in functional brain imaging data. The resulting disease-related patterns show considerable promise as clinically useful markers of disease progression and response to treatment, as well as aiding in the differential diagnosis of parkinsonian syndromes.

ACKNOWLEDGEMENTS

Supported by NIH NS R01 35069 as well as NIH RR M01 018535 awarded to the General Clinical Research Center of The Feinstein Institute for Medical Research.

REFERENCES

Abe, Y., T. Kachi, T. Kato, Y. Arahata, T. Yamada, Y. Washimi et al. 2003. Occipital hypoperfusion in Parkinson's disease without dementia: Correlation to impaired cortical visual processing. *J Neurol Neurosurg Psychiatry* 74:419–22.

Alexander, G., and J. Moeller. 1994. Application of the scaled subprofile model to functional imaging in neuropsychiatric disorders: A principal component approach to modeling brain function in disease. *Human Brain Mapping* 2:1–16.

Asanuma, K., C. Tang, Y. Ma, V. Dhawan, P. Mattis, C. Edwards, et al. 2006. Network modulation in the treatment of Parkinson's disease. *Brain* 129:2667–78.

Bell, A. J., and T. J. Sejnowski. 1995. An information-maximization approach to blind separation and blind deconvolution. *Neural Comput* 7:1129–59.

Berti, V., C. Polito, S. Ramat, E. Vanzi, M. T. De Cristofaro, G. Pellicano et al. 2010. Brain metabolic correlates of dopaminergic degeneration in de novo idiopathic Parkinson's disease. *Eur J Nucl Med Mol Imaging* 37:537–44.

Bohnen, N. I., S. Minoshima, B. Giordani, K. A. Frey, and D. E. Kuhl. 1999. Motor correlates of occipital glucose hypometabolism in Parkinson's disease without dementia. *Neurology* 52:541–6.

Brownell, A. L., K. Canales, Y. I. Chen, B. G. Jenkins, C. Owen, E. Livni et al. 2003. Mapping of brain function after MPTP-induced neurotoxicity in a primate Parkinson's disease model. *Neuroimage* 20:1064–75.

Chen, K., E. M. Reiman, Z. Huan, R. J. Caselli, D. Bandy, N. Ayutyanont et al. 2009. Linking functional and structural brain images with multivariate network analyses: A novel application of the partial least square method. *Neuroimage* 47:602–10.

Davis, K. D., E. Taub, S. Houle, A. E. Lang, J. O. Dostrovsky, R. R. Tasker et al. 1997. Globus pallidus stimulation activates the cortical motor system during alleviation of parkinsonian symptoms. *Nat Med* 3:671–4.

DeLong, M. R., and T. Wichmann. 2007. Circuits and circuit disorders of the basal ganglia. *Arch Neurol* 64:20–4.

Dhawan, V., and D. Eidelberg. 2007. PET imaging in Parkinson's disease. *Curr Med Imaging Rev* 3:233–41.

Eckert, T., K. Van Laere, C. Tang, D. E. Lewis, C. Edwards, P. Santens et al. 2007a. Quantification of Parkinson's disease-related network expression with ECD SPECT. *Eur J Nucl Med Mol Imaging* 34:496–501.

Eckert, T., C. Tang, and D. Eidelberg. 2007b. Assessment of the progression of Parkinson's disease: a metabolic network approach. *Lancet Neurol* 6:926–32.

Eckert, T., C. Tang, Y. Ma, N. Brown, T. Lin, S. Frucht, A. Feigin, and D. Eidelberg. 2008. Abnormal metabolic networks in atypical parkinsonism. *Mov Disord* 23(5):727–33.

Eidelberg, D. 2009. Metabolic brain networks in neurodegenerative disorders: A functional imaging approach. *Trends Neurosci* 32:548–57.

Eidelberg, D., J. R. Moeller, V. Dhawan, P. Spetsieris, S. Takikawa, T. Ishikawa et al. 1994. The metabolic topography of parkinsonism. *J Cereb Blood Flow Metab* 14:783–801.

Eidelberg, D., J. R. Moeller, T. Ishikawa, V. Dhawan, P. Spetsieris, T. Chaly et al. 1995. Assessment of disease severity in parkinsonism with fluorine-18-fluorodeoxyglucose and PET. *J Nucl Med* 1995; 36:378–83.

Eidelberg, D., J. R. Moeller, T. Ishikawa, V. Dhawan, P. Spetsieris, D. Silbersweig et al. 1996. Regional metabolic correlates of surgical outcome following unilateral pallidotomy for Parkinson's disease. *Ann Neurol* 39:450–9.

Eidelberg, D., J. R. Moeller, K. Kazumata, A. Antonini, D. Sterio, V. Dhawan et al. 1997. Metabolic correlates of pallidal neuronal activity in Parkinson's disease. *Brain* 120:1315–24.

Feigin, A., A. Antonini, M. Fukuda, R. De Notaris, R. Benti, G. Pezzoli et al. 2002. Tc-99m ethylene cysteinate dimer SPECT in the differential diagnosis of parkinsonism. *Mov Disord* 17:1265–70.

Feigin, A., M. Fukuda, V. Dhawan, S. Przedborski, V. Jackson-Lewis, M. J. Mentis et al. 2001. Metabolic correlates of levodopa response in Parkinson's disease. *Neurology* 57:2083–8.

Feigin, A., M. G. Kaplitt, C. Tang, T. Lin, P. Mattis, V. Dhawan et al. 2007. Modulation of metabolic brain networks after subthalamic gene therapy for Parkinson's disease. *Proc Natl Acad Sci USA* 104:19559–64.

Firbank, M. J., S. J. Colloby, D. J. Burn, I. G. McKeith, and J. T. O'Brien. 2003. Regional cerebral blood flow in Parkinson's disease with and without dementia. *Neuroimage* 20:1309–19.

Fukuda, M., A. Barnes, E. S. Simon, A. Holmes, V. Dhawan, N. Giladi et al. 2004. Thalamic stimulation for parkinsonian tremor: Correlation between regional cerebral blood flow and physiological tremor characteristics. *Neuroimage* 21:608–15.

Fukuda, M., M. Mentis, M. F. Ghilardi, V. Dhawan, A. Antonini, J. Hammerstad et al. 2001a. Functional correlates of pallidal stimulation for Parkinson's disease. *Ann Neurol* 49:155–64.

Fukuda, M., M. J. Mentis, Y. Ma, V. Dhawan, A. Antonini, A. E. Lang et al. 2001b. Networks mediating the clinical effects of pallidal brain stimulation for Parkinson's disease: A PET study of resting-state glucose metabolism. *Brain* 124:1601–9.

Ghaemi, M., J. Raethjen, R. Hilker, J. Rudolf, J. Sobesky, G. Deuschl et al. 2002. Monosymptomatic resting tremor and Parkinson's disease: A multitracer positron emission tomographic study. *Mov Disord* 17:782–8.

Guigoni, C., S. Dovero, I. Aubert, Q. Li, B. H. Bioulac, B. Bloch et al. 2005. Levodopa-induced dyskinesia in MPTP-treated macaques is not dependent on the extent and pattern of nigrostrial lesioning. *Eur J Neurosci* 22:283–7.

Gwadry, F., C. Berenstein, J. V. Horn, A. Braun. 2001. Implementation and application of principal component analysis on functional neuroimaging data: Institute for Systems Research Technical Reports, 1–27.

Habeck, C., J. W. Krakauer, C. Ghez, H. A. Sackeim, D. Eidelberg, Y. Stern et al. 2005. A new approach to spatial covariance modeling of functional brain imaging data: Ordinal trend analysis. *Neural Comput* 17:1602–45.

Habeck, C., and Y. Stern. 2010. Multivariate data analysis for neuroimaging data: overview and application to Alzheimer's disease. *Cell Biochem Biophys* 58:53–67.

Hilker, R., J. Voges, S. Weisenbach, E. Kalbe, L. Burghaus, M. Ghaemi et al. 2004. Subthalamic nucleus stimulation restores glucose metabolism in associative and limbic cortices and in cerebellum: Evidence from a FDG-PET study in advanced Parkinson's disease. *J Cereb Blood Flow Metab* 24:7–16.

Hirano, S., K. Asanuma, Y. Ma, C. Tang, A. Feigin, V. Dhawan et al. 2008. Dissociation of metabolic and neurovascular responses to levodopa in the treatment of Parkinson's disease. *J Neurosci* 28:4201–9.

Hosokai, Y., Y. Nishio, K. Hirayama, A. Takeda, T. Ishioka, Y. Sawada et al. 2009. Distinct patterns of regional cerebral glucose metabolism in Parkinson's disease with and without mild cognitive impairment. *Mov Disord* 24:854–62.

Hsu, J. L., T. P. Jung, C. Y. Hsu, W. C. Hsu, Y. K. Chen, J. R. Duann et al. 2007. Regional CBF changes in Parkinson's disease: A correlation with motor dysfunction. *Eur J Nucl Med Mol Imaging* 34:1458–66.

Huang, C., P. Mattis, K. Perrine, N. Brown, V. Dhawan, and D. Eidelberg. 2008. Metabolic abnormalities associated with mild cognitive impairment in Parkinson disease. *Neurology* 70:1470–7.

Huang, C., P. Mattis, C. Tang, K. Perrine, M. Carbon, and D. Eidelberg. 2007a. Metabolic brain networks associated with cognitive function in Parkinson's disease. *Neuroimage* 34:714–23.

Huang, C., C. Tang, A. Feigin, M. Lesser, Y. Ma, M. Pourfar et al. 2007b. Changes in network activity with the progression of Parkinson's disease. *Brain* 130:1834–46.

Imon, Y., H. Matsuda, M. Ogawa, D. Kogure, and N. Sunohara. 1999. SPECT image analysis using statistical parametric mapping in patients with Parkinson's disease. *J Nucl Med* 40:1583–9.

Jung, T.-P., S. Makeig, and M. McKeown. 2001. Imaging brain dynamics using independent component analysis. *IEEE Proceedings* 88:1107–22.

Kaasinen, V., R. P. Maguire, H. P. Hundemer, K. L. Leenders. 2006. Corticostriatal covariance patterns of 6-[18F]fluoro-L-dopa and

[18F]fluorodeoxyglucose PET in Parkinson's disease. *J Neurol* 253:340–8.

Kazumata, K., A. Antonini, V. Dhawan, J. R. Moeller, R. L. Alterman, P. Kelly et al. 1997. Preoperative indicators of clinical outcome following stereotaxic pallidotomy. *Neurology* 49:1083–90.

Kikuchi, A., A. Takeda, T. Kimpara, M. Nakagawa, R. Kawashima, M. Sugiura et al. 2001. Hypoperfusion in the supplementary motor area, dorsolateral prefrontal cortex and insular cortex in Parkinson's disease. *J Neurol Sci* 193:29–36.

Krack, P., P. Pollak, P. Limousin, D. Hoffmann, J. Xie, A. Benazzouz et al. 1998. Subthalamic nucleus or internal pallidal stimulation in young onset Parkinson's disease. *Brain* 121:451–7.

Liepelt, I., M. Reimold, W. Maetzler, J. Godau, G. Reischl, A. Gaenslen et al. 2009. Cortical hypometabolism assessed by a metabolic ratio in Parkinson's disease primarily reflects cognitive deterioration-[18F] FDG-PET. *Mov Disord* 24:1504–11.

Lin, T. P., M. Carbon, C. Tang, A. Y. Mogilner, D. Sterio, A. Beric et al. 2008. Metabolic correlates of subthalamic nucleus activity in Parkinson's disease. *Brain* 131:1373–80.

Lozza, C., J. C. Baron, D. Eidelberg, M. J. Mentis, M. Carbon, and R. M. Marie. 2004. Executive processes in Parkinson's disease: FDG-PET and network analysis. *Hum Brain Mapp* 22:236–45.

Ma, Y., V. Dhawan, C. Freed, S. Fahn, and D. Eidelberg. 2005. PET and embryonic dopamine cell transplantation in Parkinson's disease. In *Bioimaging in neurodegeneration*, eds. P. A. Broderick, D. N. Rabni, and E. H. Kolodny, 45–58. New Jersey: Humana Press.

Ma, Y., and D. Eidelberg. 2007. Functional imaging of cerebral blood flow and glucose metabolism in Parkinson's disease and Huntington's disease. *Mol Imaging* Biol 9:223–33.

Ma, Y., C. Huang, J. P. Dyke, H. Pan, D. Alsop, A. Feigin et al. 2010. Parkinson's disease spatial covariance pattern: Noninvasive quantification with perfusion MRI. *J Cereb Blood Flow Metab* 30:505–9.

Ma, Y., C. Tang, P. G. Spetsieris, V. Dhawan, and D. Eidelberg. 2007. Abnormal metabolic network activity in Parkinson's disease: Test-retest reproducibility. *J Cereb Blood Flow Metab* 27:597–605.

Ma, Y., C. Tang, J.R. Moeller, and D. Eidelberg. 2009. Abnormal regional brain function in Parkinson's disease: truth or fiction. *NeuroImage* 45:260–66.

Matsui, H., K. Nishinaka, M. Oda, N. Hara, K. Komatsu, T. Kubori et al. 2007. Heterogeneous factors in dementia with Parkinson's disease: IMP-SPECT study. *Parkinsonism Relat Disord* 13:174–81.

Miletich, R. S., M. Quarantelli, and G. Di Chiro. 1994. Regional cerebral blood flow imaging with 99mTc-bicisate SPECT in asymmetric Parkinson's disease: Studies with and without chronic drug therapy. *J Cereb Blood Flow Metab* 14 (Suppl 1):S106–14.

Minoshima, S., N.L. Foster, A.A. Sima, K.A. Frey, R.L. Albin, and D.E. Kuhl. 2001. Alzheimer's disease versus dementia with Lewy bodies: cerebral metabolic distinction with autopsy confirmation. *Ann Neurol* 50:358–65.

Mure, H., S. Hirano, C. C. Tang, I. U. Isaias, A. Antonini, Y. Ma et al. 2011. Parkinson's disease tremor-related metabolic network: Characterization, progression, and treatment effects. *Neuroimage*, 54:1244–53.

Osaki, Y., Y. Morita, M. Fukumoto, N. Akagi, S. Yoshida, and Y. Doi. 2005. Three-dimensional stereotactic surface projection SPECT analysis in Parkinson's disease with and without dementia. *Mov Disord* 20:999–1005.

Peng, S., Y. Ma, J. Flores, D. Doudet, and D. Eidelberg. 2010. Abnormal topography of cerebral glucose metabolism in parkinsonian macaques. *J Nucl Med* 51(Suppl 2):1753.

Powers, W. J., T. O. Videen, J. Markham, K. J. Black, N. Golchin, and J. S. Perlmutter. 2008. Cerebral mitochondrial metabolism in early Parkinson's disease. *J Cereb Blood Flow Metab* 28:1754–60.

Sestini, S., S. Ramat, A. R. Formiconi, F. Ammannati, S. Sorbi, and A. Pupi. 2005. Brain networks underlying the clinical effects of long-term subthalamic stimulation for Parkinson's disease: A 4-year follow-up study with rCBF SPECT. *J Nucl Med* 46:1444–54.

Spetsieris, P. G., and D. Eidelberg. 2011. Scaled subprofile modeling of resting state imaging data in Parkinson's disease: Methodological issues. *Neuroimage* 54:2899–2914.

Tang, C. C., and D. Eidelberg. 2010. Abnormal metabolic brain networks in Parkinson's disease: from blackboard to bedside. *Prog Brain Res* 184:161–76.

Tang, C. C., K. L. Poston, V. Dhawan, and D. Eidelberg D. 2010a. Abnormalities in metabolic network activity precede the onset of motor symptoms in Parkinson's disease. *J Neurosci* 30:1049–56.

Tang, C. C., K. L. Poston, T. Eckert, A. Feigin, S. Frucht, M. Gudesblatt et al. 2010b. Differential diagnosis of parkinsonism: A metabolic imaging study using pattern analysis. *Lancet Neurol* 9:149–58.

Thobois, S., M. Jahanshahi, S. Pinto, R. Frackowiak, and P. Limousin-Dowsey. 2004. PET and SPECT functional imaging studies in parkinsonian syndromes: from the lesion to its consequences. *NeuroImage* 23:1–16.

Trost, M., S. Su, P. Su, R. F. Yen, H. M. Tseng, A. Barnes et al. 2006. Network modulation by the subthalamic nucleus in the treatment of Parkinson's disease. *Neuroimage* 31:301–7.

Van Laere, K., P. Santens, T. Bosman, J. De Reuck, L. Mortelmans, and R. Dierckx. 2004. Statistical parametric mapping of (99m)Tc-ECD SPECT in idiopathic Parkinson's disease and multiple system atrophy with predominant parkinsonian features: Correlation with clinical parameters. *J Nucl Med* 45:933–42.

van Laere, K., C. van der Linden, P. Santens, V. Vandewalle, J. Caemaert, P. L. Ir et al. 2000. 99Tc(m)-ECD SPET perfusion changes by internal pallidum stimulation in Parkinson's disease. *Nucl Med Commun* 21:1103–12.

Wang, J., Y. Ma, Z. Huang, B. Sun, Y. Guan, and C. Zuo. 2010. Modulation of metabolic brain function by bilateral subthalamic nucleus stimulation in the treatment of Parkinson's disease. *J Neurol* 257:72–78.

Wu, J. C., R. Iacono, M. Ayman, E. Salmon, S. D. Lin, J. Carlson et al. 2000. Correlation of intellectual impairment in Parkinson's disease with FDG PET scan. *Neuroreport* 11:2139–44.

Wu, T., L. Wang, Y. Chen, C. Zhao, K. Li, and P. Chan. 2009. Changes of functional connectivity of the motor network in the resting state in Parkinson's disease. *Neurosci Lett* 460:6–10.

4

STRUCTURAL ABNORMALITIES IN PARKINSON'S DISEASE
MRI AND RELATED METHODS

Kathrin Reetz and Ferdinand Binkofski

INTRODUCTION

In this chapter, we review the current knowledge about structural magnetic resonance imaging (MRI) techniques in Parkinson's disease (PD) and associated disorders. PD is a neurodegenerative disorder characterized by the progressive loss of dopaminergic neurons of the substantia nigra pars compacta and clinically diagnosed on the basis of a motor symptomatology including tremor, rigidity, and bradykinesia but also a variety of non-motor signs such as mood disorders, psychotic symptoms, cognitive abnormalities, autonomic dysfunction, sensory symptoms, and sleep dysfunction. The high variability of severity and progression rates in affected individuals can be—particularly in the beginning stages and regarding the differentiation from other neurodegenerative disorders—very challenging.

The neuropathological hallmark of sporadic PD is the ongoing formation of alpha-synuclein-containing inclusions in vulnerable cells within human nervous system in association with the degeneration of pigmented dopaminergic and other brainstem nuclei. According to Braak, PD progresses in six neuropathological stages: During presymptomatic stages 1 and 2 inclusion body pathology is confined to the medulla oblongata/pontine tegmentum and the olfactory bulb/anterior olfactory nucleus. In the - probably already symptomatic - stages 3–4, the substantia nigra and other nuclear grays of the midbrain and forebrain become affected. In the final stages 5–6, the process enters the mature neocortex (Figure 1, Braak et al. 2004). Given the presymptomatic stages of suggested 5 to 20 years duration, the disease becomes manifest when nigral cell loss reaches a certain critical threshold, possibly 50 % (Fearnley and Lees 1991).

MRI has become a widely available noninvasive technique. The traditional role of MRI is to exclude symptomatic parkinsonism, but recent research efforts have been established in advanced scanning and analysis procedures, such as voxel-based morphometry, diffusion weighted and diffusion tensor imaging, inversion recovery MRI as well as MR volumetry as tools for detection of nigral and extra-nigral pathology in PD. Modern morphological and functional MRI modalities substantially contribute to the accurate diagnosis and pathophysiological understanding of PD. In view of the rapidly advancing techniques, the use of MRI in the diagnosis of PD is a highly desirable goal.

METHODS

METHODS—CONVENTIONAL, VOLUMETRIC, AND VOXEL-BASED MORPHOMETRY MRI

In traditional morphometry, the volume of the whole brain or parts of it was measured by manually drawing regions of interests (ROI) on images from brain scanning and calculating the volume enclosed. The volumes of anatomical structures assessed in this way can than become subject to statistical analysis. A more recent volumetric approach is voxel-based morphometry (VBM), which is an observer-independent computer-based neuroimaging analysis technique that allows investigation of focal brain differences in structural MRI imaging data. VBM involves a voxel-wise comparison of the local concentration of gray matter between groups of subjects or patients (Ashburner and Friston 2000). The procedure involves spatially normalizing high-resolution MR images into the same stereotactic space, segmenting the gray matter, white matter, and CSF using automated algorithms and smoothing using Gaussian kernels. Voxel-wise parametric statistical tests can then be performed. The most important prerequisite for the use of this method is, due to the large variability and age dependence of brain morphology, the careful choice of homogeneous groups of subjects as well as tight age and gender matching of the control populations. VBM is designed for analyses of large samples. Despite its faults, VBM can yield

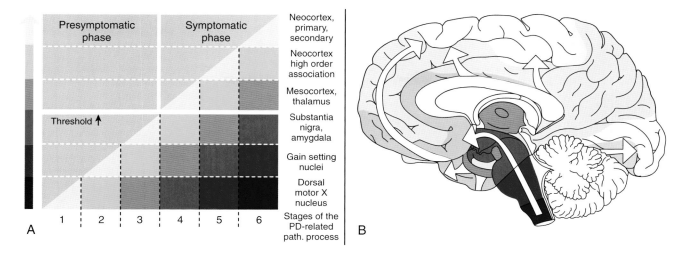

Figure 1 PD presymptomatic and symptomatic phases. (Reprinted with permission from Braak et al. 2004): The presymptomatic phase is marked by the appearance of Lewy neurites/bodies in the brains of asymptomatic persons. In the symptomatic phase, the individual neuropathological threshold is exceeded (black arrow). The increasing slope and intensity of the colored areas below the diagonal indicate the growing severity of the pathology in vulnerable brain regions (right). The severity of the pathology is indicated by darker degrees of shading in the colored arrow left (A). Diagram is showing the ascending pathological process (white arrows). The shading intensity of the colored areas corresponds to that in A (B).

valuable results originating from comparisons between groups of subjects or patients.

In the future, superior resolution and image contrast of high-field MR may provide more detailed anatomy of brain structures, and new software advances may allow improved volumetric analysis in early stages of neurodegenerative disorders. There are indeed other approaches to brain volume analysis that do not suffer the same problems as VBM. In particular, techniques that measure dimensional features directly might be also valuable scientific tools.

METHODS—DIFFUSION-WEIGHTED IMAGING (DWI) AND DIFFUSION TENSOR IMAGING (DTI)

Diffusion-weighted imaging (DWI) and diffusion tensor imaging (DTI) are MRI techniques providing quantitative measures of the microstructural integrity of nuclei and fiber tracts. DWI determines the constrained random movement of water molecules along myelinated fiber tracts in a normal brain, the so-called anisotropy of diffusion. The anisotropy in the white matter of the central nervous system reflects an organization of fiber bundles, running in parallel, and can be quantified by applying magnetic field gradients of different degrees of diffusion sensitization, allowing the calculation of apparent diffusion coefficients (ADC). Pathologic processes, including degenerative diseases, remove restrictions to water molecule movement, leading to increased mobility of water molecules, which results in reduced anisotropy and increased ADC. The integrity of tracts in white matter and,

indirectly, in neuronal connectivity in the brain can be evaluated using DTI and also diffusion tensor tractography (DTT). DWI and the calculation of the derived ADC, which is typically elevated in brain areas where neurodegeneration occurs, as well as DTI have been applied in the diagnostic evaluation of neurodegenerative disease and the discrimination of PD and other parkinsonian syndromes.

METHODS—IRON-SENSITIVE MR IMAGING

The neuropathological hallmark in PD is the presence of intracellular Lewy bodies in the substantia nigra, which are composed of alpha-synuclein, neurofilaments, ubiquitin, and iron. In the human brain, iron is stored as the biologically available and non-toxic form metalloprotein ferritin (Drayer et al. 1986). Ferritin and its degradation product, hemosiderin, affect the MR signal intensity by creating magnetic field inhomogeneities that dephase water protons passing nearby (Bizzi et al. 1990). This results in shortening of the T2 relaxation time and signal drop of the affected tissues. Several quantitative studies attempting to prove the relationship between a range of MRI parameters R2 (1/T2), R2* (1/T2*), R2' (1/T2' = R2*-R2), phase images, and brain-iron concentration have not universally agreed on the strength of the correlation (Haacke et al. 2005). Although strong linear correlations between R2 in gray-matter regions and iron concentration (Bartzokis et al. 1999; Chen et al. 1989; Gelman et al. 1999) as well as with age (Schenker et al. 1993) in healthy subjects have been demonstrated *in vitro* and *in vivo*, there are conflicting results when neurodegenerative diseases are considered (Bartzokis et al. 1999; Chen et al. 1993; Gorell et al. 1995), which may be due to the additional influence of water content of brain tissue in R2. Another approach to quantify brain iron is R2* and R2' (Ordidge et al. 1994) because of its far-reaching effects from the local fields its produces. Thus, several MRI studies using R2* and R2' were able to quantify iron levels in neurodegenerative disorders (Gorell et al. 1995; Graham et al. 2000; Ordidge et al. 1994).

METHODS—MAGNETIZATION TRANSFER MR IMAGING (MTI)

Magnetization transfer imaging (MTI) is a magnetic resonance technique developed for improving image contrast in MR imaging. It is based on application of off-resonance radio-frequency pulses and observing their effects on MR images, as well as measuring the signal intensity with and without application of the pulses. Given different tissues' different macromolecular compositions, MTI can generate very high tissue contrast that is based on well-defined physiochemical properties. This can be accomplished by combining a saturation transfer technique with standard MRI procedures (Balaban and Ceckler 1992). The technique relies on the transfer of energy between highly bound protons within structures and the very mobile protons of free water (Wolff and Balaban 1989). The degree of signal loss depends on the density of the macromolecules in the tissue. The amount of magnetization transfer correlates with the degree of myelinization (Rademacher et al. 1999) and with axonal density (van Waesberghe et al. 1999). Thus, MTI is able to indirectly image a restricted pool of protons, bound to the macromolecules (Wolff and Balaban 1989) and indexing the tissue structural integrity (Sinson et al. 2001).

STRUCTURAL MR IMAGING ABNORMALITIES IN IDIOPATHIC PARKINSON'S DISEASE

CONVENTIONAL, VOLUMETRIC, AND VOXEL-BASED MORPHOMETRY MRI TECHNIQUES IN PARKINSON'S DISEASE

Numerous MRI studies have been conducted to investigate brain alterations in PD *in vivo*. Whereas routine MRI is usually normal in PD and a number of MRI neuroimaging studies using different MRI techniques did not find any evidence for structural changes in non-demented patients

with PD compared to controls (Almeida et al. 2003; Burton et al. 2005; Cordato et al. 2002; Dalaker et al. 2009a; Ghaemi et al. 2002; Huber et al. 1989; Linder et al. 2009; Martin et al. 2009; Price et al. 2004; Schulz et al. 1999), several MRI studies have been able to reveal abnormal findings in non-demented PD patients (Table 1), often in the context of clinical variables.

Substantial work has been done to detect changes in the substantia nigra in patients with PD using MRI. As early as 1986 an MR study using T2-weighted imaging found significant changes in the substantia nigra in PD patients compared to healthy controls (Duguid et al. 1986). The pars compacta width of the substantia nigra was found to be significantly narrower in patients with PD (Stern et al. 1989). There have been several other newer approaches to measure the substantia nigra in PD. A combination of two MRI inversion-recovery pulse sequences showed an altered nigral signal (Hutchinson and Raff 1999) and a lateral-to-medial degeneration in the pars compacta of the substantia nigra (Hutchinson and Raff 2000). Based on the lateral-to-medial nigral signal gradient, PD patients could be discriminated from controls in 83% (Hu et al. 2001b). An indication of the neural loss in the substantia nigra in PD patients can be obtained from longitudinal ($T_{1\rho}$) relaxation measurements (Michaeli et al. 2007), and driven equilibrium single pulse observation of T1 (DESPOT1) detected smaller volumes of the substantia nigra in patients with PD (Menke et al. 2009). Overall, pathologic changes in the substantia nigra, in particular in the pars compacta, were found to be detectable by means of different methodological MRI techniques to differentiate PD patients from controls or other neurodegenerative disorders with parkinsonism.

Currently, the most frequently used MRI-based volumetry technique to exhibit structural abnormalities in PD, mainly due to its observer independence and user friendliness, is VBM. These studies have revealed structural alterations in the brainstem (Jubault et al. 2009), striatum (Alegret et al. 2001; Brenneis et al. 2003; Camicioli et al. 2009; Geng et al. 2006; Krabbe et al. 2005; O'Neill et al. 2002), thalamus mainly in patients with tremor-dominant PD (Cardoso et al. 2009; Kassubek et al. 2001; Kassubek et al. 2002; McKeown et al. 2008)[*], cerebellum (Benninger et al. 2009; Camicioli et al. 2009), hippocampus in non-demented PD patients (Camicioli et al. 2003; Laakso et al. 1996; Nagano-Saito et al. 2005; Ramirez-Ruiz et al. 2005; Riekkinen et al. 1998; Summerfield et al. 2005), regions

---

[*] Role of thalamus in PD tremor in metabolic PET study (Antonini Neurology 1997) and recent identification of PD network using thalamic DBS (Mure NIMG 2010).

Results	Technique	Reference
SUBSTANTIA NIGRA, MIDBRAIN		
– Smaller volumes in the SN	DESPOT1	(Menke et al. 2009)
– T1p indicated neuronal loss in the SN	Adiabatic T1p relaxation	(Michaeli et al. 2007)
– Lateral to medial hypointensity gradient in the SN	Inversion recovery	(Minati et al. 2007)
– Reduced nigral signal intensities in the ventral slice in PD and more uniform in *Parkin*-MC	SIRRIM	(Hu et al. 2006)
– Smaller volumes in the SN	MR-based volumetry	(Krabbe et al. 2005)
– Lateral to medial gradient in the SN – Discrimination PD from controls and PSP	SIRRIM	(Hutchinson et al. 2003)
– Lateral to medial gradient in the SN – Correlation with disease severity	Inversion recovery	(Hutchinson and Raff 2000)
– Thinning of the SN	Inversion recovery	(Hutchinson and Raff 1999)
– Narrower SNc width	SE pulse sequence	(Stern et al. 1989)
– Signal narrowing of the SNc	Axial T2W	(Duguid et al. 1986)
BRAIN STEM		
– WM volume reduction in the rostral part of the medulla oblongata and the caudal pons	VBM	(Jubault et al. 2009)
STRIATUM		
– Cognitive function associated with atrophy in the left putamen – Executive function associated with caudate atrophy	VBM	(Camicioli et al. 2009)
– Mild striatal GM atrophy in *Parkin*-MC and idiopathic PD patients – Correlation with disease severity and duration	VBM	(Reetz et al. 2009)
– Atrophy in the putamen in early and advanced PD – Putamen atrophy correlated negatively with disease severity	Automated segmentation MR-MS	(Geng et al. 2006)
– Smaller putaminal volumes	MRV	(Krabbe et al. 2005)
– Atrophy in the left caudate with enlargement of the left ventricle	VBM	(Brenneis et al. 2003)
– Reduced GM volume of the putamen	MRV	(O'Neill et al. 2002)
– Ventricular enlargement – Decreased putaminal volume was associated with motor impairment	MRV	(Alegret et al. 2001)
– Reduced volume in putamen and caudate	MRV using a point counting method	(Lisanby et al. 1993)
THALAMUS		
– Increased volume in mediodorsal thalamus bilaterally	VBM	(Cardoso 2009, p. 760)
– Shape differences of thalamus in PD and compared to controls	MR-MS	(McKeown et al. 2008)
– Increased gray-matter volume in the nucleus ventralis intermedius of the thalamus contralateral to PD tremor	VBM	(Kassubek et al. 2002)

(Continued)

Results	Technique	Reference
LIMBIC SYSTEM		
– Reduced GM volume in the right amygdala and right pririform cortex (when correlated with olfactory performance)	VBM	(Wattendorf et al. 2009)
– GM reductions in right hippocampus, anterior cingulate cortex	VBM	(Summerfield et al. 2005)
– Atrophy in limbic and paralimbic structures in advanced stages	VBM	(Nagano-Saito et al. 2005)
– Progressive atrophy in limbic and paralimbic regions (longitudinal study)	VBM	(Ramirez-Ruiz et al. 2005)
– Hippocampal atrophy in PD – Correlation with cognitive function	Semiautomated recursive segmentation	(Camicioli et al. 2003)
– Cognitive function is related to hippocampal atrophy	MRV	(Riekkinen et al. 1998)
– Hippocampal atrophy	MRV	(Laakso et al. 1996)
FRONTAL CORTEX		
– Left middle frontal and angular gyri	VBM	(Kostic 2010, p. 979)
– Atrophy in the prefrontal cortex in advanced stages	VBM	(Nagano-Saito et al. 2005)
– Atrophy in the frontal lobe	VBM	(Burton et al. 2004)
– Atrophy in the prefrontal cortex in PD	MRV	(O'Neill et al. 2002)
TEMPORAL CORTEX		
– WM changes in the anterior right fusiform and superior temporal gyrus	VBM	(Martin et al. 2009)
– Atrophy in the left superior temporal gyrus	VBM	(Summerfield et al. 2005)
– Atrophy in the temporal lobe	VBM	(Burton et al. 2004)
CEREBELLUM		
– Atrophy in the quadrangular lobe and decline in PD with tremor compared to those without tremor (no controls)	VBM	(Benninger et al. 2009)
– Atrophy in cerebellum – Executive function was associated with cerebellum atrophy	VBM	(Camicioli et al. 2009)
– Increased gray-matter concentrations in the VIM of the thalamus contralateral to the tremor side	VBM	(Kassubek et al. 2002)

Abbr.: DESPOT1, driven equilibrium single pulse observation of T1; GM, gray matter, MRV, MRI-based volumetry; MR-MS, manual segmentation; PD, Parkinson's disease; *Parkin*-MC, *Parkin* mutation carriers; PSP, progressive supranuclear palsy; SIRRIM, segmented inversion recovery ratio imaging; SN, substantia nigra; SNc, pars compacta of the substantia nigra; VBM, voxel-based morphometry; WM, white matter

associated with olfactory functioning in the limbic and parietal cortex (Wattendorf et al. 2009), and in frontal (Burton et al. 2004; Double et al. 1996; Hu et al. 2001a; Kostic et al. 2010), temporal (Burton et al. 2004; Hu et al. 2001a; Summerfield et al. 2005), and parietal (Hu et al. 2001a). A longitudinal approach with a between-scan interval of 25 months in patients with PD revealed progressive cortical gray-matter volume decrease in the limbic system, including the hippocampus and cingulate cortex, and paralimbic and neocortical associative temporo-occipital cortical regions (Ramirez-Ruiz et al. 2005). The findings in white matter in PD are also somewhat inconsistent: whereas one study revealed no significant differences in total volume or in the spatial distribution of white-matter hyperintensities in PD patients and controls (Dalaker et al. 2009b), another showed decreased white-matter volume in the anterior right fusiform and the superior temporal gyrus PD (Martin et al. 2009).

In summary several interesting findings exist highlighting clinical and neuropathological deficits in PD. However, the diagnostic sensitivity and specificity does not meet the current "gold standard" of radiotracer imaging.

DIFFUSION-WEIGHTED AND TENSOR MR IMAGING IN PARKINSON'S DISEASE

The substantia nigra has also been the subject of great interest in several DWI and DTI studies in PD. An early multi-shot diffusion-weighted MR-imaging study intending to measure the size of the substantia nigra found that the substantia nigra is not reduced in size in patients with PD, but was diminished in patients with secondary parkinsonism (Adachi et al. 1999).

Several DWI studies could demonstrate decreased fractional anisotropy (FA) values and increased ADC values in or around the substantia nigra in PD patients (Yoshikawa et al. 2004) and that the FA values correlated inversely with the clinical severity of PD (Chan et al. 2007). In a group of patients with early untreated PD, reduced FA values were detected in three different subregions of the substantia nigra (rostral, middle, and caudate) as compared to a respective matched control group. In the caudal subregion of interest, the sensitivity and specificity to distinguish early PD patients from healthy subjects were reported as perfect (Vaillancourt et al. 2009). Additionally, Gatellaro and colleagues found an increased mean diffusivity (MD) in the substantia nigra but unaltered MD in the thalamus, globus pallidus, putamen, and in the head of the caudate nucleus in patients with PD (Gattellaro et al. 2009). Also, DTI can yield additional valuable information concerning the pathoanatomy in PD. Using this method (Menke et al. 2009), two regions in each subject's substantia nigra were identified: an internal region that is likely to correspond with the substantia nigra pars compacta because it was mainly connected with posterior striatum, pallidum, anterior thalamus, and prefrontal cortex; and an external region that corresponds with the substantia nigra pars reticularis because it was chiefly connected with the posterior thalamus, ventral thalamus, and motor cortex. Consistent with previous studies, volumetric measurements of these regions in PD patients showed general atrophy particularly in the right substantia nigra pars reticularis.

As one of the non-motor symptoms of PD, olfactory impairment has been a focus of research in recent decades. According to the neuropathological stages of PD by Braak, the olfactory pathway is affected very early in the course of the disease (Braak et al. 2003). Interestingly, a DWI study was able to detect increased diffusivity bilaterally in the olfactory tracts in patients with mild to moderate PD (Scherfler et al. 2006). In addition, a voxel-based analysis of diffusion tensor images revealed white-matter damage bilaterally in the cerebellum and orbitofrontal cortex in patients with PD as compared to healthy controls (Zhang et al. 2009). Correlations between the FA and MD values in the cerebellum and the subject threshold for olfactory identification suggested that the disruption in the cerebellar white matter may play a role in the observed olfactory dysfunction (Zhang et al. 2009).

Also, other white-matter structures were targets of DWI and DTI investigations in PD. The ADC in the precentral and prefrontal white matter was found to be increased (Nicoletti et al. 2006); FA values were reduced in frontal areas including the supplementary motor area, prefrontal areas, and the anterior cingulate cortex (Karagulle Kendi et al. 2008) of PD patients. A whole-brain analysis using FA histograms revealed an increase of FA values in de novo PD patients, in particular in a subgroup of akinetic-rigid type (Tessa et al. 2008). MD was increased and the FA was decreased in the genu of the corpus callosum and in the superior longitudinal fasciculus; in the cingulum, only MD was altered (Gattellaro et al. 2009). It was therefore suggested that the observed widespread microstructural damage to frontal and parietal white matter occurs already in early stages of PD (Gattellaro et al. 2009). Moreover, reduced FA values in the parietal white matter correlated with executive impairment in PD (Matsui et al. 2007b).

Reports of altered FA values in the substantia nigra in PD are promising, but the exact cause of the reported FA and MD changes requires further study. Changes in tissue susceptibility—for example caused by increased iron in the degenerating brain tissue, in particular the substantia nigra—probably influence the diffusion signal in calculated FA. Advanced techniques and combination of multimodal methods will be of great interest in advancing the understanding of the observed changes.

IRON-SENSITIVE MR IMAGING IN PARKINSON'S DISEASE

Several histological studies have reported an increased iron concentration in the substantia nigra pars compacta of patients with PD (Dexter et al. 1989; Earle 1968; Jellinger et al. 1990; Riederer et al. 1989; Sofic et al. 1991; Sofic et al. 1988). It is suggested that iron facilitates the generation of free hydroxyl radicals, which are thought to play a fundamental role in causing cellular damage and death of dopamine-producing neurons in the substantia nigra (Damier et al. 1999; Kaur and Andersen 2004). Also, iron coming into contact with intracellular aggregates of alpha-synuclein may contribute to neurotoxicity and promote apoptosis

(Wolozin and Golts 2002). Studies measuring the T2 relaxation in the putamen, pallidum, and caudate nucleus in PD patients have yielded conflicting results (Antonini et al. 1993; Chen et al. 1993; Graham et al. 2000; Ryvlin et al. 1995; Vymazal et al. 1999). Nevertheless, several recent studies have demonstrated consistent elevations of iron levels in the substantia nigra of PD patients (Bartzokis et al. 1999; Gorell et al. 1995; Graham et al. 2000; Ordidge et al. 1994). In PD, significantly lower T2 hypointensity in the substantia nigra pars compacta and subthalamic nucleus has been observed, and the latter correlated with advancing disease duration (Kosta et al. 2006) and with iron content (Dormont et al. 2004). Atasoy and colleagues reported a correlation between T2 hypointensity in the substantia nigra and clinical severity in patients with PD (Atasoy et al. 2004). Using high-field-strength MRI (3T), Martin et al. also observed an increased iron content in lateral substantia nigra pars compacta even in early PD (Martin et al. 2008). Moreover, a significant increase in putaminal and pallidal iron in patients with PD was found to correlate with the severity of clinical symptomatology (Ye et al. 1996); an association between field-dependent R2 increase-based iron levels and age of onset for PD was also demonstrated (Bartzokis et al. 2004). Bartzokis et al. investigated younger-onset patients with PD, older-onset patients with PD, and controls and revealed higher iron levels among younger-onset patients, indicating that iron may be a risk factor for early age of onset in these neurodegenerative disorders (Bartzokis et al. 2004).

In conclusion, novel MRI methods and high-field-strength imaging to investigate potential substantia nigra abnormalities in PD patients may provide a noninvasive measure of iron content in PD. Recent studies are promising, but the biological and pathophysiological significance of changes in local iron content is not fully understood. The potential of MRI techniques to provide accurate and longitudinal measurements of brain iron remains to be determined.

MAGNETIC TRANSFER MR IMAGING IN PARKINSON'S DISEASE

Using magnetization transfer ratios (MTR), few studies were able to demonstrate reduced values in the substantia nigra in patients with PD relative to healthy controls (Eckert et al. 2004; Tambasco et al. 2003), especially at early disease stages (Anik et al. 2007). Regarding the substantia nigra findings in early patients with PD, the decrease in MTR was most prominent in the pars compacta of the substantia nigra but was also found in the pars reticularis (Anik et al. 2007).

Whereas Hanyu and colleagues did not find different MTR between non-demented PD patients and controls (Hanyu et al. 2001), Eckert and colleagues also observed changes of the MTR in the globus pallidus (Eckert et al. 2004), and Tambasco and colleagues as well as Anik and colleagues reported additional lower MTR values in the red nucleus and pons in PD (Anik et al. 2007; Tambasco et al. 2003) as well as in the paraventricular white matter (Tambasco et al. 2003). Reasons for these different findings may be due to different procedures in targeting the ROIs, number of areas, and clinical evaluation.

Up to now, MTI has been classified as an experimental procedure. Although the most probable explanation of the MTR changes could be gliosis and neuronal loss, the nature of these changes is still a matter of debate.

MR IMAGING IN THE DIFFERENTIAL DIAGNOSIS OF NEURODEGENERATIVE PARKINSONISM

PD is the most common neurodegenerative cause of parkinsonism, followed by progressive supranuclear palsy (PSP) and multiple system atrophy (MSA). Differential diagnosis of PD and the various atypical parkinsonian disorders such as PSP, MSA, in particular the parkinsonian variant of MSA (MSA-P), and corticobasal degeneration (CBD), can be challenging especially in early clinical stages or when the presentation is atypical. With respect to prognosis and therapy, a correct early diagnosis is of major importance in these disorders. MSA is a sporadic adult onset neurodegenerative disease presenting as a combination of parkinsonism, cerebellar ataxia, and autonomic failure (Graham and Oppenheimer 1969; Quinn 1989; Wenning et al. 2004; Wenning et al. 1997). Patients with MSA can be clinically subdivided into those with prominent parkinsonism (MSA-P) and those with prominent cerebellar ataxia (MSA-C). Progressive supranuclear palsy (PSP) and corticobasal degeneration (CBD) are sporadic parkinsonian disorders characterized by widespread degeneration with tau pathology of glial cells and neurons (Dickson et al. 2002; Hauw et al. 1994). In PSP clinical symptoms reflect dysfunction of the basal ganglia and infratentorial structures, and in CBD asymmetrical dysfunction of the basal ganglia and cortical impairment.

One of the major applications of MRI in recent years has been the differentiation of PD from other forms of parkinsonism, the potential of advanced MR imaging techniques will be summarized in the following.

CONVENTIONAL, VOLUMETRIC, AND VOXEL-BASED MORPHOMETRY MRI IN THE DIFFERENTIAL DIAGNOSIS OF NEURODEGENERATIVE PARKINSONISM

Standard non-high-field T1-, T2-weighted, and proton-density sequences typically do not show structural disease-specific abnormalities in PD. Conventional MRI, however, plays an important role excluding other pathologies and can help to distinguish between neurodegenerative diseases. In 1986, Pastakia and colleagues started investigating structural abnormalities in patients with MSA utilizing T1-weighted inversion-recovery and T2-weighted spin-echo pulse sequences (Pastakia et al. 1986). They reported atrophy of the putamen using the T1-weighted inversion-recovery sequences and an abnormal decrease in signal intensity of this structure (particularly along their lateral and posterior portions) on T2-weighted sequences (Pastakia et al. 1986). Routine MRIs in MSA (see also Figure 2) showed putaminal atrophy (100%), hypointensities (36%), and rim hyperintensities (36%) (Kraft et al. 1999; Kraft et al. 2002; Yekhlef et al. 2003). These abnormalities allowed for discrimination of MSA-P from PD, but not MSA-P from PSP and CBD (Schulz et al. 1999; Yekhlef et al. 2003). However, Paviour and colleagues reported that measuring regional brain volume in the midbrain, superior cerebellar peduncle, and pons can now also be used to distinguish between PSP and MSA-P (Paviour et al. 2006b). MSA-C can be subclassified from MSA-P by atrophy of both the pons and middle cerebellar peduncle (MCP), demonstrated

by an increased signal in the pons, MCP, and cerebellum in T2-weighted MRI (Lee et al. 2004). The increased intensity of the MCP and basis pontis is also known as "hot-cross bun" sign due to concomitant pontocerebellar degeneration.

Disease-specific findings in PSP (see also Figure 3) include atrophy of the midbrain with enlargement of the third ventricle and tegmentum, signal increase in the midbrain and in the inferior olives, as well as frontotemporal lobe atrophy (Aiba et al. 1997; Paviour et al. 2006a; Paviour et al. 2005; Savoiardo et al. 1994; Schrag et al. 2000; Seppi and Schocke 2005; Soliveri et al. 1999). The "hummingbird sign" is defined as the atrophy of the rostral and caudal midbrain tegmentum, found on sagittal T1-weighted MRI. Atrophy of the midbrain tegmentum, pons, and frontal eye field on VBM differentiated PSP from CBD with 93% accuracy (Boxer et al. 2006). MRI-based volumetry showed significant volume reduction in the pons, midbrain, thalamus, and striatum with minimal involvement of frontal gray matter (Groschel et al. 2004), and the mean midbrain volume in PSP was found to be 30% smaller than in PD and healthy controls and 15% smaller than in MSA-P (Paviour et al. 2006a; Paviour et al. 2006b). Furthermore, the superior cerebellar peduncle (SCP) was also found to be 20% smaller in PSP than in MSA and healthy controls, and 16% smaller than PD (Paviour et al. 2006b).

MRI in CBD showed marked asymmetrical atrophy in the posterior frontal and parietal regions contralateral to the more affected side (Yekhlef et al. 2003). Putaminal hypointensity

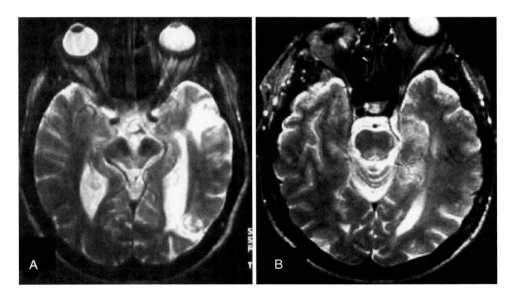

Figure 2 Structural MRI in multiple system atrophy with predominating Parkinson's-like symptoms (MSA-P) (Reprinted with permission from Csoti et al. 2004). T2-weighted MR image showing putaminal atrophy including putaminal rim hyperintensity and putaminal (dorsolateral) hypointensity (A). T1-weighted median sagittal MR image showing also cerebellar atrophy (B).

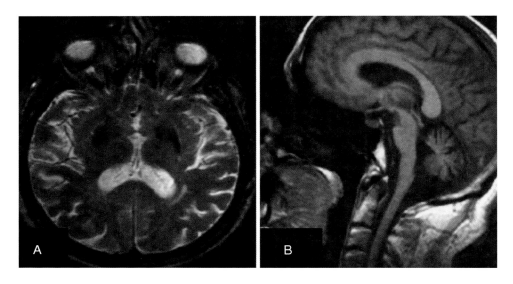

Figure 3 Structural MRI in progressive supranuclear palsy (PSP). (Reprinted with permission from Csoti et al. 2004): T2-weighted axial MR image presenting mesencephal atrophy and abnormal increased in the midbrain (A). T2-weighted axial MR image showing atrophy and diffuse increased intensity in the pontine tegmentum (B).

as well as hyperintense signal changes in the motor cortex or subcortical white matter have been noted on T2-weighted images (Hauser et al. 1996; Josephs et al. 2004; Schrag et al. 2000; Soliveri et al. 1999). VBM revealed gray-matter reduction in frontotemporal cortical areas, such as the prefrontal cortex, insular, frontal operculum, supplementary motor area, and mediotemporal area. White-matter loss was additionally reported in the midbrain including the cerebral peduncles and central midbrain (Brenneis et al. 2004). Using VBM, CBD could be differentiated from PSP (Boxer et al. 2006) based on the extent of atrophy and the regional differences.

In summary, volumetric MRI approaches are suitable to differentiate between PD and atypical parkinsonism and may also help to discriminate between atypical parkinsonism disorders (Table 2).

DIFFUSION-WEIGHTED AND TENSOR MR IMAGING IN THE DIFFERENTIAL DIAGNOSIS OF NEURODEGENERATIVE PARKINSONISM

DWI and DTI have been extensively used to identify specific diagnostic markers for PD, MSA, and PSP for a better differential diagnosis. Several DWI studies showed that putaminal diffusivity measure values can be deployed to distinguish between MSA-P, PD, and healthy subjects (Ito et al. 2007; Kollensperger et al. 2007; Nicoletti et al. 2006; Pellecchia et al. 2009; Schocke et al. 2002; Schocke et al. 2004; Seppi et al. 2003; Seppi et al. 2006b). Abnormal regional ADC/diffusivity values in the middle cerebellar peduncles (MCP) (Blain et al. 2006; Kanazawa et al. 2004; Nicoletti et al. 2006; Paviour et al. 2007; Pellecchia et al. 2009) and superior cerebellar peduncle (SCP) (Blain et al.

TABLE 2: REGIONAL ATROPHY IN ATYPICAL PARKINSONISM

DISORDER	STRUCTURAL ABNORMALITIES (REDUCED VOLUMES)						
	Striatum	Brainstem/ Midbrain	Cerebellum	Frontal cortex	Temporal cortex	Parietal cortex	Specific signs
MSA-C	+	+	+++	(+)	(+)	(+)	"Hot-cross bun" sign on T2W
MSA-P	+++	++	++	(+)	(+)	(+)	Putaminal rim hyperintensity on T2W
PSP	–	++	+	++	++	++	"Hummingbird" sign, "Penguin silhouette" sign
CDB*	–	+	–	+++'	–	+++'	Asymmetry

Abbr.: CBD, corticobasal degeneration; MSA-C, multiple system atrophy with prominent cerebellar ataxia; MSA-P, multiple system atrophy with prominent parkinsonism; PSP, progressive supranuclear palsy; T2w, T2-weighted MRI; * and in the corpus callosum; "asymmetry; + mild; ++ moderate; +++ marked.

2006; Nicoletti et al. 2008; Rizzo et al. 2008) have been shown for MSA and PSP. Given these, some studies reported differentiation of PSP from MSA (Nicoletti et al. 2008; Paviour et al. 2007) and from PD, CBD and healthy subjects (Nicoletti et al. 2006; Nicoletti et al. 2008; Rizzo et al. 2008). In some but not all studies, increased diffusivity has been found in atypical parkinsonism compared with PD patients and healthy subjects involving the caudate nucleus, globus pallidus, and thalamus (Nicoletti et al. 2006; Schocke et al. 2004; Seppi et al. 2003; Seppi et al. 2006a). In MSA-C patients, ADC values in the basis pontis and cerebellum were higher (Kanazawa et al. 2004), and FA values in the MCP, basis pontis, and internal capsule were lower than for controls (Shiga et al. 2005).

MAGNETIC TRANSFER MR IMAGING IN THE DIFFERENTIAL DIAGNOSIS OF NEURODEGENERATIVE PARKINSONISM

MTR was able to reveal abnormalities in PD, MSA, and PSP (Anik et al. 2007; Eckert et al. 2004; Hanyu et al. 2001; Naka et al. 2002; Tambasco et al. 2003). Lower MTR has been shown in the substantia nigra in PD (Anik et al. 2007; Eckert et al. 2004; Tambasco et al. 2003) and in the putamen, globus pallidus, thalamus, and subcortical white matter in PSP (Hanyu et al. 2001). Another MTI study employed this method in MSA patients and control subjects (Naka et al. 2002) and showed significant MT reduction in the putamen and in the white matter of the precentral gyrus. Eckert et al. demonstrated a good discrimination between PD and controls as well as between MSA and PSP patients using MTR (Eckert et al. 2004).

STRUCTURAL MR IMAGING ABNORMALITIES IN IDIOPATHIC PARKINSON'S DISEASE WITH NON-MOTOR CLINICAL SYMPTOMS

PARKINSON'S DISEASE WITH MILD COGNITIVE IMPAIRMENT (PD-MCI)

Even in early stages of the disease, a substantial proportion of patients with PD exhibit mild cognitive impairment (PD-MCI) (Foltynie et al. 2004; Janvin et al. 2005). MCI in PD is typically characterized by impaired attention, planning, working memory, executive and visuospatial functions (Owen et al. 1992). MCI behaves as an independent non-motor feature of the disorder that has an important impact on functional outcome. As the disease progresses

there is an apparent increase in the severity and broadening of cognitive impairment affecting other domains (Owen et al. 1992). The neuropsychological and clinical heterogeneity of cognitive impairment in PD has been tied to dopaminergic dysfunction, manifesting as deficits in flexibility, planning, working memory, and reinforcement learning (Kehagia et al. 2010). It is generally believed that these mild cognitive changes represent early stages of dementia (Janvin et al. 2006; Levy et al. 2002). A few studies have recently investigated structural abnormalities using MRI in PD-MCI patients (Table 3). A recent VBM study suggested the presence of different neuroanatomic substrates in PD patients with amnestic MCI (aMCI), including involvement of posterior-medial cortical areas, compared to those without MCI (Lee et al. 2010b). Several studies found similar structural findings in PD patients with dementia (PDD), with atrophy in the temporal lobe, including the hippocampus, and frontal cortex (Beyer et al. 2007a; Jokinen et al. 2009). Atrophy in the hippocampus was—again similar to findings in PDD—related to mild cognitive impairment in PD patients (Jokinen et al. 2009). An association between cognitive impairment in patients with PD and structural atrophy (Alegret et al. 2001; Camicioli et al. 2009) as well as ventricular enlargement (Alegret et al. 2001; Dalaker et al. 2011) was observed in some MRI studies. Nevertheless, there are also studies reporting no regional gray-matter atrophy in PD-MCI (Dalaker et al. 2010). Interesting in this context, MCI in PD seems to be independent from damage of white-matter hyperintensities (Burton et al. 2006; Dalaker et al. 2009b).

PARKINSON'S DISEASE WITH DEMENTIA (PDD)

Patients with PD are at high risk for the development of dementia; the range of incidence rates for dementia is between 4.2% and 9.4% per year (Aarsland et al. 2001; Hughes et al. 2000). Based on relevant socioeconomic concerns, it becomes evident that early and accurate diagnosis as well as disease-modifying treatment if effective, is of value. The literature on the structural MRI abnormalities underlying PDD is heterogeneous; an overview of the findings is given in Table 3. Several MRI investigations were performed to determine whether similarities in neurostructural pathology existed between PDD and dementia with Lewy bodies (DLB) (Lee et al. 2010a). DLB is a spectrum of disorders characterized pathologically by alpha-synuclein inclusions in the brainstem, subcortical nuclei, and limbic and neocortical areas, and clinically by attentional disturbance, parkinsonism, dementia, and visual hallucinations (McKeith et al. 2005). Because DLB and PDD have a considerable clinical overlap,

Results	Technique	Reference
PARKINSON'S DISEASE WITH MILD COGNITIVE IMPAIRMENT (PD-MCI)		
– Ventricular enlargement	Volumetric segmentation	(Dalaker et al. 2011)
– Reduced GM density in the precuneus and left prefrontal and primary motor areas compared to controls and in the bilateral precuneus – Left primary motor, and right parietal areas#	VBM	(Lee et al. 2010b)
– Mild left caudate atrophy	Radial distance mapping and MR-based volumetry	(Apostolova et al. 2010)
– Hippocampal atrophy – Hippocampal atrophy was related to cognitive function	MR-based volumetry	(Jokinen et al. 2009)
– Cortical atrophy in bilateral temporal and left frontal lobes	VBM	(Beyer et al. 2007a)
PARKINSON'S DISEASE WITH DEMENTIA (PDD)		
– Reduced FA values in bilateral frontal, left temporal, and left parietal WM	DTI	(Lee et al. 2010a)
– Left medial and lateral as well as right medial caudate atrophy, ventricular enlargement	Radial distance mapping and MR-based volumetry	(Apostolova et al. 2010)
– Increased white matter hyperintensities	Semiquantitative visual rating	(Lee et al. 2010c)
– Reduced volume in the right cuneus and left inferior parietal cortex	VBM	(Sanchez-Castaneda et al. 2009)
– Reduced GM density in the bilateral DLPFC, temporal, occipital, posterior cingular, and right parietal cortical areas – Reduced WM density in the left posterior temporal, occipital, and prefrontal areas	VBM	(Lee et al. 2010b)
– Reduced volume of the entorhinal cortex	MR-based volumetry	(Kenny et al. 2008)
– Bilateral hippocampal GM atrophy	ROI, VBM	(Ibarretxe-Bilbao et al. 2008)
– Hippocampal atrophy	Manual segmentation	(Bouchard et al. 2008)
– FA reduction in the bilateral posterior cingulate'	DTI	(Matsui et al. 2007b)
– Cortical atrophy in bilateral temporal and frontal lobes as well as left parietal lobe	VBM	(Beyer et al. 2007a)
– Increased white-matter hyperintensities in deep white-matter and periventricular'	VSR-S	(Beyer et al. 2006)
– Increased rates of atrophy in PDD compared to PD and controls	Serial volumetric MRI	(Burton et al. 2005)
– Cortical atrophy in the limbic/paralimbic system including the anterior cingulate cortex and hippocampus and in the temporal lobe, dorsolateral prefrontal cortex, thalamus, and caudate'	VBM	(Nagano-Saito et al. 2005)
– In follow-up (25 months) increased atrophy in the right temporo-occipital regions including the hippocampus	VBM	(Ramirez-Ruiz et al. 2005)
– Atrophy in the amygdala and hippocampus	MRI-based volumetry	(Junque et al. 2005)
– Medial temporal lobe atrophy	VSR-S	(Tam et al. 2005)
– Atrophy in bilateral putamen, accumbens nuclei, hippocampus, parahippocampal region, anterior cingulate, left thalamus	VBM	(Summerfield et al. 2005)

(Continued)

Results	Technique	Reference
– Atrophy in bilaterally temporal lobe including hippocampus and parahippocampus, and the occipital lobe, the right frontal lobe and left parietal lobe, amygdala, striatum, claustrum, and thalamus	VBM	(Burton et al. 2004)
– Smaller hippocampal volume – Correlation with cognitive impairment	MRI-based volumetry	(Camicioli et al. 2003)
– Smaller hippocampal volume	MRI-based volumetry	(Laakso et al. 1996)
PARKINSON'S DISEASE WITH DEPRESSION		
– FA value reduction in bilateral mediodorsal thalamic regions*	DTI	(Li et al. 2010)
– WM loss in the right frontal lobe, anterior cingulate, and the inferior OFC*	VBM	(Kostic et al. 2010)
– Increased volume in bilateral thalami	Roi guided VBM	(Cardoso et al. 2009)
– Atrophy in the bilateral orbitofrontal and rectus gyrus, right superior temporal pole*	VBM	(Feldmann et al. 2008)
– FA value reduction in bilateral frontal ROIs possibly representing ACC*	DTI	(Matsui et al. 2007a)

Abbr.: ACC, anterior cingulate cortex; DLB, dementia with Lewy bodies; DLPFC, dorsolateral prefrontal cortex; DTI, diffusion tensor imaging; FA, fractional anisotropy; GM, gray matter; OFC, orbitofrontal cortex; PD, Parkinson's disease; PDD, Parkinson's disease with dementia; ROI, region of interest analysis; VBM, voxel-based morphometry; VSR-S, visual standardized rating (Scheltens); WM, white matter; * compared to PD patients without depression; # compared to patients with mild cognitive impairment without PD, 'compared to PD patients without dementia

the distinction becomes based on the timing of the onset of cognitive symptoms relative to extrapyramidal symptoms. Thus, it has been argued that DLB and PDD represent the same entity. Although it was reported that the pattern of gray-matter atrophy in PDD resembles more closely DLB than Alzheimer's Disease (AD) (Burton et al. 2004), other studies suggested—based on subtle clinical and neurobiological differences—that PDD and DLB are not identical entities (Beyer et al. 2007b; Lee et al. 2010a) and that PDD exhibits less cortical atrophy than DLB (Beyer et al. 2007b). The predominant structural abnormalities associated with PDD involve hippocampus, caudate nucleus, cingulum and frontal cortex. It is not known whether inconsistencies in these regions are due to small samples, poorly matched groups, and the neuropsychological and clinical heterogeneity of PDD.

PARKINSON'S DISEASE WITH DEPRESSION

Depression is the most common psychiatric disease in PD occurring in approximately half of patients. In 12%–37% of PD patients, depressive symptoms are seen before motor symptoms (Taylor et al. 1986). In the debate that depression in PD might merely be reactive to physical limitations and loss of independent function, several studies have shown that patients with PD have higher levels of depression than people with similar levels of disability from other causes, and that levels of depression are not related to the severity of PD symptoms. The occurrence of depression in PD might be due to a reactive process to the chronic, disabling symptoms of PD or, alternatively, associated with neuroanatomical and brain functional changes referrable to the neurodegenerative process. Recent neuropsychological and functional imaging studies indicate that monoaminergic mechanisms in structures of the limbic system are related to depression in PD (Bowers et al. 2006; Remy et al. 2005; Tessitore et al. 2002). Structural abnormalities in PD patients with depression have been found mainly in the limbic and thalamic regions. White-matter loss has been reported within the cortical-limbic circuit (Kostic et al. 2010). Microstructural changes have been noted within the white matter in the thalamus in PD patients with depression (Li et al. 2010). A ROI-guided VBM analysis showed increased volume of the mediodorsal thalamic nuclei in PD patients with depression (Cardoso et al. 2009). Further, whole-brain VBM revealed a decrease in gray-matter density in the bilateral orbitofrontal and right temporal regions as well as the limbic system (Feldmann et al. 2008). DTI revealed FA reductions in the anterior cingulate bundles in PD patients with depression (Matsui et al. 2007a).

STRUCTURAL MR IMAGING ABNORMALITIES IN GENETIC DETERMINED PARKINSON'S DISEASE

In the past decade, genetic studies of PD families from different geographical regions have strengthened the hypothesis that PD has a substantial genetic component.

Since 1997, a total of 18 PD loci have been discovered through linkage analysis (PARK1-15) or genome-wide association studies (PARK16-18) (Bekris et al. 2010; Farrer 2006; Pankratz et al. 2003). Mutations in the genes for *LRRK2, Parkin,* and *PINK1* are the most common ones and account for about 3% of all PD patients (Klein and Schlossmacher 2006). While the duration of the premotor

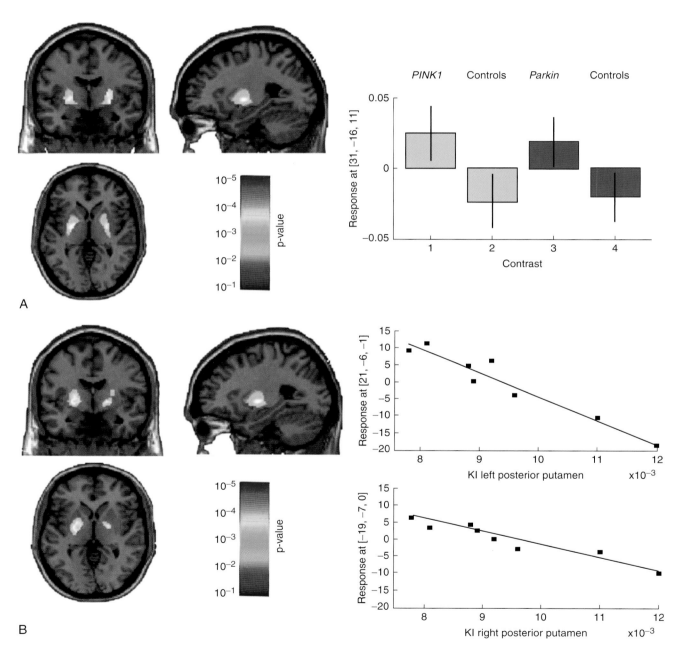

Figure 4 Striatal changes in gray-matter volume in asymptomatic carriers with a single mutant *Parkin* or *PINK1* allele and metabolic-morphometric regression analysis (modified from Binkofski et al. 2007): Main contrast between the VBM data of the asymptomatic heterozygous *Parkin* and *PINK1* mutation carriers and matched controls without a *Parkin* or *PINK1* mutation revealing an increase of the volume of the striatum and GPI in both groups (A). Simple regression analysis between the individual gray-matter images of asymptomatic heterozygous *Parkin* mutation carriers and the individual Ki values, obtained from the posterior putamen at the voxel-by-voxel level. The Ki values showed a linear decrease with increasing gray-matter volume mainly in the left posterior putamen and to a lesser extent in the right putamen (B). The color scale represents the p-values.

Paviour, D. C., S. L. Price, M. Jahanshahi, A. J. Lees, and N. C. Fox. 2006a. Longitudinal MRI in progressive supranuclear palsy and multiple system atrophy: Rates and regions of atrophy. *Brain* 129: 1040–9.

Paviour, D. C., S. L. Price, M. Jahanshahi, A. J. Lees, and N. C. Fox. 2006b. Regional brain volumes distinguish PSP, MSA-P, and PD: MRI-based clinico-radiological correlations. *Mov Disord* 21: 989–996.

Paviour, D. C., S. L. Price, J. M. Stevens, A. J. Lees, and N. C. Fox. 2005. Quantitative MRI measurement of superior cerebellar peduncle in progressive supranuclear palsy. *Neurology* 64:675–9.

Paviour, D. C., J. S. Thornton, A. J. Lees, and H. R. Jager. 2007. Diffusion-weighted magnetic resonance imaging differentiates Parkinsonian variant of multiple-system atrophy from progressive supranuclear palsy. *Mov Disord* 22:68–74.

Pellecchia, M. T., P. Barone, C. Mollica, E. Salvatore, M. Ianniciello, K. Longo et al. 2009. Diffusion-weighted imaging in multiple system atrophy: A comparison between clinical subtypes. *Mov Disord* 24: 689–96.

Price, S., D. Paviour, R. Scahill, J. Stevens, M. Rossor, A. Lees et al. 2004. Voxel-based morphometry detects patterns of atrophy that help differentiate progressive supranuclear palsy and Parkinson's disease. *Neuroimage* 23:663–9.

Quinn, N. 1989. Multiple system atrophy—the nature of the beast. *J Neurol Neurosurg Psychiatry* Supp l:78–89.

Rademacher, J., V. Engelbrecht, U. Burgel, H. Freund, and K. Zilles. 1999. Measuring in vivo myelination of human white matter fiber tracts with magnetization transfer MR. *Neuroimage* 9:393–406.

Ramirez-Ruiz, B., M. J. Marti, E. Tolosa, D. Bartres-Faz, C. Summerfield, P. Salgado-Pineda et al. 2005. Longitudinal evaluation of cerebral morphological changes in Parkinson's disease with and without dementia. *J Neurol* 252:1345–52.

Reetz, K., C. Gaser, C. Klein, J. Hagenah, C. Buchel, S. Gottschalk et al. 2009. Structural findings in the basal ganglia in genetically determined and idiopathic Parkinson's disease. *Mov Disord* 24: 99–103.

Reetz, K., R. Lencer, S. Steinlechner, C. Gaser, J. Hagenah, C. Buchel et al. 2008. Limbic and frontal cortical degeneration is associated with psychiatric symptoms in PINK1 mutation carriers. *Biol Psychiatry.* 64: 214–7.

Reetz, K., V. Tadic, M. Kasten, N. Bruggemann, A. Schmidt, J. Hagenah et al. 2010. Structural imaging in the presymptomatic stage of genetically determined parkinsonism. *Neurobiol Dis* 39:402–8.

Remy, P., M. Doder, A. Lees, N. Turjanski, and D. Brooks. 2005. Depression in Parkinson's disease: Loss of dopamine and noradrenaline innervation in the limbic system. *Brain* 128:1314–22.

Riederer, P., E. Sofic, W. D. Rausch, B. Schmidt, G. P. Reynolds, K. Jellinger et al. 1989. Transition metals, ferritin, glutathione, and ascorbic acid in parkinsonian brains. *J Neurochem* 52:515–20.

Riekkinen, P. Jr., K. Kejonen, M. P. Laakso, H. Soininen, K. Partanen, and M. Riekkinen. 1998. Hippocampal atrophy is related to impaired memory, but not frontal functions in non-demented Parkinson's disease patients. *Neuroreport* 9:1507–11.

Rizzo, G., P. Martinelli, D. Manners, C. Scaglione, C. Tonon, P. Cortelli et al. 2008. Diffusion-weighted brain imaging study of patients with clinical diagnosis of corticobasal degeneration, progressive supranuclear palsy and Parkinson's disease. *Brain* 131:2690–700.

Ryvlin, P., E. Broussolle, H. Piollet, F. Viallet, Y. Khalfallah, and G. Chazot. 1995. Magnetic resonance imaging evidence of decreased putaminal iron content in idiopathic Parkinson's disease. *Arch Neurol* 52:583–8.

Sanchez-Castaneda, C., R. Rene, B. Ramirez-Ruiz, J. Campdelacreu, J. Gascon, C. Falcon et al. 2009. Correlations between gray matter reductions and cognitive deficits in dementia with Lewy bodies and Parkinson's disease with dementia. *Mov Disord* 24:1740–6.

Savoiardo, M., F. Girotti, L. Strada, E. Ciceri. 1994. Magnetic resonance imaging in progressive supranuclear palsy and other parkinsonian disorders. *J Neural Transm Suppl* 42:93–110.

Schenker, C., D. Meier, W. Wichmann, P. Boesiger, and A. Valavanis. 1993. Age distribution and iron dependency of the T2 relaxation time in the globus pallidus and putamen. *Neuroradiology* 35: 119–24.

Scherfler, C., M. F. Schocke, K. Seppi, R. Esterhammer, C. Brenneis, W. Jaschke et al. 2006. Voxel-wise analysis of diffusion weighted imaging reveals disruption of the olfactory tract in Parkinson's disease. *Brain* 129:538–42.

Schocke, M. F., K. Seppi, R. Esterhammer, C. Kremser, W. Jaschke, W. Poewe et al. 2002. Diffusion-weighted MRI differentiates the Parkinson variant of multiple system atrophy from PD. *Neurology* 58:575–80.

Schocke, M. F., K. Seppi, R. Esterhammer, C. Kremser, K. J. Mair, B. V. Czermak et al. 2004. Trace of diffusion tensor differentiates the Parkinson variant of multiple system atrophy and Parkinson's disease. *Neuroimage* 21:1443–51.

Schrag, A., C. D. Good, K. Miszkiel, H. R. Morris, C. J. Mathias, A. J. Lees et al. 2000. Differentiation of atypical parkinsonian syndromes with routine MRI. *Neurology* 54:697–702.

Schulz, J. B., M. Skalej, D. Wedekind, A. R. Luft, M. Abele, K. Voigt et al. 1999. Magnetic resonance imaging-based volumetry differentiates idiopathic Parkinson's syndrome from multiple system atrophy and progressive supranuclear palsy. *Ann Neurol* 45:65–74.

Seppi, K., and M. Schocke. 2005. An update on conventional and advanced magnetic resonance imaging techniques in differential diagnosis of neurodegenerative parkinsonism. *Curr Opin Neurobiol* 18:370–375.

Seppi, K., M. F. Schocke, R. Esterhammer, C. Kremser, C. Brenneis, J. Mueller et al. 2003. Diffusion-weighted imaging discriminates progressive supranuclear palsy from PD, but not from the parkinson variant of multiple system atrophy. *Neurology* 60:922–7.

Seppi, K., M. F. Schocke, K. J. Mair, R. Esterhammer, C. Scherfler, F. Geser et al. 2006a. Progression of putaminal degeneration in multiple system atrophy: A serial diffusion MR study. *Neuroimage* 31:240–5.

Seppi, K., M. F. Schocke, K. Prennschuetz-Schuetzenau, J. K. Mair, R. Esterhammer, C. Kremser et al. 2006b. Topography of putaminal degeneration in multiple system atrophy: A diffusion magnetic resonance study. *Mov Disord* 21:847–52.

Shiga, K., K. Yamada, K. Yoshikawa, T. Mizuno, T. Nishimura, M. Nakagawa. 2005. Local tissue anisotropy decreases in cerebello-petal fibers and pyramidal tract in multiple system atrophy. *J Neurol* 252:589–96.

Sinson, G., L. J. Bagley, K. M. Cecil, M. Torchia, J. C. McGowan, R. E. Lenkinski et al. 2001. Magnetization transfer imaging and proton MR spectroscopy in the evaluation of axonal injury: Correlation with clinical outcome after traumatic brain injury. *AJNR Am J Neuroradiol* 22:143–51.

Sofic, E., W. Paulus, K. Jellinger, P. Riederer, M. B. Youdim. 1991. Selective increase of iron in substantia nigra zona compacta of parkinsonian brains. *J Neurochem* 56:978–82.

Sofic, E., P. Riederer, H. Heinsen, H. Beckmann, G. P. Reynolds, G. Hebenstreit et al. 1988. Increased iron (III) and total iron content in post mortem substantia nigra of parkinsonian brain. *J Neural Transm* 74:199–205.

Soliveri, P., D. Monza, D. Paridi, D. Radice, M. Grisoli, D. Testa et al. 1999. Cognitive and magnetic resonance imaging aspects of corticobasal degeneration and progressive supranuclear palsy. *Neurology* 53: 502–7.

Steinlechner, S., J. Stahlberg, B. Volkel, A. Djarmati, J. Hagenah, A. Hiller et al. 2007. Co-occurrence of affective and schizophrenia spectrum disorders with PINK1 mutations. *J Neurol Neurosurg Psychiatry* 78:532–5.

Stern, M. B., B. H. Braffman, B. E. Skolnick, H. I. Hurtig, and R. I. Grossman. 1989. Magnetic resonance imaging in Parkinson's disease and parkinsonian syndromes. *Neurology* 39:1524–6.

Summerfield, C., C. Junque, E. Tolosa, P. Salgado-Pineda, B. Gomez-Anson, M. J. Marti et al. 2005. Structural brain changes in Parkinson disease with dementia: A voxel-based morphometry study. *Arch Neurol* 62:281–5.

Tam, C. W., E. J. Burton, I. G. McKeith, D. J. Burn, and J. T. O'Brien. 2005. Temporal lobe atrophy on MRI in Parkinson disease with dementia: A comparison with Alzheimer disease and dementia with Lewy bodies. *Neurology* 64:861–5.

Tambasco, N., G. P. Pelliccioli, P. Chiarini, G. E. Montanari, F. Leone, M. L. Mancini et al. 2003. Magnetization transfer changes of grey and white matter in Parkinson's disease. *Neuroradiology* 45:224–30.

Taylor, A. E., J. A. Saint-Cyr, A. E. Lang, and F. T. Kenny. 1986. Parkinson's disease and depression. A critical re-evaluation. *Brain* 109 (Pt 2): 279–92.

Tessa, C., M. Giannelli, R. Della Nave, C. Lucetti, C. Berti, A. Ginestroni et al. 2008. A whole-brain analysis in de novo Parkinson disease. *AJNR Am J Neuroradiol* 29:674–80.

Tessitore, A., A. R. Hariri, F. Fera, W. G. Smith, T. N. Chase, T. M. Hyde et al. 2002. Dopamine modulates the response of the human amygdala: A study in Parkinson's disease. *J Neurosci* 22:9099–103.

Vaillancourt, D. E., M. B. Spraker, J. Prodoehl, I. Abraham, D. M. Corcos, X. J. Zhou et al. 2009. High-resolution diffusion tensor imaging in the substantia nigra of de novo Parkinson disease. *Neurology* 72:1378–84.

van Waesberghe, J. H., W. Kamphorst, C. J. De Groot, M. A. van Walderveen, J. A. Castelijns, R. Ravid et al. 1999. Axonal loss in multiple sclerosis lesions: Magnetic resonance imaging insights into substrates of disability. *Ann Neurol* 46:747–54.

Vymazal, J., A. Righini, R. A. Brooks, M. Canesi, C. Mariani, M. Leonardi et al. 1999. T1 and T2 in the brain of healthy subjects, patients with Parkinson disease, and patients with multiple system atrophy: Relation to iron content. *Radiology* 211:489–95.

Wattendorf, E., A. Welge-Lussen, K. Fiedler, D. Bilecen, M. Wolfensberger, P. Fuhr et al. 2009. Olfactory impairment predicts brain atrophy in Parkinson's disease. *J Neurosci* 29:15410–3.

Wenning, G. K., C. Colosimo, F. Geser, W. Poewe. 2004. Multiple system atrophy. *Lancet Neurol* 3:93–103.

Wenning, G. K., F. Tison, Y. Ben Shlomo, S. E. Daniel, and N. P. Quinn. 1997. Multiple system atrophy: A review of 203 pathologically proven cases. *Mov Disord* 12:133–47.

Wolff, S. D., and R. S. Balaban. 1989. Magnetization transfer contrast (MTC) and tissue water proton relaxation in vivo. *Magn Reson Med* 10:135–44.

Wolozin, B., and N. Golts. 2002. Iron and Parkinson's disease. *Neuroscientist* 8:22–32.

Ye, F. Q., P. S. Allen, and W. R. Martin. 1996. Basal ganglia iron content in Parkinson's disease measured with magnetic resonance. *Mov Disord* 11:243–9.

Yekhlef, F., G. Ballan, F. Macia, O. Delmer, C. Sourgen, and F. Tison. 2003. Routine MRI for the differential diagnosis of Parkinson's disease, MSA, PSP, and CBD. *J Neural Transm* 110:151–69.

Yoshikawa, K., Y. Nakata, K. Yamada, and M. Nakagawa. 2004. Early pathological changes in the parkinsonian brain demonstrated by diffusion tensor MRI. *J Neurol Neurosurg Psychiatry* 75:481–4.

Zhang, K., C. Yu, Y. Zhang, X. Wu, C. Zhu, P. Chan et al. 2009. Voxel-based analysis of diffusion tensor indices in the brain in patients with Parkinson's disease. *Eur J Radiol* 77:269–73.

5

TRANSCRANIAL SONOGRAPHY IN PARKINSONIAN SYNDROMES

Daniela Berg

INTRODUCTION

More than 15 years ago, the first paper on a specific ultrasound feature in Parkinson's disease (PD) detected by transcranial sonography (TCS) was published (Becker et al. 1995). This initial description of substantia nigra (SN) hyperechogenicity gave rise to astonishment in some and skepticism in others. Most of all, however, it was the basis for a multitude of further investigations and a spreading of the method, not only to related disorders but also to many places all over the world. The method of TCS is easy to perform, even in anxious patients, free of side effects and relatively inexpensive. Therefore, interest in the estimation of its value is great.

A neuroimaging tool valuable for the diagnostic workup of PD should fulfill at least some of the following requirements. It should be useful

- in the diagnosis and differential diagnosis of parkinsonian syndromes, especially with regard to the differentiation of atypical parkinsonian syndromes (aPS) and secondary parkinsonian syndromes (sPS)

- in the early diagnosis of PD, in which clinical symptoms are often insufficient to make a clear diagnosis—i.e., constitute a biomarker for the diagnosis of PD

- in monitoring progression of PD

- to detect subjects at risk for PD, as it is known that the occurrence of motor symptoms is anteced by a neurodegenerative process over a long time period

- in the delineation of pathophysiological processes causative for the disease to help understanding the etiology of the disease

So far, there is no neuroimaging tool that suffices all points raised.

In the following, the method of TCS and its limitations are described, as is its value concerning the named requirements.

METHOD

For the proper depiction of parenchymal structures, a high-end ultrasound machine equipped with a 1–4 MHz transducer needs to be applied. The patient is posed in a supine position and the probe is placed consecutively at both temporal bone windows by the examiner, who is usually sitting at the head of the examination table. For the evaluation of brain structures relevant for the differential diagnosis of parkinsonian syndromes, two standardized scanning planes are used: the mesencephalic scanning plane and the third ventricular scanning plane (Figure 1). For B-mode imaging of the brain in these planes, a penetration depth of 14–16 cm and a dynamic range of 45–55 dB are applied, and the contour amplification is set to medium or high. In the post-processing parameters low echo signals are moderately suppressed. Time gain compensation and image brightness is adjusted as needed. Setting the probe in parallel to the imagined orbitomeatal line leads to a nearly axial section through the midbrain (mesencephalic scanning plane) in which the butterfly-shaped hypoechogenic midbrain can easily be delineated from the highly echogenic basal cisterns (Figure 2). Within the hypoechogenic brainstem, some hyperechogenic structures can clearly be delineated: the hyperechogenic midline (brainstem raphe), a usually comma-shaped thin or spotted line in the anatomical area of the substantia nigra (SN) and the often only partly visible red nucleus (RN), medial of the SN (Figure 3). For visualization of the third ventricular plane, the probe is tilted 15–20° upward. Here the usually calcified and therefore hyperechogenic pineal gland is a landmark for orientation at the posterior end of the third ventricle.

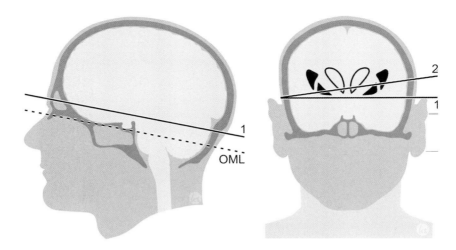

Figure 1 Standardized planes of B-mode sonography in movement disorders. The probe is placed at the temporal bone window. From there the two typical scanning planes for Parkinsonian syndromes are depicted. For visualization of the mesencephalic plane (1) the probe is placed in parallel to the orbitomeatal line (OML). The third ventricular plane (2) is reached by tilting the probe 15°–20° upward.

The hyperechogenic ependyma of the third ventricle and the anterior horns helps in the demarcation of the hypoechogenic CSF-system. The adjacent basal ganglia are normally also hypoechogenic and can therefore usually not be separated (Figure 3).

Because of the ultrasound characteristics (long waves with inferior resolution close to the probe) structures close to the midline (SN, raphe, and RN) are assessed from the ipsilateral, whereas structures more distant from the midline (side-ventricles, basal ganglia) are assessed from the contralateral side. When the method was started to be used for movement disorders, all structures except the ventricular system were assessed semiquantitatively. To overcome subjectivity inherent in this approach, the SN and sometimes even the extension of hyperechogenicity in the area of the basal ganglia are now also measured. So far, there exists

no satisfying possibility to quantify the brightness of the echosignal at certain structures. However, it has been found that planimetric measurement of the brain structures of interest mirrors extremely well the visual impression of the degree of hyper- or hypoechogenicity and the clinical state. Therefore, certain structures are encircled manually and the area of hyperechogenicity is measured planimetrically.

The best known and most commonly assessed structure is the SN. Here cut-off values for increased or decreased SN echogenicity have been established. It is important to notice that these cut-off values may vary depending on the ultrasound system used. Therefore, percentile ranks of the normal population assessed with the specific system are taken as reference points. For the SN, areas above the 90th percentile of the healthy population are classified as markedly hyperechogenic, and areas

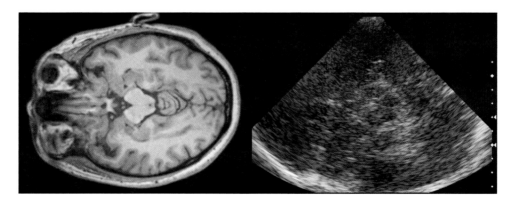

Figure 2 Mesencephalic scanning plane obtained by TCS on the right side and corresponding MRI scan on the left side. The hypoechogenic butterfly-shaped mesencephalic brain stem is well demarcated by the surrounding hyperechogenic basal cisterns. Within the brainstem a thin hyperechogenic line can be seen on both sides in the anatomical area of the substantia nigra. The mesencephalic midline raphe can be seen as a continuous line. Echogenicity of both the substantia nigra and the raphe are normal in this case.

IMAGING IN PARKINSON'S DISEASE

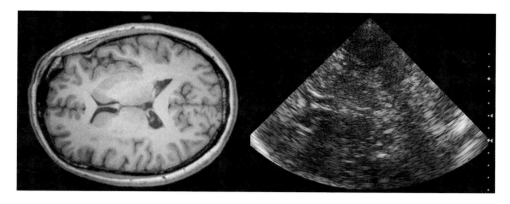

Figure 3 Third ventricular plane obtained by TCS on the right side and corresponding MRI scan on the left side. The third ventricle and the anterior horns are well delineable, as the ependyma of the ventricular system is markedly hyperechogenic. The basal ganglia are normally hypoechogenic with no specific structure to be separated.

between the 75th and 90th percentile as moderately hyperechogenic (see also Berg et al. 2006a; Walter et al. 2007a; Berg et al. 2008) (Figure 4a and 4b). Besides the SN, the third ventricle as well as the anterior horns are quantified. For the whole system, the transverse diameter at the inner layer of the ependyma is measured perpendicularly (see Figure 5). Here reference values exist, which need to be interpreted in relation to age. For subjects younger than 60 years, the diameter of the third ventricle should not exceed 7mm and the anterior horns should not

exceed 17mm. For subjects older than 60 years, the respective maximum values are 10mm and 20mm (Berg et al. 2006a; Berg et al. 2008).

The other structures of importance for the application of TCS in parkinsonian syndromes are still usually rated semiquantitatively. For example, the raphe nowadays is rated, in general, on a two-point system with 0 = midline interrupted or missing and 1 = normal hyperechogenic midline, or the structures of the basal ganglia (caudate nucleus and lentiform nucleus) as isoechogenic to the

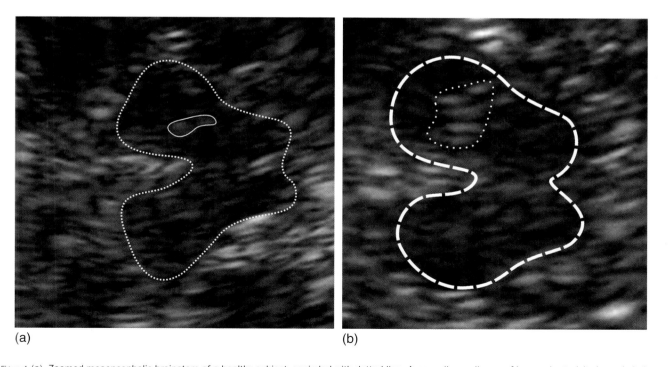

(a)   (b)

Figure 4 (a). Zoomed mesencephalic brainstem of a healthy subject, encircled with dotted line. A normally small area of hyperechogenicity is encircled ipsilateral to the insonating probe with a continuous line. The midline raphe is only slightly visible but continuous. The hyperechogenic structure at the dorsal end of the midline raphe is the aqueduct. (b). Zoomed mesencephalic brainstem of a PD patient. An increased area of hyperechogenicity is encircled ipsilateral to the insonating probe with a dotted line. The midline raphe is continuous.

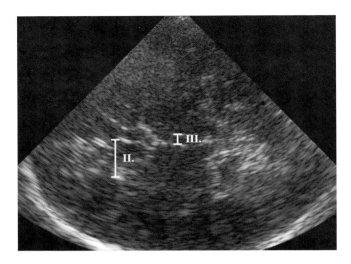

Figure 5 Measurement of the width of the ventricular system in the third ventricular scanning plane. The third ventricle (III) is measured perpendicularly from the inner layer of the ependyma of one side to the inner layer of the ependyma of the other side. The anterior horn of the side ventricle (II) is measured contralaterally to the insonating probe perpendicularly from the septum pellucidum to the tip of the side ventricle. At the posterior end of the third ventricle, the hyperechogenic structure of the pineal gland can be seen.

surrounding brain parenchyma (grade 1) or moderately (grade 2) or markedly (grade 3) hyperechogenic. Encircling of the hyperechogenic areas in the anatomical region of the lentiform nucleus is also done, as well as determination of the anatomical localization, by measuring the distance from landmark structures such as the ventricular system, but there exist no reference values so far.

To apply the method and interpret studies published so far, it is important to understand pitfalls and limitations of the method. Besides adhering to the cut-off values, the major issues are

(i) the applied ultrasound machine—only high-end ultrasound machines with ultrasound specific cut-offs should be used.

(ii) the quality of the temporal bone window—in about 10% of the Caucasian population the transtemporal bone window is not sufficient to depict the relevant structures. This percentage is even higher in other ethnicities, for example the Asian population.

(iii) the experience of the investigator—as the method is quick, side-effect free, and seemingly easy to apply, it is sometimes forgotten that similar to all other neuroimaging techniques proper training and experience is essential for good data acquisition and interpretation.

ULTRASOUND FEATURES IN IDIOPATHIC AND MONOGENETIC PARKINSON'S DISEASE

Since the first description of SN hyperechogenicity in idiopathic Parkinson's disease, numerous independent groups from all over the world have confirmed this finding (Berg et al. 2001c; Walter et al. 2002; Huang et al. 2007; Kim et al. 2007; Okawa et al. 2007; Ressner et al. 2007; Tsai et al. 2007; Mijajlovic et al. 2008; Budisic et al. 2009), showing that this ultrasound feature is visible in 68% to 99% of the PD subjects investigated (Vlaar et al. 2009). The difference in prevalence is mainly due to the definition of cut-off values, the difference in ultrasound machines, and the ethnic background of the population studied (for example, lower prevalence in a Taiwanese cohort (Huang et al. 2007)). Similar findings have been reported in *monogenetic forms* of PD. So far there exist investigations of patients with PD caused by mutations in the alpha-synuclein, Parkin, PINK1, DJ1, LRRK2, and ATP13A2 gene (Walter et al. 2004b; Berg et al. 2005b; Hedrich et al. 2006; Hagenah et al. 2007; Schweitzer et al. 2007b; Hagenah et al. 2008).

In all but ATP13A2 mutation carriers with the clinical presentation of Parkinson's disease, SN hyperechogenicity is found in general, though sometimes the echosignal is not as striking as in idiopathic PD (Schweitzer et al. 2007b) but still pathological. Concerning ATP13A2, so far only one family has been investigated. No hyperechogenic SN was found in a compound heterozygous affected carrier of this mutation (Brüggemann, Hagenah et al. 2010). Further families need to be studied to determine whether normal SN echogenicity is the rule in this form of PD. Of note is that hyperechogenicity is also found in other subtypes of PD, such as Perry's syndrome (Saka et al. 2010).

A number of studies indicate that there is some relation of the extension of ultrasound signal and clinical findings. In general, the area of hyperechogenicity is larger contralateral to the side that is clinically first affected and that persists to be the more impaired side (Berg et al. 2001c; Berg et al. 2006a; Walter et al. 2007a; Walter et al. 2007b). The predictive value of SN hyperechogenicity is quite high, as shown in a study in which the sonographer investigating either PD patients or controls was completely blinded, and the subject to be investigated was veiled and examined in a darkened room to avoid any bias due to clinical impression. In this study, the positive predictive value for PD solely derived from the TCS finding was 85.7%. Only in 6 of 42 subjects with clinically presenting

PD was SN hyperechogenicity not found. As selection of subjects was done only clinically, the differential diagnosis in these subjects needs to be determined in follow-up investigations, but it can be assumed that the predictive value for PD may even be higher (Prestel et al. 2006).

As the structure assessed is small, there has been a lot of debate concerning the validity of the method. This concern has been addressed by a recent study with four experienced sonographers investigating the same patients and controls in a blinded fashion. The results revealed a substantial intra- (ICC 0.96 and 0.93, respectively, for both hemispheres) and inter-rater reliability (ICC 0.84 and 0.89) for quantitative computerized SN planimetry (van de Loo et al., 2010). Therefore, the value of the ultrasound signal in the diagnosis of PD is high and the reliability of assessment is good according to the published literature.

In contrast to the diagnostic value, the issue of a potential use to monitor disease progression has not been completely solved. Most of the studies published so far indicate that extension of the echosignal is not related to disease severity (Berg et al. 2001c; Spiegel et al. 2006; Walter et al. 2007a). Still there are some reports claiming an association of echosignal extension and disease severity (Kolevski et al. 2007; Tsai et al. 2007; Weise et al. 2009). Moreover, prevalence of SN hyperechogenicity seems to increase in the "elderly", healthy subjects older than 80 years (Behnke et al. 2007) and there are observations of a positive correlation with age (Hagenah et al. 2010). However, a small five-year follow-up study showed that there is no noteworthy change in the extension of SN hyperechogenicity in PD patients over a time interval of five years (Berg et al. 2005a). Therefore, it may be hypothesized that in the diseased, neurodegenerative state, SN hyperechogenicity constitutes a stable marker, while in healthy subjects, a slight increase in the area of echogenicity may be found with increasing age. Thinking this hypothesis through a bit further, one may speculate that compensating mechanisms like cell loss in neurodegenerative processes on the one hand and increasing iron accumulation and microglia activation on the other hand may keep the signal stable, while in the aging but not neurodegeneratively affected brain, age-related processes may lead to a slight increase in signal extension. Hence, SN hyperechogenicity does not seem suitable as a progression marker in PD. However, the fact that the same signal extension seen in later stages of the disease can already be documented at very early stages gives the marker an enormous diagnostic value in the early disease phase, in which clinical diagnosis is often difficult.

The diagnostic value of hyperechogenicity has been demonstrated in a study including 60 patients with first signs indicative of a parkinsonian syndrome. Patients were evaluated at an early stage, and a clinical diagnosis could not be made at baseline in 63% of cases. Follow-up one year later, when diagnosis was established by clinical and, in unclear cases, functional neuroimaging investigations, showed that the TCS findings from baseline allowed the diagnosis of PD with a sensitivity of 90.7%, a specificity of 82.4%, and a positive predictive value of 92.9% (Gaenslen et al. 2008).

TCS IN THE DIFFERENTIAL DIAGNOSIS OF PARKINSONIAN SYNDROMES

TCS FINDINGS IN SECONDARY PARKINSONIAN SYNDROMES

Secondary parkinsonian syndromes (sPS) clinically mimic idiopathic PD because they are associated with typical motor features, including bradykinesia, rigidity, and/or tremor. However, these symptoms are not caused by degeneration of the nigrostriatal system as in idiopathic PD or in atypical PS (see below). Instead, other well-distinguishable causes are the reason for the parkinsonian phenotype. With regard to neuroimaging, the common causes of sPS can be divided on the one hand into those in which structural neuroimaging techniques, like CCT or MRI, can depict the cause of the movement disorder (e.g., vascular or posttraumatic parkinsonism, hydrocephalus, or metabolic disorders like Wilson's or Fahr's disease). On the other hand, the clinical picture of parkinsonism can be mimicked by diseases with no distinct structural alteration, like depression or essential tremor. In the case of uncertainty concerning these diagnoses, the function of the nigrostriatal system can be evaluated by visualization of the presynaptic dopaminergic system. In contrast to the aforementioned methods, the technique of TCS combines the capability to detect specific structural changes of most of the sPS and to depict SN hyperechogenicity as typical structural alteration for PD. Therefore, this one technique may be used for most of the above-mentioned differential diagnoses. In the following, TCS findings in the most common sPS will be discussed.

TCS findings in secondary PS with (typical) findings on routine structural neuroimaging methods

a. **Hydrocephalus**—The most striking finding is the at-once-visible enlargement of the ventricular system (Figure 6), which can be measured and compared

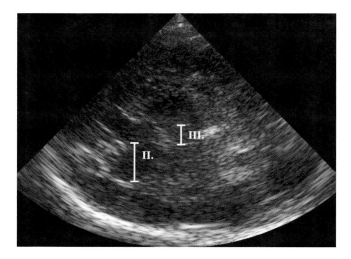

Figure 6 Enlarged ventricular system, scanned in the third ventricular scanning plane. The third ventricle (III) is measured perpendicularly from the inner layer of the ependyma of one side to the inner layer of the ependyma of the other side. The anterior horn of the side ventricle (II) is measured contralaterally to the insonating probe perpendicularly from the septum pellucidum to the tip of the side ventricle. At the posterior end of the third ventricle, the hyperechogenic structure of the pineal gland can be seen.

with the established normal values (see above). Additionally, application of the M-mode allows the visualization of undulation of the septum pellucidum for estimation of intraventricular pressure (Becker et al. 1994). In contrast to idiopathic PD, the area of hyperechogenicity at the SN is generally not enlarged. However, importantly, hydrocephalus may also develop in idiopathic PD. The easy applicability of TCS allows a frequent and quick use whenever the question of hydrocephalus as a cause of a parkinsonian syndrome or an additional hydrocephalus to the already diagnosed PD arises.

b. **Vascular parkinsonism**—This diagnosis is a challenge for all neuroimaging techniques. For the structural neuroimaging techniques, no cut-off of lesion load to make the diagnosis of vascular parkinsonism is defined. For functional neuroimaging it needs to be considered that vascular lesions may affect the nigrostriatal system, which may lead to a reduced uptake of radiotracer on SPECT or PET images, which, however, are in general differently located compared to idiopathic PD. Concerning TCS, no typical B-mode finding allows the diagnosis of vascular parkinsonism. However, evidence of atherosclerosis determined by Doppler or Duplex sonography of the intracerebral vessels make a vascular cause of parkinsonism likely. Moreover, according to the literature, patients with a sole vascular cause of

parkinsonism display, in general, normal SN echogenicity (Tsai et al. 2007). However, the comorbidity of vascular diseases and PD in the elderly population needs to be considered. Only in the case of normal SN echogenicity (and possibly additional Doppler or Duplex findings suggestive for atherosclerosis) is the differential diagnosis of vascular parkinsonism very likely. In the case of SN hyperechogenicity, either (additional) idiopathic PD or the occurrence of SN hyperechogenicity in about 10% of healthy subjects needs to be considered, a percentage that seems to increase in the elderly (Behnke et al. 2007).

c. **Parkinsonism in disorders with heavy metal or calcium accumulation**—

   c1. *Wilson's disease (WD)*—One of the most important differential diagnoses of movement disorders, including parkinsonism, especially in younger subjects, is Wilson's disease, as specific treatment options are at hand. Neurological symptoms are caused by copper accumulation within the brain, predominantly in the basal ganglia. Accordingly, the most striking ultrasound finding in WD is a distinct hyperechogenicity of the lentiform nucleus (Figure 7). Extension of the area of echogenicity is associated with severity of symptoms and can extend into the thalamus and other structures. This may be evident before

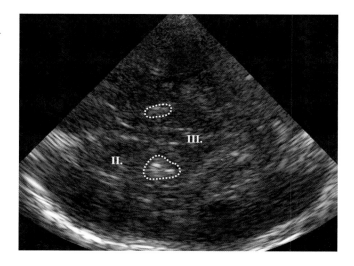

Figure 7 Hyperechogenicity on both sides within the lentiform nucleus, encircled with dotted lines. This finding is typical for Wilson's disease, calcification of the basal ganglia, and dystonia and is frequently found in atypical parkinsonian syndromes. The third ventricle (III) and the anterior horn of the side ventricle (II) are marked.

structural changes can be detected by MRI (Walter et al. 2005). However, the SN may also be affected. In a study investigating 21 patients with Wilson's disease with (n = 18) and without (n = 3) neurologic symptoms, 47.5% had SN hyperechogenicity (Walter et al. 2005).

TCS findings in secondary PS with no abnormality on routine structural neuroimaging methods

a. **Essential tremor**—Similar to other routine structural neuroimaging methods, no typical B-mode features are found on TCS. Also, the SN is generally normal, allowing the diagnosis of "non-PD" tremor. In different studies TCS has been shown to differentiate tremor-dominant PD from ET with a sensitivity of 75% to 86%, a specificity of 84% to 93%, and a positive predictive value of 91% to 95% (Stockner et al. 2007; Doepp et al. 2008). However, prevalence of SN hyperechogenicity is higher in ET (16%) compared to the normal population. As patients with ET have a three- to fourfold increased risk for developing PD during their lifetime (Benito-Leon et al. 2009), it may be hypothesized that ET patients with SN hyperechogenicity will be the ones who are at higher risk for additional PD in the future.

b. **Depression**—In general, a high percentage of patients exhibiting parkinsonism due to severe depression shows raphe hypoechogenicity as an important diagnostic feature and normal SN echogenicity (Figure 8). However, it needs to be noted that in depressed subjects, SN hyperechogenicity is found more often (up to 40% (Walter et al. 2007c)) than in the non-depressed healthy population. This may be due to the fact that depression may antecede PD as a premotor marker. In fact, the conversion to PD is about 2–3 times higher in individuals with depression than in non-depressed subjects (Schuurman et al. 2002; Leentjens et al. 2003). The fact that SN hyperechogenicity in depressed subjects is associated with mild motor asymmetry also seems to indicate that there might be an increased risk for PD in this subgroup of depressed subjects. Still, longitudinal follow-up studies are necessary to confirm this hypothesis. For clinical differential diagnosis it can be stated that depressed subjects with normal SN echogenicity can easily be

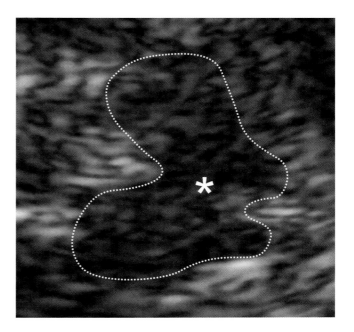

Figure 8 Zoomed mesencephalic brainstem of a patient with depression. The normally continuous midline is missing (asterisk). The hyperechogenic structure dorsal of the asterisk is the aqueduct. SN echogenicity is normal.

separated. If SN hyperechogenicity is present, it cannot be differentiated whether it is a marker for PD, a premotor marker, or of other so-far-unknown or no relevance.

TCS FINDINGS IN ATYPICAL PARKINSONIAN SYNDROMES

The exact pathophysiology leading to the neurodegeneration responsible for atypical parkinsonian syndromes (aPS) is still unclear. Clinically, aPS are characterized by a parkinsonian syndrome with additional features like gaze palsy or autonomic symptoms, little or no L-dopa responsiveness, and a more rapid progression.

The term atypical parkinsonian syndromes (aPS) is used today as an umbrella term for multiple system atrophy (MSA), progressive supranuclear palsy (PSP), corticobasal degeneration (CBD), and diffuse Lewy body disease (DLBD). Underlying pathology and overlap to idiopathic PD is quite different in these disease entities. Whereas DLBD is regarded by some as a sub-form of iPD, PSP is a tauopathy with completely different neuropathological changes. For differentiation on TCS, the SN, the basal ganglia, and the ventricular system need to be evaluated.

a. **DLBD**—In accordance with the clinical presentation and the neuropathological findings, TCS in DLBD is strikingly similar to idiopathic PD, underscoring the hypothesis that iPD and DLBD have a common pathogenesis. SN hyperechogenicity is found with a similar prevalence and extension of area as in idiopathic PD (Walter et al. 2006), although lateralization of SN hyperechogenicity, which is usually observed in iPD, is often not present. Ultrasound findings of the basal ganglia are as unspectacular as in iPD. However, in subjects with DLBD, a larger width of the ventricular system can be measured—at least when compared to non-demented PD patients. This sign of progressive brain atrophy is also evident in patients with Parkinson's disease and dementia (Walter et al. 2006), especially in the later stages.

b. **MSA**—Clinically, the differentiation of the parkinsonian type of MSA (MSA-P) from idiopathic PD is more challenging than the classification of subjects presenting with additional ataxia as cerebellar type of MSA (MSA-C). Importantly, even at early stages of the disease, hyperechogenicity of the lentiform nucleus is found in more than 70% of MSA patients; this finding is unusual for iPD. Concerning echogenicity of the SN, the literature is not completely consistent, which is primarily due to the fact that different cut-offs for SN hyperechogenicity were used, and in some studies different forms of aPS—mainly MSA and PSP—were investigated in relation to iPD. Behnke and colleagues (Behnke et al. 2005), for example, classified subjects with an area of SN hyperechogenicity between the 40th and 80th percentile derived from two large cohorts of healthy subjects as moderately hyperechogenic. This grouping is not in line with the consensus criteria published later (Berg et al. 2006a; Walter et al. 2008), as areas of echogenicity between the 75th and 90th percentile are defined as moderately hyperechogenic. Extracting only MSA patients from the studies published so far and keeping the cut-off of the 75th percentile as moderately and the 90th as markedly hyperechogenic, the prevalence of SN hyperechogenicity in MSA varies between 0% and 25% (Behnke et al. 2005; Okawa et al. 2007; Walter et al. 2007b; Gaenslen et al. 2008). The combined consideration of typical SN and lentiform nucleus echogenicity has been shown to differentiate iPD from MSA-P (and PSP) with a positive predictive value of 0.91 (i.e., in the case of iPD, hyperechogenicity of the SN and normal echogenicity of the lentiform nucleus, in contrast to normal SN and

hyperechogenicity of the lentiform nucleus in MSA-P) (Behnke et al. 2005). Very encouraging is the predictive value of TCS findings for diagnosis in patients presenting at very early disease stages, not allowing a clinical diagnosis with certainty. In the prospective study of 60 de novo patients (Gaenslen et al. 2008) (see above), eight subjects were finally diagnosed as MSA or PSP. In all of them, the baseline examination showed normal echogenicity of the SN, indicating that this single feature is already valuable for diagnosis in the very early disease stages.

c. **PSP**—The recent description of different subtypes of PSP (for review see Williams and Lees 2009) has not only lead to rethinking in the diagnosis of patients with parkinsonian syndromes but also to a re-evaluation of neuroimaging findings. Before the subtypes were acknowledged, TCS findings in PSP were considered similar to MSA with regard to the basal ganglia and the SN. Frequently, hyperechogenicity of the lentiform nucleus is detected while the SN, taking the same problems with cut-off values into account as explained above for MSA, is described with an overall prevalence of hyperechogenicity of 0%–41% according to the guideline criteria (Behnke et al. 2005; Okawa et al. 2007; Walter et al. 2007b; Gaenslen et al. 2008). First, new publications differentiating subtypes of PSP, however, indicate that SN hyperechogenicity can be found in a non-negligible percentage in a specific PSP subtype—i.e., the PSP-Parkinsonian subtype (PSP-P). Initial studies indicate that this subtype involves SN hyperechogenicity in over 80% of subjects, while the Richardson subtype (RS) generally shows normal echogenicity. A further imaging parameter, the dilated third ventricle, can often be seen in PSP (Walter et al. 2004a), particularly in patients with the RS subtype (Ebentheuer et al. 2010; Bouwmans et al., 2010).

d. **CBD**—In MSA and PSP (at least in the RS subtype) normal echogenicity of the SN with hyperechogenicity of the lentiform nucleus are the typical findings, which can help in the differential diagnosis of these disorders from PD. By contrast, in CBD, echogenicity of the SN is found similar to idiopathic PD. In fact, SN hyperechogenicity is very common (88%) in CBD, and the echogenic area is often larger than in idiopathic PD

(Walter et al. 2004a). The pathomechanisms leading to abnormal echogenicity of the SN in CBD may be similar or different from those in PD. Nonetheless, more than 80% of CBD subjects described so far exhibited hyperechogenicity of the lentiform nucleus, which is in general not present in PD (Walter et al. 2004a). In contrast to PSP (especially RS), which can be difficult to discern clinically from CBD because of overlapping features, the ventricular system is normally not enlarged in CBD.

SPECIFICITY OF TCS FINDINGS

The best described ultrasound features in the diagnosis and differential diagnosis of parkinsonian syndromes are SN and lentiform nucleus hyperechogenicity. However, as seen above, neither of the two is specific for one diagnosis. Moreover, other disorders affecting the basal ganglia like Huntington's disease (Postert et al. 2004; Lambeck et al. 2008), SCA 2 (Mijajlovic et al. 2008), and spinocerebellar ataxia type 3 (Postert et al. 2004), and attention-deficit/hyperactivity disorder (ADHD) (Krauel et al. 2010) may also be associated with a change in echogenicity of one of these structures. Therefore, neither a hyperechogenicity of the SN nor an increased echogenicity of the lentiform nucleus predicts the diagnosis of a specific parkinsonian syndrome with 100% specificity. However, the combination of ultrasound features (especially regarding the SN, the lentiform nucleus, and the ventricular system) has been shown to be extremely helpful in the differential diagnosis even at early disease stages in the clinical routine. Therefore, employment of this fast-to-perform, easy-to-apply, and cheap technique can be useful as an additional tool in the diagnostic workup of parkinsonian syndromes.

In addition to the diagnostic use, TCS findings have prompted research in new directions and have lead to promising findings for our understanding of some movement disorders and further applications.

REASONS FOR CHANGES IN BRAIN TISSUE ECHOGENICITY

Ultrasound waves are reflected at tissue interfaces. This is why the ventricular system is well delineated. One of the major reasons for hyperechogenicity in movement disorders is an accumulation of heavy metals—leading to differences in tissue composition when compared to the surrounding brain parenchyma. This can easily be understood with regard to the hyperechogenicity of the basal ganglia in Wilson's disease or welding-associated parkinsonism (see above). Also, increased amounts of calcium, like in Fahr's disease (see above), likely lead to a different tissue structure and therefore to strong reflection of the ultrasound waves.

The typical hyperechogenicity of the lentiform nucleus in dystonia, an area in which no structural alterations had been seen on MRI or CCT up to that time, lead to the biochemical workup of that region in patients who died and suffered from dystonia during their lifetime. Interestingly, an increased amount of copper and consecutive changes in copper transporting proteins were found in dystonic patients (Becker et al. 1999; Berg et al. 2000; Becker et al. 2001). These findings could not have been prompted without the identification and workup of the hyperechogenicity of the lentiform nucleus.

In Parkinson's disease, a number of postmortem studies have discovered histological and biochemical alterations associated with the disease (reviewed for example in Gerlach et al. 1994; Double et al. 2000; Berg et al. 2001a). Of these, increased tissue iron content and microglia activation have been shown to be associated with the increased area of echogenicity detected by TCS (Berg et al. 2006b; Berg 2007). Especially for iron, several lines of evidence show the association of an increased ultrasound signal and elevated tissue iron levels. First in an animal experiment (Berg et al. 1999b) and then in human postmortem studies (Berg et al. 1999a; Berg et al. 2002), it could be shown that larger areas of hyperechogenicity correspond to increased tissue iron content. Interestingly, from the animal experiment, it could be derived that it is not the ferritin-bound form of iron that leads to the increased echosignal. So far it is not clear in which form or bound to what macromolecule iron is responsible for the increased reflection of ultrasound waves. Different mechanisms may contribute to increased iron levels within the SN. One study based on the TCS findings showed that specific mutations in the ceruloplasmin gene (ceruloplasmin is involved in cellular iron import and export as well as intracellular iron metabolism) are associated with SN hyperechogenicity and PD (Hochstrasser et al. 2004; Hochstrasser et al. 2005). Moreover, a recent study demonstrated that microglia activation may additionally contribute to the enhanced echosignal of the SN in PD (Berg et al., 2010). More research needs to be done in this field. The relative ease of access to the ultrasound signal will help to obtain cohorts of patients and controls for further studies.

SN HYPERECHOGENICITY AS A RISK MARKER FOR PD?

The fact that SN hyperechogenicity can already be found in the very early stages of PD, as well as the observation that the area of hyperechogenicity is similarly large in early and late disease stages and does not grossly change in the course of the disease (at least not within five years, as shown in a first rather small five-year follow-up study, see above), indicates that this marker is rather stable. Therefore, it is not suitable to measure disease progression.

However, already in the first study of PD patients (Becker et al., 1995), a promising new perspective for the method became evident—i.e., its application in the premotor diagnosis of PD.

It is well known that in PD diagnosis can be made only when more than half of the neurons at the PD-vulnerable site of the SN have degenerated (Fearnley and Lees 1991). Many clinical and neuroimaging studies indicate that several years (if not decades) of neurodegeneration antecede the clinically obvious presentation of motor symptoms (for review see Hawkes 2008). Therefore, the following questions are at hand: Does SN hyperechogenicity—the typical sonographic sign for PD—occur in healthy subjects and, if so, does it indicate subjects at risk for this neurodegenerative disorder?

DOES SN HYPERECHOGENICITY OCCUR IN HEALTHY SUBJECTS AND WHAT IS THE PREVALENCE?

Already in the first TCS study on PD patients, it was obvious that SN hyperechogenicity may also occur in healthy subjects—in that study, 2 out of 30 subjects displayed the increased SN echosignal (Becker et al. 1995). Only two years later, one of these two subjects was diagnosed with incident PD. Consecutive investigations on the prevalence of SN hyperechogenicity revealed that in adults up to about 70 years of age, an increased area of echogenicity can be found with the same prevalence. According to the cut-off for hyperechogenicity (see above) cross-sectional data revealed SN hyperechogenicity in about 10% of healthy adult subjects in all age groups up to about 70 years (Berg et al. 1999a; Berg et al. 2002). However, in some studies the percentage is slightly higher (Behnke et al. 2007; Liepelt et al. 2009). This is dependent on the age of the included subjects (see above—SN hyperechogenicity seems to be more prevalent in the elderly) and on the family history of PD, as it has been shown that first-degree relatives of

patients with idiopathic PD display SN hyperechogenicity in more than 40% (Ruprecht-Dorfler et al. 2003; Schweitzer et al. 2007a).

IS THERE A FUNCTIONAL RELEVANCE OF THE ULTRASOUND FEATURE IN YET HEALTHY SUBJECTS?

Since the first conversion to PD has been observed in an at-baseline healthy subject with SN hyperechogenicity, numerous studies have proven that SN hyperechogenicity does indeed disclose a vulnerability of the nigrostriatal system in at least some of the healthy persons in whom the echosignal is found. Moreover, an association of the ultrasound abnormality with most of the currently known risk and premotor markers has been shown. According to a number of studies, subjects with SN hyperechogenicity but without the clinical picture of PD may show

(i) a reduced presynaptic tracer uptake in PET and SPECT examinations of the nigrostriatal system in about 60% (Berg et al. 1999a; Berg et al. 2002)

(ii) signs of motor retardation, sole resting tremor, and other slight extrapyramidal symptoms with increasing age (Behnke et al. 2007)

(iii) more often and more severe extrapyramidal features following administration of neuroleptics (Berg et al. 2001b)

(iv) unilateral motor slowing when performing demanding motor tasks (Ruprecht-Dorfler et al. 2003)

(v) more often premotor symptoms, like

    a. RBD (Stockner et al. 2009; Unger et al. 2009)

    b. olfactory dysfunction (Haehner et al. 2007; Liepelt et al. 2009)

    c. depression (Walter et al. 2007b)

    d. specific neuropsychological deficits known to be primarily affected in PD (Liepelt et al. 2008)

compared to healthy subjects without this ultrasound signal.

Even more convincing evidence can be derived from the fact that yet healthy mutation carriers for different kinds of monogenetic PD also show SN hyperechogenicity on TCS.

Prospective follow-up studies of these subjects with regard to the TCS finding has not been done yet. However, the risk of PD in the asymptomatic mutation carriers is well known for the specific mutations. For idiopathic PD, a first prospective longitudinal study on subjects older than 50 years reports the exciting finding of a more than 17-fold increased relative risk for the development of PD in initially healthy subjects with SN hyperechogenicity (Berg et al.,In Press). Further studies are needed to confirm this finding. If it holds true that SN hyperechogenicity discloses such a highly increased risk for PD, new research strategies for premotor batteries and consecutively neuroprotective treatment strategies will follow.

CONCLUSIONS AND PERSPECTIVES

Since the first description of transcranial sonography in Parkinson's disease in 1995, application of the method has multiplied manifold. Due to the easy and quick applicability, it has been established as a supplementary diagnostic tool in many places all over the world. Moreover, the spectrum of diseases in which the method adds valuable additional information in the diagnostic workup has broadened a lot. For parkinsonian syndromes it is especially in the early disease stages, in which clinical criteria are often insufficient, that the method can be applied with great benefit.

Several groups work at an optimization of the method, concerning aspects such as measuring signal intensity, expert systems to compare findings, automatic quantification of areas of hyperechogenicity, and still better resolution. With further improvement of the method, more information on the pathophysiological basis of ultrasound changes, and thereby a better understanding of the cause and development of parkinsonian syndromes, may be elucidated.

Moreover, new fields of applications are constantly arising. First publications indicate that intra- and postoperative monitoring of the placement of brain electrodes is one promising field for increasing application in the future (Walter et al. 2009).

One of the most promising fields, however, seems to be the application of TCS in the premotor diagnosis of PD. Short investigation times, easy handling, and low costs of the side effect free method make it very likely that, if the finding of a markedly increased risk for PD in yet healthy subjects with SN hyperechogenicity can be confirmed, TCS may be implemented as a screening instrument in premotor test batteries.

REFERENCES

Becker, G., U. Bogdahn, H. M. Strassburg, A. Lindner, W. Hassel, J. Meixensberger, and E. Hofmann. 1994. Identification of ventricular enlargement and estimation of intracranial pressure by transcranial color-coded real-time sonography. *J Neuroimaging* 4:17–22.

Becker, G., J. Seufert, U. Bogdahn, H. Reichmann, and K. Reiners. 1995. Degeneration of substantia nigra in chronic Parkinson's disease visualized by transcranial color-coded real-time sonography. *Neurology* 45:182–184.

Becker, G., D. Berg, W. D. Rausch, H. K. Lange, P. Riederer, and K. Reiners. 1999. Increased tissue copper and manganese content in the lentiform nucleus in primary adult-onset dystonia. *Ann Neurol* 46:260–263.

Becker, G., D. Berg, M. Francis, M. Naumann. 2001. Evidence for disturbances of copper metabolism in dystonia: From the image towards a new concept. *Neurology* 57:2290–2294.

Behnke, S., D. Berg, M. Naumann, and G. Becker. 2005. Differentiation of Parkinson's disease and atypical parkinsonian syndromes by transcranial ultrasound. *J Neurol Neurosurg Psychiatry* 76:423–425.

Behnke, S., K. L. Double, S. Duma, G. A. Broe, V. Guenther, G. Becker, and G. M. Halliday. 2007. Substantia nigra echomorphology in the healthy very old: Correlation with motor slowing. *Neuroimage* 34:1054–1059.

Benito-Leon, J., E. D. Louis, and F. Bermejo-Pareja. 2009. Risk of incident Parkinson's disease and parkinsonism in essential tremor: A population based study. *J Neurol Neurosurg Psychiatry* 80:423–425.

Berg, D., G. Becker, B. Zeiler, O. Tucha, E. Hofmann, M. Preier, P. Benz, W. Jost, K. Reiners, and K. W. Lange. 1999a. Vulnerability of the nigrostriatal system as detected by transcranial ultrasound. *Neurology* 53:1026–1031.

Berg, D., C. Grote, W. D. Rausch, M. Maurer, W. Wesemann, P. Riederer, and G. Becker. 1999b. Iron accumulation in the substantia nigra in rats visualized by ultrasound. *Ultrasound Med Biol* 25:901–904.

Berg, D., A. Weishaupt, M. J. Francis, N. Miura, X. L. Yang, I. D. Goodyer, M. Naumann, M. Koltzenburg, K. Reiners, and G. Becker. 2000. Changes of copper-transporting proteins and ceruloplasmin in the lentiform nuclei in primary adult-onset dystonia. *Ann Neurol* 47:827–830.

Berg, D., M. Gerlach, M. B. Youdim, K. L. Double, L. Zecca, P. Riederer, and G. Becker. 2001a. Brain iron pathways and their relevance to Parkinson's disease. *J Neurochem* 79:225–236.

Berg, D., B. Jabs, U. Merschdorf, H. Beckmann, and G. Becker. 2001b. Echogenicity of substantia nigra determined by transcranial ultrasound correlates with severity of parkinsonian symptoms induced by neuroleptic therapy. *Biol Psychiatry* 50:463–467.

Berg, D., C. Siefker, and G. Becker. 2001c. Echogenicity of the substantia nigra in Parkinson's disease and its relation to clinical findings. *J Neurol* 248:684–689.

Berg, D., W. Roggendorf, U. Schroder, R. Klein, T. Tatschner, P. Benz, O. Tucha, M. Preier, K. W. Lange, K. Reiners, M. Gerlach, and G. Becker. 2002. Echogenicity of the substantia nigra: Association with increased iron content and marker for susceptibility to nigrostriatal injury. *Arch Neurol* 59:999–1005.

Berg, D., B. Merz, K. Reiners, M. Naumann, and G. Becker. 2005a. Five-year follow-up study of hyperechogenicity of the substantia nigra in Parkinson's disease. *Mov Disord* 20:383–385.

Berg, D., K. Schweitzer, P. Leitner, A. Zimprich, P. Lichtner, P. Belcredi, T. Brussel, C. Schulte, S. Maass, and T. Nagele. 2005b. Type and frequency of mutations in the LRRK2 gene in familial and sporadic Parkinson's disease*. *Brain* 128:3000–3011.

Berg, D., S. Behnke, and U. Walter. 2006a. Application of transcranial sonography in extrapyramidal disorders: updated recommendations. *Ultraschall Med* 27:12–19.

Berg, D., H. Hochstrasser, K. J. Schweitzer, and O. Riess. 2006b. Disturbance of iron metabolism in Parkinson's disease—ultrasonography as a biomarker. *Neurotox Res* 9:1–13.

Berg, D. 2007. Disturbance of iron metabolism as a contributing factor to SN hyperechogenicity in Parkinson's disease: Implications for idiopathic and monogenetic forms. *Neurochem Res* 32:1646–1654.

Berg, D., J. Godau, and U. Walter. 2008. Transcranial sonography in movement disorders. *Lancet Neurol* 7:1044–1055.

Berg, D., J. Godau, P. Riederer, M. Gerlach, and T. Arzberger. 2010. Microglia activation is related to substantia nigra echogenicity. *J Neural Transm* 117(11):1287–1292.

Berg, D., K. Seppi, S. Behnke, I. Liepelt, K. Schweitzer, H. Stockner, F. Wollenweber, A. Gaenslen, P. Mahlknecht, J. Spiegel, J. Godau, H. Huber, K. Srulijes, S. Kiechl, M. Bentele, A. Gasperi, T. Schubert, T. Hiry, M. Probst, V. Schneider, J. Klenk, M. Sawires, J. Willeit, W. Maetzler, K. Fassbender, T. Gasser, and W. Poewe. In Press. Enlarged substantia nigra hyperechogenicity and risk for Parkinson disease-37 months three-centre study of 1847 elderly. *Arch Neurol*.

Bouwmans, A. E., A. M. Vlaar, K. Srulijes, W. H. Mess, and W. E. Weber. 2010. Transcranial sonography for the discrimination of idiopathic Parkinson's disease from the atypical parkinsonian syndromes. *Int Rev Neurobiol* 90:121–146.

Brüggemann, N., J. Hagenah, K. Reetz, A. Schmidt, M. Kasten, I. Buchmann, S. Eckerle, M. Bähre, A. Münchau, A. Djarmati, J. van der Vegt, H. Siebner, F. Binkofski, A. Ramirez, M. I. Behrens, and C. Klein. 2010. Recessively inherited parkinsonism: Effect of ATP13A2 mutations on the clinical and neuroimaging phenotype. *Arch Neurol* 67(11):1357–1363.

Budisic, M., Z. Trkanjec, J. Bosnjak, A. Lovrencic-Huzjan, V. Vukovic, and V. Demarin. 2009. Distinguishing Parkinson's disease and essential tremor with transcranial sonography. *Acta Neurol Scand* 119: 17–21.

Doepp, F., M. Plotkin, L. Siegel, A. Kivi, D. Gruber, E. Lobsien, A. Kupsch, and S. J. Schreiber. 2008. Brain parenchyma sonography and 123I-FP-CIT SPECT in Parkinson's disease and essential tremor. *Mov Disord* 23:405–410.

Double, K. L., M. Gerlach, M .B. Youdim, and P. Riederer. 2000. Impaired iron homeostasis in Parkinson's disease. *J Neural Transm Suppl* (60):37–58.

Ebentheuer, J., M. Canelo, E. Trautmann, C. Trenkwalder. 2010. Substantia nigra echogenicity in progressive supranuclear palsy. *Mov Disord* 25:765–768.

Fearnley, J. M., A. J. Lees. 1991. Ageing and Parkinson's disease: Substantia nigra regional selectivity. *Brain* 114 (Pt 5): 2283–2301.

Gaenslen, A., B. Unmuth, J. Godau, I. Liepelt, A. Di Santo, K. J. Schweitzer, T. Gasser, H. J. Machulla, M. Reimold, K. Marek, and D. Berg. 2008. The specificity and sensitivity of transcranial ultrasound in the differential diagnosis of Parkinson's disease: A prospective blinded study. *Lancet Neurol* 7:417–424.

Gerlach, M., D. Ben-Shachar, P. Riederer, and M. B. Youdim. 1994. Altered brain metabolism of iron as a cause of neurodegenerative diseases? *J Neurochem* 63:793–807.

Haehner, A., T. Hummel, C. Hummel, U. Sommer, S. Junghanns, and H. Reichmann. 2007. Olfactory loss may be a first sign of idiopathic Parkinson's disease. *Mov Disord* 22:839–842.

Hagenah, J., I. R. Konig, J. Sperner, L. Wessel, G. Seidel, K. Condefer, R. Saunders-Pullman, C. Klein, and N. Bruggemann. 2010. Life-long increase of substantia nigra hyperechogenicity in transcranial sonography. *Neuroimage* 51:28–32.

Hagenah, J. M., I. R. Konig, B. Becker, R. Hilker, M. Kasten, K. Hedrich, P. P. Pramstaller, C. Klein, and G. Seidel. 2007. Substantia nigra hyperechogenicity correlates with clinical status and number of Parkin mutated alleles. *J Neurol* 254:1407–1413.

Hagenah, J. M., B. Becker, N. Bruggemann, A. Djarmati, K. Lohmann, A. Sprenger, C. Klein, and G. Seidel. 2008. Transcranial sonography findings in a large family with homozygous and heterozygous PINK1 mutations. *J Neurol Neurosurg Psychiatry* 79:1071–1074.

Hawkes, C. H. 2008. The prodromal phase of sporadic Parkinson's disease: Does it exist and if so how long is it? *Mov Disord*. 23: 1799–1807.

Hedrich, K., S. Winkler, J. Hagenah, K. Kabakci, M. Kasten, E. Schwinger, J. Volkmann, P. P. Pramstaller, V. Kostic, P. Vieregge, and C. Klein. 2006. Recurrent LRRK2 (Park8) mutations in early-onset Parkinson's disease. *Mov Disord* 21:1506–1510.

Hochstrasser, H., P. Bauer, U. Walter, S. Behnke, J. Spiegel, I. Csoti, B. Zeiler, A. Bornemann, J. Pahnke, G. Becker, O. Riess, and D. Berg. 2004. Ceruloplasmin gene variations and substantia nigra hyperechogenicity in Parkinson disease. *Neurology* 63:1912–1917.

Hochstrasser, H., J. Tomiuk, U. Walter, S. Behnke, J. Spiegel, R. Kruger, G. Becker, O. Riess, and D. Berg. 2005. Functional relevance of ceruloplasmin mutations in Parkinson's disease. *Faseb J* 19:1851–1853.

Huang, Y. W., J. S. Jeng, C. F. Tsai, L. L. Chen, and R. M. Wu. 2007. Transcranial imaging of substantia nigra hyperechogenicity in a Taiwanese cohort of Parkinson's disease. *Mov Disord* 22:550–555.

Jankovic, J. 2005. Searching for a relationship between manganese and welding and Parkinson's disease. *Neurology* 64:2021–2028.

Kim, J. Y., S. T. Kim, S. H. Jeon, and W. Y. Lee. 2007. Midbrain transcranial sonography in Korean patients with Parkinson's disease. *Mov Disord* 22:1922–1926.

Kolevski, G., I. Petrov, and V. Petrova. 2007. Transcranial sonography in the evaluation of Parkinson disease. *J Ultrasound Med* 26:509–512.

Krauel, K., H. C. Feldhaus, A. Simon, C. Rehe, M. Glaser, H. H. Flechtner, H. J. Heinze, and L. Niehaus. 2010. Increased echogenicity of the substantia nigra in children and adolescents with attention-deficit/hyperactivity disorder. *Biol Psychiatry* 68(4): 352–358.

Lambeck, J., W. Niesen, and B. Zucker. 2008. Substantia nigra hyperechogenicity in Huntington's disease. *Akt Neurologie* 35:152 (abstract).

Leentjens, A. F., M. Van den Akker, J. F. Metsemakers, R. Lousberg, and F. R. Verhey. 2003. Higher incidence of depression preceding the onset of Parkinson's disease: A register study. *Mov Disord* 18: 414–418.

Liepelt, I., A. Wendt, K. J. Schweitzer, B. Wolf, J. Godau, A. Gaenslen, T. Bruessel, and D. Berg. 2008. Substantia nigra hyperechogenicity assessed by transcranial sonography is related to neuropsychological impairment in the elderly population. *J Neural Transm* 1 15: 993–999.

Liepelt, I., S. Behnke, K. Schweitzer, B. Wolf, J. Godau, F. Wollenweber, U. Dillmann, A. Gaenslen, A. Di Santo, W. Maetzler, and D. Berg. 2009. Pre-motor signs of PD are related to SN hyperechogenicity assessed by TCS in an elderly population. *Neurobiol Aging* (Epub ahead of print).

Mijajlovic, M., N. Dragasevic, E. Stefanova, I. Petrovic, M. Svetel, V. S. Kostic. 2008. Transcranial sonography in spinocerebellar ataxia type 2. *J Neurol* 255:1164–1167.

Okawa, M., H. Miwa, Y. Kajimoto, K. Hama, S. Morita, I. Nakanishi, and T. Kondo. 2007. Transcranial sonography of the substantia nigra in Japanese patients with Parkinson's disease or atypical parkinsonism: Clinical potential and limitations. *Intern Med* 46:1527–1531.

Postert, T., J. Eyding, D. Berg, H. Przuntek, G. Becker, M. Finger, and L. Schols. 2004. Transcranial sonography in spinocerebellar ataxia type 3. *J Neural Transm Suppl* (68):123–133.

Prestel, J., K. J. Schweitzer, A. Hofer, T. Gasser, and D. Berg. 2006. Predictive value of transcranial sonography in the diagnosis of Parkinson's disease. *Mov Disord* 21:1763–1765.

Ressner, P., D. Skoloudik, P. Hlustik, and P. Kanovsky. 2007. Hyperechogenicity of the substantia nigra in Parkinson's disease. *J Neuroimaging* 17:164–167.

Ruprecht-Dorfler, P., D. Berg, O. Tucha, P. Benz, M. Meier-Meitinger, G. L. Alders, K. W. Lange, and G. Becker. 2003. Echogenicity of the substantia nigra in relatives of patients with sporadic Parkinson's disease. *Neuroimage* 18:416–422.

Saka, E., M. A. Topcuoglu, A. U. Demir, and B. Elibol. 2010. Transcranial sonography in Perry syndrome. *Parkinsonism Relat Disord* 16:68–70.

Schuurman, A. G., M. van den Akker, K. T. Ensinck, J. F. Metsemakers, J. A. Knottnerus, A. F. Leentjens, and F. Buntinx. 2002. Increased risk of Parkinson's disease after depression: A retrospective cohort study. *Neurology* 58:1501–1504.

Schweitzer, K. J., S. Behnke, I. Liepelt, B. Wolf, C. Grosser, J. Godau, A. Gaenslen, T. Bruessel, A. Wendt, F. Abel, A. Muller, T. Gasser, and D. Berg. 2007a. Cross-sectional study discloses a positive family history for Parkinson's disease and male gender as epidemiological risk factors for substantia nigra hyperechogenicity. *J Neural Transm* 114:1167–1171.

Schweitzer, K. J., T. Brussel, P. Leitner, R. Kruger, P. Bauer, D. Woitalla, J. Tomiuk, T. Gasser, and D. Berg. 2007b. Transcranial ultrasound in different monogenetic subtypes of Parkinson's disease. *J Neurol* 254:613–616.

Spiegel, J., D. Hellwig, M. O. Mollers, S. Behnke, W. Jost, K. Fassbender, S. Samnick, U. Dillmann, G. Becker, and C. M. Kirsch. 2006. Transcranial sonography and [123I]FP-CIT SPECT disclose complementary aspects of Parkinson's disease. *Brain* 129:1188–1193.

Stockner, H., M. Sojer, K KS, J. Mueller, G. K. Wenning, C. Schmidauer, and W. Poewe. 2007. Midbrain sonography in patients with essential tremor. *Mov Disord* 22:414–417.

Stockner, H., A. Iranzo, K. Seppi, M. Serradell, V. Gschliesser, M. Sojer, F. Valldeoriola, J. L. Molinuevo, B. Frauscher, C. Schmidauer, J. Santamaria, B. Hogl, E. Tolosa, and W. Poewe. 2009. Midbrain hyperechogenicity in idiopathic REM sleep behavior disorder. *Mov Disord* 24:1906–1909.

Tsai, C. F., R. M. Wu, Y. W. Huang, L. L. Chen, P. K. Yip, and J. S. Jeng. 2007. Transcranial color-coded sonography helps differentiation between idiopathic Parkinson's disease and vascular parkinsonism. *J Neurol* 254:501–507.

Unger, M. M., J. C. Moller, T. Ohletz, K. Stiasny-Kolster, W. H. Oertel, and G. Mayer. 2009. Transcranial midbrain sonography in narcoleptic subjects with and without concomitant REM sleep behaviour disorder. *J Neurol* 256:874–877.

van de Loo, S., U. Walter, S. Behnke, J. Hagenah, M. Lorenz, M. Sitzer, R. Hilker, and D. Berg. 2010. Reproducibility and diagnostic accuracy of substantia nigra sonography for the diagnosis of Parkinson's disease. *J Neurol Neurosurg Psychiatry* 81(10):1087–1092.

Vlaar, A. M., A. Bouwmans, W. H. Mess, S. C. Tromp, and W. E. Weber. 2009. Transcranial duplex in the differential diagnosis of parkinsonian syndromes: A systematic review. *J Neurol* 256:530–538.

Walter, U., M. Wittstock, R. Benecke, and D. Dressler. 2002. Substantia nigra echogenicity is normal in non-extrapyramidal cerebral disorders but increased in Parkinson's disease. *J Neural Transm* 109: 191–196.

Walter, U., D. Dressler, A. Wolters, T. Probst, A. Grossmann, R. Benecke. 2004a. Sonographic discrimination of corticobasal degeneration vs progressive supranuclear palsy. *Neurology* 63:504–509.

Walter, U., C. Klein, R. Hilker, R. Benecke, P. P. Pramstaller, and D. Dressler. 2004b. Brain parenchyma sonography detects preclinical parkinsonism. *Mov Disord* 19:1445–1449.

Walter, U., K. Krolikowski, B. Tarnacka, R. Benecke, A. Czlonkowska, and D. Dressler. 2005. Sonographic detection of basal ganglia lesions in asymptomatic and symptomatic Wilson disease. *Neurology* 64:1726–1732.

Walter, U., D. Dressler, A. Wolters, M. Wittstock, B. Greim, and R. Benecke. 2006. Sonographic discrimination of dementia with Lewy bodies and Parkinson's disease with dementia. *J Neurol* 253: 448–454.

Walter, U., S. Behnke, J. Eyding, L. Niehaus, T. Postert, G. Seidel, and D. Berg. 2007a. Transcranial brain parenchyma sonography in movement disorders: State of the art. *Ultrasound Med Biol* 33:15–25.

Walter, U., D. Dressler, A. Wolters, M. Wittstock, and R. Benecke. 2007b. Transcranial brain sonography findings in clinical subgroups of idiopathic Parkinson's disease. *Mov Disord* 22:48–54.

Walter, U., J. Hoeppner, L. Prudente-Morrissey, S. Horowski, S. C. Herpertz, and R. Benecke. 2007c. Parkinson's disease-like midbrain sonography abnormalities are frequent in depressive disorders. *Brain* 130:1799–1807.

Walter, U., D. Dressler, C. Lindemann, A. Slachevsky, and M. Miranda. 2008. Transcranial sonography findings in welding-related Parkinsonism in comparison to Parkinson's disease. *Mov Disord* 23:141–145.

Walter, U., A. Wolters, M. Wittstock, R. Benecke, H. W. Schroeder, J. U. Muller. 2009. Deep brain stimulation in dystonia: Sonographic monitoring of electrode placement into the globus pallidus internus. *Mov Disord* 24:1538–1541.

Weise, D., R. Lorenz, M. Schliesser, A. Schirbel, K. Reiners, and J. Classen. 2009. Substantia nigra echogenicity: A structural correlate of functional impairment of the dopaminergic striatal projection in Parkinson's disease. *Mov Disord* 24:1669–1675.

Williams, D. R., and A. J. Lees. 2009. Progressive supranuclear palsy: Clinicopathological concepts and diagnostic challenges. *Lancet Neurol* 8:270–279.

6

PARKINSONIAN TREMOR

Ioannis U. Isaias and Angelo Antonini

CLINICAL AND PATHOPHYSIOLOGICAL FEATURES OF TREMOR IN PD

Tremor in Parkinson's disease (PD) is characterized by 4–6 Hz activity at rest in the limbs with distal predominance. Tremor can be triggered or increased in amplitude by maneuvers such as voluntary movement of other body parts, walking, anxiety, or stress (i.e., arithmetic calculations are commonly used to induce tremor).

PD tremor is neither a consistent nor a homogeneous feature across patients or within an individual patient's disease course. The most common way to clinically rate tremor is with the Unified Parkinson's Disease Rating Scale (UPDRS), which has only a single patient rating of tremor (0–4 scale on question 16) and two examiner ratings of tremor amplitude at rest for each limb and during posture/action limb for each arm (0–32 total rating scale for questions 20 and 21). Data regarding tremor ratings from large PD studies relying only on the UPDRS are at times in conflict with smaller, but tremor-specific studies using more sophisticated methods such as accelerometry or quantitative EMG (Koller et al. 1986; Koller and Herbster 1987). Finally, many studies did not consistently assess re-emergent resting tremor with sustained posture and fail to distinguish it from postural tremor (Henderson et al.1994; Kraus et al. 2006).

The physiology of resting tremor remains not completely understood, and aspects of parkinsonian tremor are in apparent contradiction with our understanding of motor symptoms of PD as a reflection of an underlying dopamine deficiency (Joffroy 1969; Hallet 2003). Early animal models of PD, based on lesions of midbrain areas in monkeys, suggest that dopaminergic nigral loss alone is not sufficient to produce resting tremor. Indeed, structural lesions of the substantia nigra produce akinetic syndromes but not tremor, which is rather the result of damage to the nigrostriatal dopaminergic projections in combination with damage to the rubro-olivo-cerebello-rubral and cerebello-thalamic pathways (Péchadre et al. 1976; Lamarre et al. 1975; Jenner and Marsden 1984; Lenz et al. 1993). Moreover, chemical animal models of PD, like those following injection of 6-hydroxydopamine and MPTP, primarily induced damage of dopaminergic neurons, mainly reproducing akinetic-rigid features but only occasionally tremor (Burns et al. 1983; Bergman et al. 1994, 1998; Wilms et al. 1999; Raz et al. 2000). In humans, structural lesions resulting in predominately resting tremor are rarely reported (Gonzalez-Alegre 2007), and the presence or absence of resting tremor was proposed in the context of clinical criteria to distinguish idiopathic PD from other forms of parkinsonism (Kulisevsky et al. 1996; Krauss et al. 1995; Lee et al. 1993; Thanvi et al. 2005).

The frequency of tremor in subjects with PD is often remarkably similar within one body part (e.g., a limb) (Hunker et al. 1990). However, tremor in different extremities, even on the same body side, is almost never coherent (Raethjen et al. 2000; Ben-Pazi et al. 2001). The absence of tremor coherence could hint at mechanical or spinal reflex mechanisms rather than a single central oscillator. Nevertheless, several studies failed to demonstrate a frequency reduction of tremor as a result of load addition to the trembling limb, and resetting experiments—in which the tremulous limb is reset by mechanical perturbation—have been even less conclusive (Elble and Koller 1990; Deuschl et al. 2000).

In line with a central nervous system (CNS) hypothesis, lesions within the CNS can suppress parkinsonian tremor (Machado et al. 2006), and brain lesions were in the past considered a therapeutic option to suppress tremor in PD patients. In addition, rhythmic and synchronous neuronal firing, recorded in the ventral intermediate nucleus (Vim) of the thalamus, subthalamic nucleus (STN), and globus pallidus internus (GPi), correlates with tremor in the limbs in both MPTP monkeys and in patients with PD (Rodriguez-Oroz et al. 1998; Hurtado et al. 2005; Reck et al. 2009). The Vim is the surgical target with the most established record of efficacy to reduce tremor in PD (Lenz et al. 1993; Koller et al. 1997). Recent studies established that deep brain stimulation (DBS) of the Vim is at least equally efficacious as thalamotomy for the reduction in tremor (Tasker et al. 1998; DBS-Study Group 2001; Putzke et al. 2003). Several trials also described improvement in parkinsonian tremor after DBS of the STN (Rodriguez-Oroz et al. 1998; Krack et al. 1998; Patel et al. 2003; Sturman et al. 2004; Blahak 2007) and the GPi (Taha et al. 1977; Vitek et al. 2003). Taken together, the results of comparable effects on tremor reduction by lesioning or stimulating (DBS) different brain areas further puzzle the role of independent oscillating circuits within a widespread tremor-generating network (Timmermann et al. 2003; Hurtado et al. 2005; Reck et al. 2009).

Understanding the neurotransmitter abnormalities involved in parkinsonian tremor is also complicated by the variable response to medications (Navan et al. 2003; Schrag et al. 2002; Olanow et al. 1994; Lieberman et al. 1997; Kunig et al. 1999). Anticholinergic agents, which were the first drugs available for the symptomatic treatment of PD, tend to have better effects on tremor than on akinetic-rigid symptoms (Doshay et al. 1956; Brumlik et al. 1964). However, the effectiveness of anticholinergics in the treatment of tremor as well as the need to use them given the large number of therapeutic strategies is debated (Koller 1986; Schrag et al. 1999; Katzenschlager et al. 2003). Dopamine agonists are superior to L-dopa in the treatment of tremor (Navan et al. 2003; Schrag et al. 2002; Olanow et al. 1994; Lieberman et al. 1997; Kunig et al. 1999), but evidence comes primarily from studies with patients with L-dopa refractory tremor rather than from direct comparisons with L-dopa. Clozapine also shows some efficacy on L-dopa refractory parkinsonian tremor (Bonuccelli et al. 1997; Friedman et al. 1997; Binder et al. 2003), and budipine, a possible glutamate antagonist, ameliorates resting tremor when added to L-dopa (Jellinger and Bliesath 1987; Spieker 1995, 1999; Przuntek et al. 2002; Reichmann 2006).

REGIONAL BRAIN CHANGES ASSOCIATED WITH PD TREMOR

Only a few articles used imaging techniques to investigate the pathophysiological basis of parkinsonian tremor. Several studies instead addressed the differential diagnosis between parkinsonian tremor and essential tremor (ET). To this regard, Brooks and colleagues measured striatal ^{18}F-dopa influx constants (Ki) for 20 subjects with isolated predominantly postural tremor and 11 subjects with predominantly rest tremor in comparison with 30 controls and 16 PD patients. They reported a 10%–13% lower ^{18}F-dopa uptake in the basal ganglia of ET patients, but the difference did not reach statistical significance. An overlap was also described between different forms of tremor: two of the patients with sporadic postural tremor showed subnormal putamen ^{18}F-dopa Ki, with one subject (who later became akinetic) falling in the PD range, and all 11 subjects with rest tremor had significantly reduced putamen ^{18}F-dopa uptake contralateral to the more affected limbs. Interestingly, the rest tremor responded to L-dopa in only four of the nine patients for whom the drug was prescribed (Brooks et al. 1992). Following studies did not confirm the presence of dopaminergic defects in subjects with ET. In particular, both [^{123}I]β-CIT and SPECT (Asenbaum et al. 1998) and [^{11}C]d-threo-methylphenidate and PET (Breit et al. 2006) did not discriminate ET from healthy controls. Benamer and colleagues (Benamer et al. 2003) also failed to find any [^{123}I]FP-CIT binding differences between healthy controls and ET patients. However, Lee and colleagues (Lee et al. 1999) using [^{123}I]IPT and SPECT and Schwarz and colleagues (Schwarz et al. 2004) with [^{123}I]FP-CIT and SPECT reported reduced striatal binding in ET with clinical features suggestive of PD (i.e., isolated rest tremor and visual-motor coordination failure, respectively). More recent dopamine receptor binding studies also revealed a mild dopaminergic loss, especially in the caudate nucleus, in subjects with ET (Jankovic et al. 1993; Lee et al. 1999; Isaias et al. 2008, 2010). Similarly, the caudate nucleus was more affected in PD subjects with tremor when compared to a matched cohort of patients without clinically evident tremor (Isaias et al. 2007; Eggers et al. 2010). Nonetheless, although PD and ET may share a common dopaminergic base for tremor onset, the two diseases are fundamentally different pathological entities. Indeed, besides the clinically evident differences between the parkinsonian rest tremor and the predominant action tremor in ET subjects, PD and ET are clearly differentiated by the dopaminergic content in the putamen (Isaias et al. 2008), and ET subjects do not manifest a PD-like progressive dopaminergic loss in the basal ganglia (Isaias et al. 2010). Furthermore, we recently demonstrated, by means of SPECT and ECD, that ET subjects do not manifest a typical parkinsonian brain network (PDRP) (Isaias et al. 2010).

The role of caudate nucleus in the pathophysiology of tremor is not well established and, besides imaging studies, there is only indirect clinical and pathophysiological evidence of its role in tremor genesis. Tremor can be induced by intracaudate injections of bretylium, tetrabenazine, mescaline, chlorpromazine, or acepromazine and further suppressed by local injections of catecholamines (Lalley et al. 1973; Buzsaki et al. 1990). Electrical stimulation of the head of the caudate nucleus in rats also determined the onset of tremor (Buzsaki et al. 1990). Patients with contralateral infarction of the caudate nucleus showed delayed onset of parkinsonian tremor but not of bradykinesia or rigidity (Kim et al. 1992), and a more prominent degeneration of the medial substantia nigra pars compacta, which projects mainly to the caudate nucleus, was described in tremulous variant PD (Jellinger et al. 1999). Therefore, patients with tremor dominant PD, and possibly ET, may have a very selective dysfunction of the caudate nucleus-thalamic pathway. Eventually, with dopamine depletion in the caudate nucleus, thalamic targets fire in a burst oscillatory fashion and act as a pacemaker (Berezovskii et al. 1977; Kopell et al. 2006; Caretti et al. 2008). Moreover, the caudate nucleus, as well as the motor and premotor cortex, hand and lower-limb sensory, supplementary motor area (SMA), motor vermis, and cerebellar gray nuclei showed normalized cerebral blood flow increases during tremor on the electrode side (Vim DBS). Interestingly, apart from the caudate nucleus, all other regions are also activated during execution of repetitive voluntary movements in man (Chollet et al. 1991; Colebatch et al. 1991; Seitz et al. 1990; Fox et al. 1985), thus confirming similarities of brain structures between parkinsonian tremor and voluntary movement (Duffau et al. 1996).

The caudate-cerebellar pathway, via the inferior olive (Sedgwick et al. 1967; Fox et al. 1968), may also play a role in tremor development. In this case, the loss of inhibitory dopaminergic innervation of the caudate nucleus will determine a release of the excitatory caudate-olive pathway and trigger abnormal oscillations of the inferior olive (Lorenz and Deuschl 2007). This "trigger" effect may also explain the lack of correlation between resting tremor and loss of dopamine transporter ligand binding (Priker et al. 2003; Spiegel et al. 2007; Isaias et al. 2007) and loss of ^{18}F-dopa uptake at PET imaging (Benamer et al. 2003). Further supporting a role of the caudate-cerebellar pathway in tremor onset, six patients with tremor following an upper peduncular lesion showed a marked decrease of ^{18}F-dopa uptake in the striatum ipsilateral to the lesion without significant changes in D_2-specific binding measured by [^{76}Br]bromolisuride and PET. The decrease in ^{18}F-dopa uptake was even more marked in both the caudate nucleus and the putamen than in patients with PD, and all subjects showed some benefit from L-dopa therapy (Remy et al. 1995). Finally, increased metabolic activity was found in the cerebellum (vermis and cerebellar gray nuclei) in two studies investigating parkinsonian tremor with PET and FDG or $H_2^{15}O$ (Parker et al. 1992 and Kassubek et al. 2001, respectively). Despite the evidence of cerebellar activation in subjects with PD and tremor, its distinctive role in parkinsonian tremor has not yet been elucidated (see later). The first step to identify a putative complementary role for the basal ganglia (e.g., caudate nucleus) and the cerebellum would be to elucidate the interactions at a thalamic level. This, however, may not be clear in that tremor-related hypermetabolism, mainly located in a thalamic subnucleus receiving input from the basal ganglia (VLa or Vop), might also be modulated by stereotactic modulation of a thalamic area receiving cerebellar input (VLp or Vim).

As mentioned, Vim DBS has been used to suppress tremor in PD patients, and a few imaging studies also investigated tremor changes during Vim stimulation (Davis et al. 1997; Deiber et al. 1993; Parker et al. 1992; Fukuda et al. 2004). Deiber and colleagues (Deiber et al. 1993) examined six subjects with unilateral parkinsonian tremor and Vim DBS in three situations: (i) absence of tremor following effective stimulation; (ii) tremor in presence of ineffective stimulation; and (iii) tremor with no stimulation. In summary, $H_2^{15}O$ and PET showed, during effective stimulation compared with noneffective stimulation, a major decrease in activity in the rostral cerebellum medially and paramedially with no significant lateralization. Compared with the standard tremor state without stimulation, the ventral intermediate nucleus stimulation at the ineffective 50–65 Hz frequency caused a decrease of activity in the homolateral cerebral hemisphere without any effect on the cerebellum. The cerebral structures involved were in the left inferior precentral cortex and in the anterior cingulate gyrus. The main result of the study was that the suppression of tremor caused by high-frequency stimulation is specifically associated with depressed activity medially and paramedially in the rostral cerebellum. Also of interest, stimulation of the ventral intermediate nucleus at a frequency ineffective at suppressing tremor (a condition of virtually no motor or proprioceptive change) was associated with a decrease of activity in the ipsilateral cerebral hemisphere, including precentral and medial cortical areas. Davis and colleagues (Davis et al. 1997), using a similar design, associated tremor suppression with flow decrements in the contralateral cerebellum, the supplementary motor, and the cingulate. A similar reduction in motor cortical cerebral perfusion was reported in a SPECT study of Vim DBS in PD that employed a simple off–on design (Wielepp et al. 2001). These studies suggest that Vim DBS mediates tremor relief in PD through a reduction in cerebello-thalamocortical synaptic activity, as proposed in stereotaxic thalamotomy (Boecker et al. 1997).

Although this PET and DBS combined approach has provided insight into the pathophysiological mechanism of parkinsonian tremor, the main drawback is the presence of multiple variables that are difficult to separate in the interpretation of the results. Indeed, the subtraction of a baseline condition, characterized by the presence of active resting tremor with DBS turned off, from a test condition with no tremor and DBS turned on, changes two variables: activation of the stimulator and reduction or elimination of resting tremor. To partially overcome this problem, Duffau and colleagues investigated seven subjects with hemi-parkinsonian tremor using $H_2^{15}O$ and PET both before and after tremor arrest induced by administration of L-dopa as well as during voluntary repetitive movements of the hand contralateral to tremor side. In this study, the precentral gyrus and paracentral gyrus contralateral to tremor, the SMA and the cerebellar vermis showed an increase in blood flow during rest without L-dopa as compared to rest under L-dopa (Duffau et al. 1996).

Finally, Fukuda and colleagues investigated the relationship between regional cerebral blood flow (rCBF) and specific physiological tremor characteristics during Vim stimulation, showing that the rCBF changes in motor regions and cerebellum had different physiological correlates. In particular, the sensorimotor cortex and SMA were preferentially modeled by tremor amplitude and the cerebellum by tremor frequency. In addition, the authors also revealed functional changes after DBS in brain regions not typically associated with motor pathways such as increased occipital cortical blood flow during tremor suppression (Fukuda et al. 2004) (Figure 1). Indeed, in an overlapping area of visual cortex, residual rCBF changes presented a negative correlation with tremor amplitude (Davis et al. 1997).

Despite the aforementioned evidence, the role of the cerebellum in the genesis of parkinsonian tremor has been overall questioned by a multitracer PET study. Ghaemi and colleagues investigated eight subjects with monosymptomatic resting tremor (mRT), eight patients with PD that showed all three classic parkinsonian symptoms, and seven age-matched healthy subjects. Subjects underwent cerebral magnetic resonance imaging (MRI) and multitracer PET with ^{18}F-dopa (FDOPA), ^{18}F-FDG, and ^{11}C-raclopride (RAC). PD and mRT patients did not show significant differences in ^{18}F-dopa-, RAC-, or FDG-PET scans. In FDOPA- and RAC-PET, significant differences between the pooled patient data and control subjects were found in the anterior

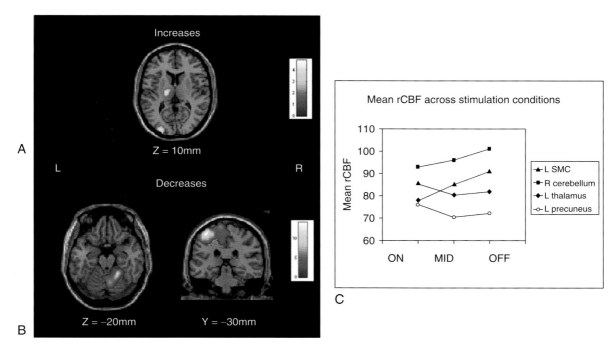

Figure 1 Main effects of Vim stimulation on regional cerebral blood flow (rCBF). Significant voxels thresholded at $P_u < 0.01$ (height uncorrected) and $P_k < 0.05$ (extent corrected) are superimposed onto the SPM99 T1 MRI template of a single individual to facilitate anatomical localization. Stimulation resulted in rCBF increases (A) in the ipsilateral thalamus and occipital association area (BA 18, 19), and decreases (B) in the ipsilateral primary sensorimotor cortex (BA 1-3/4), caudal supplementary motor area (SMA), and contralateral cerebellum. Mean normalized rCBF values for each of these voxels (maxima) are displayed for each stimulation condition (C).

and posterior putamen ipsilateral and contralateral to the more affected body side. In addition, the authors reported a difference for the normalized glucose metabolism values for the whole cerebellum between PD patients and healthy controls, but no abnormalities were seen in the mRT group. This suggests that at least part of the cerebellar hyperactivation seen in tremulous PD might be related to akinesia and rigidity rather than tremor (Ghaemi et al. 2002).

BRAIN NETWORKS RELATED TO PD TREMOR

In a prior FDG-PET study (Antonini et al. 1998) comparing tremor predominant and atremulous PD patients, Antonini and colleagues used FDG and PET to map the functional topography of PD tremor (tremor-specific network). They utilized a multiregional principal component analysis and a cross-sectional design to identify a distinct ponto-thalamocortical covariance pattern in tremor-predominant PD patients, further supporting the knowledge of different metabolic networks for hypo- and hyperkinetic symptoms in PD. The activity of this metabolic network has been shown to decrease after Vim stimulation (Trost et al. 2003). Kassubek and colleagues (Kassubek et al. 2001) also used FDG and PET to identify a tremor-specific metabolic network with focal hypermetabolism in the thalamus, approximately corresponding to VLa according to Jones or Vop according to Hassler (Macchi et al. 1997).

Recent advances in imaging analytical techniques, such as the ordinal trends canonical variates analysis (OrT/CVA) (Habeck et al. 2005), allowed for the identification

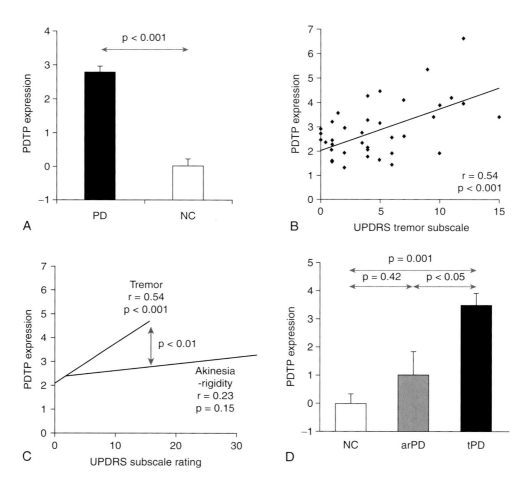

Figure 2 Validation of PDTP expression as a network correlate of parkinsonian tremor. (A) Bar graph showing mean PDTP (± SE) in a prospective group of 41 PD patients (*black bars*) and 20 age-matched healthy control subject (*white bars*). The expression of this disease-related pattern in this testing group (p < 0.001, relative to controls). (B) PDTP expression correlated (r = 0.54, p < 0.001) with UPDRS subscale ratings for tremor in the PD group. (C) The correlation of PDTP scores with tremor was significantly greater in magnitude (p < 0.01; multiple regression analysis) than with subscale ratings for akinesia-rigidity (see text). (D) Bar graph showing mean PDTP subject scores (± SE) in tremor dominant and akinesia-rigidity dominant PD patients (arPD and tPD, respectively), and in normal control (NC) subjects undergoing perfusion imaging with ECD SPECT (see text). PDTP expression was significantly higher in the tPD patients than in the arPD (p < 0.05) and NC groups (p = 0.001).

of functional brain networks within individual subjects. Utilizing this approach, Mure and colleagues (Mure et al. 2010) studied nine tremor-dominant PD patients who underwent FDG-PET at baseline and during Vim DBS. They identified a specific PD tremor-related metabolic pattern (PDTP) characterized by covarying metabolic increases in the cerebellum/dentate nucleus, the primary motor cortex, and the caudate/putamen. In the absence of Vim stimulation, PDTP expression correlated significantly with concurrent accelerometric measurement of tremor amplitude. With stimulation, consistent reductions in pattern expression were evident in the patients. In prospective PD populations, PDTP network activity exhibited an excellent test–retest reproducibility and a significant correlation with UPDRS tremor subscales, but not akinesia-rigidity (Figure 2 and 3).

Tremor generation has been linked to abnormal activity in the cerebello-thalamocortical (CbTC) pathway (Timmermann et al. 2003). That said, the role of the basal ganglia in mediating this symptom has remained the subject of debate (Deuschl et al. 2000; Timmermann et al. 2003; Mure et al. 2011; Helmich et al. 2011). In a magnetoencephalography study, Timmermann and colleagues reported a tremor-coherent oscillatory network involving the primary motor cortex, thalamus, and cerebellum (Timmermann et al. 2003). Prior imaging studies showed that both thalamotomy and Vim DBS suppressed neural activity in the primary motor cortex and the anterior cerebellum (Deiver et al. 1993; Boecker et al. 1997; Wielepp et al. 2001; Fukuda et al. 2004). These regions constitute key nodes of the PDTP topography. Interestingly, the PDTP also includes a significant contribution from the striatum, albeit of lower magnitude

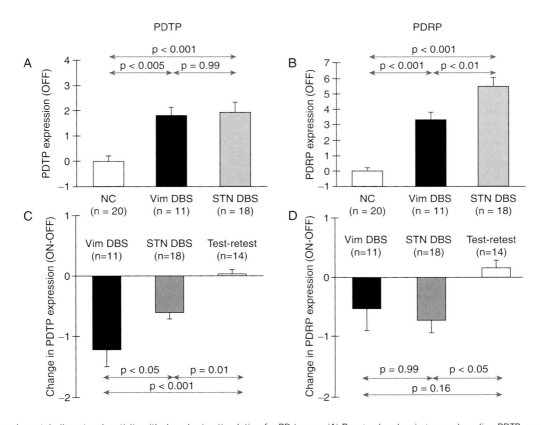

Figure 3 Changes in metabolic network activity with deep brain stimulation for PD tremor. (A) Bar graphs showing mean baseline PDTP expression (± SE) in the Vim DBS patients (*black*), the STN DBS patients (*gray*), and the healthy control subjects (*white*). There was a significant difference in PDTP expression across the three groups (p < 0.001; one-way ANOVA), with comparable elevations in baseline pattern expression in both the Vim DBS (p < 0.005) and STN DBS groups (p < 0.001) relative to controls. (B) Baseline PDRP expression also differed across the three groups (p < 0.001), with higher expression in both treatment groups relative to controls (p < 0.001). Nonetheless, PDRP expression was higher in the STN than in the Vim DBS groups (p < 0.01). (C) Treatment-mediated changes (ON-OFF) in mean PDTP expression (± SE) in the Vim DBS patients (*black*), the STN DBS patients (*gray*), and the test-retest PD control subjects (*white*). Changes in PDTP expression were different across the three groups (p < 0.001; one-way ANOVA), with stimulation-mediated declines in network activity in both DBS groups (Vim: p < 0.001; STN: p = 0.001, relative to the test-retest control group). PDTP modulation was greater with Vim than STN stimulation (p < 0.05). (D) There was also a significant group difference in treatment-mediated PDRP modulation (p = 0.02). Treatment-mediated reductions in PDRP expression reached significance (p < 0.05) with STN stimulation, but not with Vim stimulation (p = 0.16).

than the other nodes of this network. Metabolic activity in the putamen was found to correlate with tremor ratings in another FDG-PET study (Lozza et al. 2002, HBM, 2004). In the primate, the striatum receives cerebellar output via the ventrolateral and intralaminar thalamic nuclear groups (Hoshi et al. 2005). Thus, while the observed tremor-related network changes are most prominent in the primary motor cortex and cerebellum, these regions may interconnect through the Vim thalamus and putamen.

CONCLUSION

There are two possible mechanisms for parkinsonian tremor currently under discussion (Rodriguez-Oroz et al. 2009). Firstly, increased basal ganglia output may lead to increased excitability of the primary motor cortex and synchronous basal ganglia firing, thereby facilitating oscillatory activity in the motor loop. Secondly, the neuronal network underlying tremor may not lie in the basal ganglia. This possibility is supported by the association between the Vim and cerebellar activation and tremor and by the exquisite sensitivity of Vim manipulations to cessation of tremor. In this case, extrastriatal dopamine denervation, or loss of other transmitters such as catecholaminergic neurons, could facilitate synchronous oscillatory activity within the thalamus and basal ganglia. Nonetheless, a specific pattern of neurodegeneration accounting for tremor and differentiating PD-dominant tremor from akinetic-rigid forms has not been found. Indeed, parkinsonian tremor behaves in a more complex and heterogeneous manner than the other cardinal signs of bradykinesia and rigidity, and there is converging evidence of independent oscillating circuits within a widespread tremor-generating network (Timmerman et al. 2003; Hurtado et al. 2005; Reck et al. 2009). The relative contribution of non-dopaminergic (e.g., cholinergic, serotonergic, and noradrenergic) systems to these circuits has not yet been investigated and should be clarified. Indeed, one study correlated parkinsonian tremor with decreased serotonergic function measured by midbrain raphe binding of a 5-HT(1A) ligand (Doder et al. 2003).

REFERENCES

Antonini, A., J. R. Moeller, T. Nakamura, P. Spetsieris, V. Dhawan, and D. Eidelberg. 1998. The metabolic anatomy of tremor in Parkinson's disease. *Neurology* 51:803–810.

Asenbaum, S., W. Pirker, P. Angelberger, G. Bencsits, M. Pruckmayer, T. Brücke et al. 1998. [123I]b-CIT and SPECT in essential tremor and Parkinson's disease. *J Neural Transm* 105:1213–1228.

Benamer, H. T. S., W. H. Oertel, J. Patterson, D. M. Hadley, O. Pogarell, H. Höffken et al. 2003. Prospective study of presynaptic dopaminergic imaging in patients with mild parkinsonism tremor disorders: Part 1. Baseline and 3-month observation. *Mov Disord* 9:977–984.

Ben-Pazi, H., H. Bergman, J. A. Goldber, N. Giladi, D. Hansel, A. Reches, and E. S. Simon. 2001. Synchrony of rest tremor in multiple limbs in Parkinson's disease: Evidence for multiple oscillators. *J Neural Transm* 108:287–296.

Berezovskii, V. K., and N. N. Oleshko. 1977. Electrophysiological characteristics of caudate-thalamic connections. *Neurophysiology* 9: 431–435.

Bergman, H., A. Raz, A. Feingold, A. Nini, I. Nelken, D. Hansel et al. 1998. Physiology of MPTP tremor. *Mov Disord* 13:29–34.

Bergman, H., T. Wichmann, B. Karmon, and M. R. DeLong. 1994. The primate subthalamic nucleus. II. Neuronal activity in the MPTP model of parkinsonism. *J Neurophysiol* 72:507–520.

Binder, D. K., G. Rau, and P. A. Starr. 2003. Hemorrhagic complications of microelectrode-guided deep brain stimulation. *Stereotact Funct Neurosurg* 80:28–31.

Blahak, C., J. C. Wohrle, H. H. Capelle et al. 2007. Tremor reduction by subthalamic nucleus stimulation and medication in advanced Parkinson's disease. *J Neurol* 254:169–178.

Boecker, H., A. J. Wills, A. Ceballos-Baumann, M. Samuel, D. G. Thomas, C. D. Marsden, and D. J. Brooks. 1997. Stereotactic thalamotomy in tremor-dominant Parkinson's disease: An H2(15)O PET motor activation study. *Ann Neurol* 41:108–111.

Bonucelli, U., R. Cervolo, S. Salvetti, C. D'Avino, P. Dell Dotto, G. Rossi, and L. Murri. 1997. Clozapine in Parkinson's disease tremor. Effects of acute and chronic administration. *Neurology* 49:1587–1590.

Breit, S., M. Reimold, G. Reischl, T. Klockgether, U. Wüllner. 2006. [C]D-threo-methylphenidate PET in patients with Parkinson's disease and essential tremor. *J Neural Transm* 113:187–193.

Brooks, D. J., E. D. Playford, V. Ibanez et al. 1992. Isolated tremor and disruption of the nigrostriatal dopaminergic system: An 18F-dopa PET study. *Neurology* 42:1554–1560.

Brumlik, J., G. Canter, R. LaTorre et al. 1964. A critical analysis of the affects of trihexiphnidyl (Artane) on the components of the parkinsonian syndrome. *J Nerv Ment Dis* 138:424–431.

Burns, R. S., C. C. Chiueh, S.P. Markey, M. H. Ebert, D. M. Jacobowitz, and I. J. Kopin. 1983. A primate model of parkinsonism: Selective destruction of dopaminergic neurons in the pars compacta of the substantia nigra by N-methyl-4-phenyl-1,2,3,6-tetrahydropyridine. *Proc Natl Acad Sci USA* 80:4546–4550.

Buzsaki, G., A. Smith, S. Berger, L. J. Fisher, and F. H. Gage. 1990. Petit mal epilepsy and Parkinsonian tremor. *Neuroscience* 36:1–14.

Caretti, V., D. Stoffers, A. Winogrodzka et al. 2008. Loss of thalamic serotonin transporters in early drug-naïve Parkinson's disease patients is associated with tremor: An [(123)I]beta-CIT SPECT study. *J Neural Transm* 115:721–729.

Chollet, F., V. Dipierro, R. J. S. Wise, D. J. Brooks, R. S. Dolan, and R. S. J. Frackowiak. 1991. The functional anatomy of motor recovery after stroke in humans: A study with positron emission tomography. *Ann. Neurol* 29:63–71.

Colebatch, J. G., M. P. Deiber, K. J. Passingham, J. Friston, and R. S. J. Frackowiak. 1991. Regional cerebral blood flow during voluntary arm and hand movements in normal subjects. *J. Neurophysiol* 65:1392–1401.

Davis, K. D., E. Taub, S. Houle, A. E. Lang, J. O. Dostrovsky, R. R. Tasker, and A. M. Lozano. 1997. Globus pallidus stimulation activates the cortical motor system during alleviation of parkinsonian symptoms. *Nat Med* 3:671–674.

Deep-Brain Stimulation for Parkinson's Disease Study Group. 2001. Deep-brain stimulation of the subthalamic nucleus or the pars interna of the globus pallidus in Parkinson's disease. *N Engl J Med* 345: 956–963.

Deiber, M. P., P. Pollak, R. Passingham, P. Landais, C. Gervason, L. Cinotti et al. 1993. Thalamic stimulation and suppression of parkinsonian tremor. Evidence of a cerebellar deactivation using positron emission tomography. *Brain* 116:267–279.

Deuschl, G., J. Raethjen, R. Baron, M. Lindemann, H. Wilms, and P. Krack. 2000. The pathophysiology of parkinsonian tremor: A review. *J Neurol* 247(5):33–48.

Doder, M., E. A. Rabiner, N. Turjanski, A. J. Lees, and D. J. Brook. 2003. Tremor in Parkinson's disease and serotonergic dysfunction: An 11C-WAY 100635 PET study. *Neurology* 60:601–605.

Doshay, L. J. 1956. Five year study of benztropine (Cogentin)methane sulfonate. *JAMA* 162:1031–1034.

Duffau, H., Tzourio, N., Caparros-Lefebvre, D, Parker F, and B. Mazoyer. 1996. Tremor and voluntary repetitive movement in Parkinson's disease: comparison before and after L-dopa with positron emission tomography. *Exp Brain Res* 107:453–62.

Elble, R. J., W. C. Koller. 1990. *Tremor*. The Johns Hopkins University Press, U.S.A.

Eggers, C., Kahraman, D., Fink, G.R., Schmidt, M., and L. Timmermann. 2011. Akinetic-Rigid and Tremor-Dominant Parkinson's Disease Patients Show Different Patterns of FP-CIT Single Photon Emission Computed Tomography. *Mov Disord* 26:416–23.

Fox, M., and T. D. Williams. 1968. Responses evoked in the cerebellar cortex by stimulation of the caudate nucleus in the cat. *J Physiol* 198:435–449.

Fox, P. T., M. E. Raichle, and W. T. Thach. 1985. Functional mapping of the human cerebellum with positron emission tomography. *Proc Natl Acad Sci USA* 82:7462–7466.

Friedman, J. H., Koller, W. C., M. C. Lannon, K. Busenbark, E. Swanson-Hyland, and D. Smith. 1997. Benztropine versus clozapine for the treatment of tremor in Parkinson's disease. *Neurology* 48:1077–1081.

Fukuda, M., A. Barnes, E. S. Simon, A. Holmes, V. Dhawan, N. Giladi, H. Fodstad, Y. Ma, and D. Eidelberg. 2004. Thalamic stimulation for parkinsonian tremor: correlation between regional cerebral blood flow and physiological tremor characteristics. *Neuroimage* 21(2):608–15.

Ghaemi, M., J. Raethjen, R. Hilker et al. 2002. Monosymptomatic resting tremor and Parkinson's disease: A multitracer P Positron emission tomographic study. *Mov Disord* 17:782–788.

Gonzalez-Alegre, P. 2007. Monomelic parkinsonian tremor caused by contralateral substantia nigra stroke. *Parkinsonism Relat Disord* 13:182–184.

Habeck C., Krakauer JW., Ghez C., Sackeim HA., Eidelberg D., Stern Y., Moeller J.R. 2005. A new approach to spatial covariance modeling of functional brain imaging data: ordinal trend analysis. *Neural Comput* 17:1602-45.

Hallet, M. 2003. Parkinson revisited: Pathophysiology of motor signs. *Adv Neurol* 91:19–28.

Helmich, R. C., M. J. R. Janssen, W. J. G. Oyen, B. R. Bloem, and I. Toni. 2011. Pallidal dysfunction drives a cerebellothalamic circuit into Parkinson tremor. *Ann Neurol* 69:269–81.

Henderson, J. M., C. Yiannikas, J. G. Morris, R. Einstein, D. Jackson, and K. Byth. 1994. Postural tremor of Parkinson's disease. *Clin Neuropharmacol* 17:277–285.

Hoshi, E., Tremblay, L., Féger, J., Carras, P.L., and P. L. Strick. 2005. The cerebellum communicates with the basal ganglia. *Nat Neurosci* 8(11):1491–1493.

Hunker, C. J., and J. H. Abbs. 1990. Uniform frequency of parkinsonian resting tremor in the lips, jaw, tongue, and index finger. *Mov Disord* 5:71–77.

Hurtado, J. M., L. L. Rubchinsky, K. A. Sigvardt et al. 2005. Temporal evolution of oscillations and synchrony in GPi/muscle pairs in Parkinson's disease. *J Neurophysiol* 93:1569–1584.

Isaias, I. U., R. Benti, R. Cilia, M. Canesi, G. Marotta, P. Gerundini, G. Pezzoli, and A. Antonini. 2007. [123I]FP-CIT striatal binding in early Parkinson's disease patients with tremor vs. akinetic-rigid onset. *Neuroreport* 14:1499–1502.

Isaias, I. U., M. Canesi, R. Benti, P. Gerundini, R. Cilia, G. Pezzoli, and A. Antonini. 2008. Striatal dopamine transporter abnormalities

in patients with essential tremor. *Nucl Med Commun* 29:349–53.

Isaias, I. U., M. Marotta, S. Hirano, M. Canesi, R. Benti, A. Righini et al. 2010 Imaging essential tremor. *Mov Disord* 25(6):679–686.

Jankovic, J., C. Contant, J. Perlmutter. 1993. Essential tremor and Parkinson's disease. *Neurology* 43:1447–1448.

Jellinger, K., and H. Bliesath. 1987. Adjuvant treatment of Parkinson's disease with budipine: A double-blind trial versus placebo. *J Neurol* 234:280–282.

Jellinger, K. A. 1999. Post mortem studies in Parkinson's disease—is it possible to detect brain areas for specific symptoms? *J Neural Transm Suppl* 56:1–29.

Jenner, P., and C. D. Marsden. 1984. Neurochemical basis of parkinsonian tremor. In *Movement disorders: Tremor*, ed. L. J. Findley and R. Capildeo R, 305–319. Oxford University Press, Oxford.

Joffroy, A. J. 1969. Pathophysiology of parkinsonian tremor. *N Engl J Med* 281:446–447.

Kassubek, J., F. D. Juengling, B. Hellwig, M. Knauff, J. Spreer, H. Carl, C. H. Lücking. 2001. Hypermetabolism in the ventrolateral thalamus in unilateral Parkinsonian resting tremor: A positron emission tomography study. *Neuroscience Letters* 304:17–20.

Katzenschlager, R., C. Sampaio, J. Costa, and A. Lees. 2003. Anticholinergics for symptomatic management of Parkinson's disease. *Cochrane Database Syst Rev* 2:CD003735.

Kim, J. S. 1992. Delayed onset hand tremor caused by cerebral infarction. *Stroke* 23:292–294.

Koller, W., R. Pahwa, K. Busenbark, J. Hubble, S. Wilkinson, A. Lang et al. 1997. High-frequency unilateral thalamic stimulation in the treatment of essential and parkinsonian tremor. *Ann Neurol* 42:292–299.

Koller, W. C., G. Herbster. 1987. Adjuvant therapy of parkinsonian tremor. *Arch Neurol* 44:921–923.

Koller, W. C. 1986. Pharmacologic treatment of parkinsonian tremor. *Arch Neurol* 43:126–127.

Kopell, B. H., A. R. Rezai, J. W. Chang, and J. L. Vitek. 2006. Anatomy and physiology of the basal ganglia: Implications for deep brain stimulation for Parkinson's disease. *Mov Disord* 21:238–246.

Krack, P., A. Benazzouz, P. Pollak et al. 1998. Treatment of tremor in Parkinson's disease by subthalamic nucleus stimulation. *Mov Disord* 13:907–914.

Kraus, P. H., M. R. Lemke, and H. Reichmann. 2006. Kinetic tremor in Parkinson's disease—an underrated symptom. *J Neural Transm* 113:845–853.

Krauss, J. K., T. Paduch, F. Mundinger, W. Seeger. 1995. Parkinsonism and rest tremor secondary to supratentorial tumours sparing the basal ganglia. *Acta Neurochir* 133:22–29.

Kulisevsky, J., M. L. Berthier, A. Avila, and C. Roig. 1996. Unilateral parkinsonism and stereotyped movements following a right lenticular infarction. *Mov Disord* 11:752–754.

Kunig, G., O. Pogarell, J. C. Moller, M. Delf, amd W. H. Oertel. 1999. Pramipexole, a nonergot dopamine agonist, is effective against rest tremor in intermediate to advanced Parkinson's disease. *Clin Neuropharmacol* 22:301–305.

Lalley, F. M., G. V. Rossi, and W. W. Baker. 1973. Tremor induction by intracaudate injections of bretylium, tetrabenazine, or mescaline: Functional deficits in the caudate dopamine. *J Pharm Sci* 62:1302–1307.

Lamarre, Y., A. J. Joffroy, M. Dumont, C. De Montigny, F. Grou, and J. P. Lund. 1975. Central mechanisms of tremor in some feline and primate models. *Can J Neurol Sci* 2(3):227–33.

Lee, M. S., Y. D. Kim, J. H. Im, H. J. Kim, J. O. Rinne, K. P. Bhatia et al. 1999. 123I-I PT brain SPECT study in essential tremor and Parkinson's disease. *Neurology* 52:1422–1426.

Lee, M. S., S. A. Lee, J. H. Heo, and I. S. Choi. 1993. A patient with a resting tremor and a lacunar infarction at the border between the thalamus and the internal capsule. *Mov Disord* 8:244–246.

Lenz, F. A., J. L. Vitek, and M. R. DeLong. 1993. Role of the thalamus in parkinsonian tremor: Evidence from studies in patients and primate models. *Stereotact Funct Neurosurg* 60:94–103.

Lieberman, A., A. Ranhosky, and D. Korts. 1997. Clinical evaluation of pramipexole in advanced Parkinson's disease: Results of double-blind, placebo-controlled, parallel-group study. *Neurology* 49:162–168.

Lorenz, D. and G. Deuschl. 2007. Update on pathogenesis and treatment of essential tremor. *Curr Opin Neurol* 20:447–452.

Lozza, C., R. M. Marie, and J. C. Baron. 2002. The metabolic substrates of bradykinesia and tremor in uncomplicated Parkinson's disease. *Neuroimage* 17:688–699.

Macchi, G. and E. G. Jones. 1997. Toward an agreement on terminology of nuclear and subnuclear divisions of the motor thalamus. *J. Neurosurg* 86:670–685.

Machado, A., A. R. Rezai, B. H. Kopell, R. E. Gross, A. D. Sharan, A. L. Benabid. 2006. Deep brain stimulation for Parkinson's disease: Surgical technique and perioperative management. *Mov Disord* 21:247–258.

Mure, H., Hirano, S., Tang, C. C., Isaias, I. U., Antonini, A., Ma, Y., Dhawan, V., and D. Eidelberg. 2010. Parkinson's disease tremor-related metabolic network: characterization, progression, and treatment effects. *Neuroimage* 54:1244-53.

Navan, P., L. J. Findley, J. A. Jeffs, R. K. Pearce, and P. G. Bain. 2003. Randomized, double-blind, 3-month parallel study of the effects pramipexole, pergolide, and placebo on parkinsonian tremor. *Mov Disord* 18:1324–1331.

Olanow, C. W., S. Fahn, M. Muenter et al. 1994. A multicenter double-blind placebo-controlled trial of pergolide adjunct to Sinemet in Parkinson's disease. *Mov Disord* 9:40–47.

Parker, F., N. Tzourio, S. Blond, H. Petit, and B. Mazoyer. 1992. Evidence for a common network of brain structures involved in parkinsonian tremor and voluntary repetitive movement. *Brain Res* 1992 584: 11–17.

Patel, N. K., P. Heywood, K. O'Sullivan, R. McCarter, S. Love, S. S. Gill. 2003. Unilateral subthalamotomy in the treatment of Parkinson's disease. *Brain* 125(4):1136–1145.

Péchadre, J. C., L. Larochelle, and L. J. Poirier. 1976. Parkinsonian akinesia, rigidity and tremor in the monkey. Histopathological and neuropharmacological study. *J Neurol Sci* 28(2):147–57.

Peng, S., Y. Ma, J. Flores, D. Doudet, and D. Eidelberg. 2010. Abnormal topography of cerebral glucose metabolism in parkinsonian macaques. *J Nucl Med* 51(Suppl 2):1753.

Przuntek, H., S. Bittkau, H. Bliesath et al. 2002. Budipine provides additional benefit in patients with Parkinson disease receiving a stable optimum dopaminergic drug regimen. *Arch Neurol* 59: 803–806.

Putzke, J. D., R. E. Wharen Jr, Z. K. Wszolek, M. F. Turk, A. J. Strongosky, and R. J. Uitti. 2003. Thalamic deep brain stimulation for tremor-predominant Parkinson's disease. *Parkinonism Relat Disord* 10: 81–88.

Raethjen, J., M. Lindemann, H. Schmaljohann, R. Wenzelburger, G. Pfister, and G. Deuschl. 2000. Multiple oscillators are causing parkinsonian and essential tremor. *Mov Disord* 15:84–94.

Raz, A., E. Vaadia, and H. Bergman. 2000. Firing patterns and correlations of spontaneous discharge of pallidal neurons in the normal and the tremulous 1-methyl-4-phenyl-1,2,3,6-tetrahydropyridine vervet model of parkinsonism. *J Neurosci* 20:8559–8571.

Reck, C., E. Florin, L. Wojtecki et al. 2009. Characterisation of tremor-associated local field potentials in the subthalamic nucleus in Parkinson's disease. *Eur J Neurosci* 29:599–612.

Reichmann, H. 2006. Budipine in Parkinson's tremor. *J Neurol Sci* 248: 53–55.

Remy, P., A. de Recondo, G. Defer, C. Loc'h, P. Amarenco, V. Plante-Bordeneuve et al. 1995. Peduncular "rubral" tremor and dopaminergic denervation: A PET study. *Neurology* 45:472–477.

Rodriguez-Oroz, M. C., O. J. Guridi, L. Alvarez et al. 1998. The subthalamic nucleus and tremor in Parkinson's disease. *Mov Disord* 13(3): 111–118.

Rodriguez-Oroz, M. C., M. Jahanshahi, P. Krack, R. Litvan, R. Marcias, E. Bezard, J. A. Obeso. 2009. Initial clinical manifestations of Parkinson's disease: Features and pathophysiological mechanisms. *Lancet Neurol* 8:1128–39.

Schrag, A., J. Keens, and J. Warner. Ropinorole Study Group. 2002. Ropinirole for the treatment of tremor in early Parkinson's disease. *Eur J Neurol* 9:253–257.

Schrag, A., L. Schelosky, U. Scholz, and W. Poewe. 1999. Reduction of Parkinsonian signs in patients with Parkinson's disease by dopaminergic versus anticholinergic single-dose challenges. *Mov Disord* 14:252–255.

Schwarz, M., D. Groshar, R. Inzelberg, and S. Hockerman. 2004. Dopamine-transporter imaging and visuo-motor testing in essential tremor, practical possibilities for detection of early stage Parkinson's disease. *Parkinsonism Relat Disord* 10:385–389.

Sedgwick, E. M., and T. D. Williams. 1967. Responses of single units in the inferior olive to stimulation of the limb nerves, peripheral skin receptors, cerebellum, caudate nucleus and motor cortex. *J Physiol* 189:261–279.

Seitz, R. J., P. E. Roland, C. Bohm, T. Greitz, and S. Stone-Elanders. 1990. Motor learning in man: A positron emission tomography study. *Neuroreport* 1:17–20.

Spiegel, J., D. Hellwig, S. Samnick, W. Jost, M. O. Mollers, K. Fassbender et al. 2007. Striatal FP-CIT uptake differs in the subtypes of early Parkinson's disease. *J Neural Transm* 114:331–335.

Spieker, S., P. Loschmann, C. Jentgens, A. Boose, T. Klockgether, and J. Dichgans). 1995. Tremorlytic activity of budipine: A quantitative study with long-term tremor recordings. *Clin Neuropharmacol* 18:266–272.

Sturman, M. M., D. E. Vaillancourt, L. V. Metman, R. A. Bakay, and D. M. Corcos. 2004. Effects of subthalamic nucleus stimulation and medication on resting and postural tremor in Parkinson's disease. *Brain* 127(9):2131–2143.

Taha, J. M., J. Favre, T. K. Baumann, and K. J. Burchiel. 1977. Tremor control after pallidotomy in patients with Parkinson's disease: Correlation with microrecording findings. *J Neurosurg* 86:642–647.

Tasker, R. R. 1998. Deep brain stimulation is preferable to thalamotomy for tremor suppression. *Surg Neurol* 49:145–153.

Thanvi, B., N. Lo, and T. Robinson. 2005. Vascular Parkinsonism—an important cause of Parkinsonism in older people. *Age Ageing* 34: 114–119.

Timmermann, L., J. Gross, M. Dirks, J. Volkmann, H. J. Freund, and A. Schnitzler. 2003. The cerebral oscillatory network of parkinsonian resting tremor. *Brain* 126(1):199–212.

Trost, M., A. Barnes, E. Simon, V. Dhawan, D. Eidelberg, and H. Fodstad. 2003. Changes in activity of abnormal metabolic brain networks in Parkinson's disease patients treated with Vim DBS. Communications of the European Neurological Society. *J Neurol* 250:93.

Vitek, J. L., A. E. Bakay, A. Freeman et al). 2003. Randomized trial of pallidotomy versus medical therapy for Parkinson's disease. *Ann Neurol* 53:558–569.

Wielepp, J. P., J. M. Burgunder, T. Pohle, E. P. Ritter, J. A. Kinser, and J. K. Krauss. 2001. Deactivation of thalamocortical activity is responsible for suppression of parkinsonian tremor by thalamic stimulation: A 99mTc-ECD SPECT study. *Clin Neurol Neurosurg* 103(4): 228–31.

Wilms, H., J. Sievers, and G. Deuschl. 1999. Animal models of tremor. *Mov Disord* 14:557–571.

7

ATYPICAL PARKINSONIAN SYNDROMES

Kathleen L. Poston

INTRODUCTION

Parkinsonism is defined by symptoms of bradykinesia, rigidity, and tremor and can be classified as primary (idiopathic Parkinson's disease [PD], or IPD), secondary, or caused by a multiple system degenerative disorder other than IPD (Fahn and Jankovic 2007). In these multiple system degenerative disorders, patients exhibit parkinsonian symptoms along with other motor and cognitive features. Collectively, these disorders are often referred to as "atypical parkinsonism," "atypical parkinsonian syndrome," or "Parkinson's plus syndromes". However, they actually represent several specific disease entities that differ in clinical presentation, pathology, and treatment strategies. Multiple system atrophy (MSA), progressive supranuclear palsy (PSP), corticobasal degeneration (CBD), and dementia with Lewy bodies (DLB) are the most common atypical parkinsonian syndromes and account for almost 15% of parkinsonian patients evaluated in academic subspecialty movement disorder clinics (Fahn and Jankovic 2007).

MSA is characterized by autonomic failure associated with either parkinsonism or variable cerebellar symptoms along with other atypical features (Gilman et al. 2008). Historically, patients with predominant autonomic, parkinsonian, or cerebellar symptoms were classified as Shy-Drager syndrome, striatonigral degeneration, or spontaneous olivopontocerebellar atrophy, respectively. However, in 1989 Pap et al. (1989) demonstrated glial cytoplasmic inclusions as the common underlying pathology in patients with these three clinical syndromes, thus unifying them under MSA, a single disease entity. The subclassification of MSA is determined by the predominant presenting motor symptom, which is parkinsonism in 80% of patients (designated MSA-P subtype) and cerebellar ataxia in the other 20% (designated MSA-C subtype) (Gilman et al. 2008; Wenning and Stefanova 2009). PSP is classically characterized by early postural instability and falls, vertical supranuclear gaze palsy, frontal subcortical dementia, and levodopa-unresponsive parkinsonism (Williams and Lees 2009;

Litvan et al. 2003). However, clinical variants have recently been identified, and the term Richardson's syndrome is used to describe patients with classic findings, including falls, cognitive dysfunction, abnormalities of gaze, and postural instability early in the disease, while the term PSP-Parkinsonism is used to describe patients with asymmetric onset, early bradykinesia, and a limited response to levodopa treatment (Williams et al. 2005). By contrast, CBD is an asymmetric neurodegenerative disorder characterized by rigidity and limb apraxia, often with limb dystonia, bradykinesia, and stimulus-sensitive myoclonus (Litvan et al. 2003; Boeve, Lang, and Litvan 2003), which can also present with predominant cognitive dysfunction (Mahapatra et al. 2004). Finally, DLB is characterized by dementia with parkinsonism, recurrent visual hallucinations, and fluctuating cognition (Litvan et al. 2003; McKeith et al. 2005). Typically, the dementia in patients with DLB develops either before or within one year of the onset of parkinsonian motor symptoms.

While these atypical syndromes can readily be distinguished on postmortem examination, non-pathological diagnosis currently relies on clinical identification of disease-specific signs and symptoms (Gilman et al. 2008; Litvan et al. 2003). However, there is substantial clinical overlap between syndromes, particularly in patients with early symptoms, as many disease-defining characteristics develop later in the disease course. Therefore, early distinction between IPD and these atypical syndromes, as well as distinction among atypical syndromes, can be extremely challenging for the clinician. Indeed, the positive predictive value (PPV) of an initial clinical diagnosis of IPD is only 75%, and many  patients identified as having atypical parkinsonian disorders on autopsy are initially given a diagnosis of IPD (Hughes et al. 2002). While the PPV for a clinical diagnosis of IPD improves to almost 99% after clinical follow-up, the PPV for a clinical diagnosis of MSA and PSP is only 85.7% and 80%, respectively. For CBD, the PPV of a clinical diagnosis is less than 40%. These atypical parkinsonian syndromes are more aggressive and less treatable than PD (O'Sullivan et al. 2008). Therefore, accurate diagnosis is critical for patient counseling and treatment decisions. In addition, disease-specific treatments for these neurodegenerative conditions will likely require early intervention; thus early, accurate diagnosis is essential for clinical trials.

Several structural and functional neuroimaging techniques have been developed to help the clinician and researcher make a more accurate diagnosis in patients with MSA, PSP, CBD, and DLB. However, most imaging studies are conducted with patients later in the disease course, who have a clinically determined possible or probable diagnosis at the time of imaging. While this approach ensures that all patients enrolled into research studies are likely to have a correct diagnosis, the results cannot be generalized to patients with early disease who have not yet developed the characteristic symptoms included in the diagnostic criteria. However, it is early patients who cannot be diagnosed by consensus criteria (Litvan et al. 2003) that are the most challenging for the clinician and would most benefit from further objective evaluation with imaging. Indeed, a few studies have addressed this problem by examining patients with an uncertain diagnosis at the time of imaging and then using the diagnosis on clinical follow-up as the comparative "gold standard" (Tang et al. 2010; Gaenslen et al. 2008; Estorch et al. 2008; Coulier et al. 2003). While not always practical to achieve, research studies should also include patients with an unknown diagnosis at the time of imaging and true diagnostic confirmation at autopsy (Tang et al. 2010; Poston et al. 2009b; Walker et al. 2007). Nonetheless, sufficient data does exist from more limited studies to suggest that certain techniques can aid the clinician in difficult-to-diagnose patients. Specifically, imaging findings are now included in the revised consensus criteria as additional features supporting a diagnosis of possible MSA (Gilman et al. 2008), including putamen or pontine atrophy on magnetic resonance imaging (MRI) and putamen or cerebellar hypometabolism on brain [18F]fluorodeoxyglucose (FDG) positron emission tomography (PET). In addition, imaging techniques are currently being developed and validated as objective biomarkers for disease progression in these atypical syndromes, which will be invaluable for assessing disease progression in future clinical trials specifically targeting these currently untreatable disorders.

STRUCTURAL IMAGING

In patients with parkinsonism, standard T2-weighted and T1-weighted MRI is primarily used to exclude underlying pathologies, such as vascular parkinsonism, normal pressure hydrocephalus, brain tumors, or demyelinating lesions. Other rare etiologies of parkinsonism can also be excluded on MRI, such as Wilson's disease, manganese-induced parkinsonism, and neurodegeneration associated with brain iron accumulation.

MRI can also be useful when characteristic abnormalities of specific atypical parkinsonian syndromes are present. For instance, researchers have described several characteristic abnormal findings in patients with MSA (Bhattacharya et al. 2002; Schrag et al. 1998; Abe et al. 2006; Ito, Shirai, and Hattori 2007). Specifically, T2-weighted MRI has revealed cerebellar and middle cerebellar peduncle (MCP) atrophy as well as infratentorial signal hyperintensities within the pons

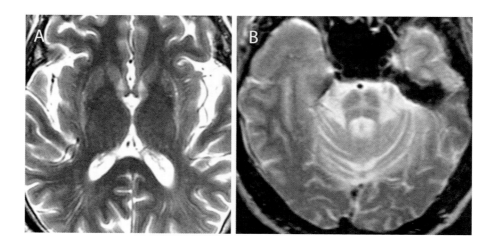

Figure 1 Magnetic resonance imaging in multiple system atrophy. (A) Patient with MSA-P with bilateral putamen atrophy and slit-like hyperintense putaminal rim on T2-weighted MRI (1.5 Tesla). (B) Patient with MSA-C with classic "hot-cross bun" sign in the pons. [Reprinted from Poston 2010]

and MCP, referred to as the "hot cross bun" sign (Figure 1). Putaminal atrophy and a hyperintense putaminal rim, with or without hypointensity in the dorsolateral part of the putamen, are also seen on T2-weighted MRI and are associated with MSA when using a 1.5 Tesla (T) field strength magnet. However, the hyperintense putaminal rim is nonspecific on the higher field 3 T MRI and has been documented in normal subjects at this field strength (Lee et al. 2005). When present at 1.5 T, these MRI findings have a high specificity for distinguishing clinically possible or probable MSA patients from IPD patients and normal controls (Schrag et al. 1998). However, most MSA patients have a normal MRI, particularly in early disease since signal abnormalities become more pronounced as the disease progresses (Brooks and Seppi 2009; Horimoto et al. 2002). Further, the presence of these findings does not distinguish MSA from other atypical parkinsonian syndromes (Brooks and Seppi 2009; Kraft et al. 1999).

Characteristic structural MRI findings have also been described in patients with PSP and CBD (Savoiardo et al. 1994; Oba et al. 2005; Slowinski et al. 2008; Soliveri et al. 1999). Specific MRI abnormalities associated with PSP include midbrain atrophy, dilation of the third ventricle and aqueduct, increased signal in the midbrain and in the inferior olives, and atrophy of the superior cerebellar peduncle (SCP). Atrophy of the midbrain tegmentum with preservation of the pons can best be seen on the mid-sagittal view and is often referred to as the "penguin" or "hummingbird" sign (Graber and Staudinger 2009). Visual assessment of SCP atrophy has been shown to separate patients with clinically probable PSP from those with MSA, IPD, and from controls on a group level. When applied to individual

subjects, this technique achieves 94% specificity but only 74% sensitivity due to significant overlap between PSP patients and non-PSP patients (Paviour et al. 2007). Similarly, signal changes in the SCP have been associated with patients with PSP, but not patients with MSA-P or IPD. However, this finding is present in only 25% of probable PSP patients and has not been described in early subjects (Hiroshi et al. 2008). When present, these findings can aid in the diagnosis of PSP. Nevertheless, they are not sensitive for detecting PSP, particularly in patients early in the disease course since atrophy and signal changes develop as the disease progresses and are not typically present at symptom onset (Schrag et al. 2000). MRI findings described in CBD patients include asymmetric atrophy of the premotor and parietal cortex with dilation of the lateral ventricle (Figure 2) (Soliveri et al. 1999; Hauser et al. 1996). However, these findings are not sensitive for differentiating CBD from other neurodegenerative disorders. Indeed, the most common MRI finding in CBD is nonspecific global atrophy, and in many cases the MRI is initially normal (Mahapatra et al. 2004; Josephs et al. 2004).

Several MRI-based analysis techniques, including quantitative volumetric assessment and diffusion-weighted imaging, have been shown to successfully distinguish patients with different parkinsonian disorders (Seppi and Poewe 2010; Hotter et al. 2009). Although most of these techniques have only been shown to separate patients by disease group (i.e., IPD, MSA, PSP, CBD), some have demonstrated accurate classification in individual clinically diagnosed patients (Brooks and Seppi 2009). Quattrone et al. (2008) has shown using volumetric MRI and quantitative analysis that midbrain area and SCP width are reduced in PSP and that this

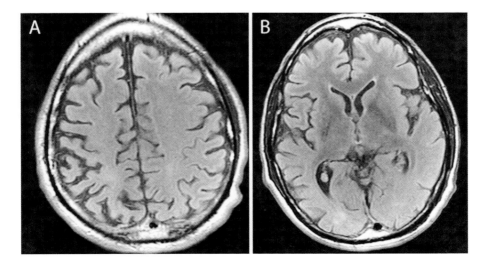

Figure 2 Magnetic resonance imaging in corticobasal degeneration. Note the asymmetric cortical atrophy in the (A) parietal and (B) temporal lobes with ventricular dilation. [Reprinted from Poston 2010]

approach is more sensitive than visual analysis in differentiating PSP from MSA-P. In this study, the researchers developed an index using a ratio of the pontine-midbrain area and a ratio of the MCP-SCP width to accurately diagnose established PSP patients with 100% sensitivity and specificity. Increased regional apparent diffusion coefficient (rADC) in the globus pallidus and caudate measured using diffusion-weighted imaging (DWI) MRI can also be used to differentiate PSP and IPD by group, but this technique needs to be validated prospectively in individual patients (Nicoletti et al. 2006). In patients with a clinically established diagnosis, quantitative voxel-based analysis of MRI can differentiate CBD from PSP (Boxer et al. 2006). Similar to conventional MRI, these studies include patients in advanced stages when atrophy and signal changes are more likely to be found on MRI, thus limiting the generalizability of these findings. Therefore, the role of these quantitative MRI techniques in clinical practice remains to be seen and will be clarified only with prospective studies in early, undiagnosed patients and diagnostic confirmation by subsequent long-term clinical follow-up or autopsy.

FUNCTIONAL IMAGING

Positron emission tomography (PET) and single photon emission computed tomography (SPECT) are functional imaging techniques that use various radioligands to provide quantitative assessment of glucose metabolism, blood flow, nigrostriatal dysfunction, and changes in receptor availability in neurodegenerative disorders. Using these techniques, both resting state and task-related cerebral activation patterns have been described in IPD and atypical parkinsonian syndromes. SPECT is more widely available, less costly, and usually does not require an on-site cyclotron because most SPECT radioisotopes have a long half-life. PET has the advantage of higher resolution and thus greater power to differentiate between different pathological disorders. Although many PET radiotracers require an on-site cyclotron, FDG does not and is available commercially. The following section will discuss the use of PET and SPECT for studying underlying disease processes and diagnosing atypical parkinsonian disorders.

METABOLIC AND PERFUSION IMAGING

FDG PET imaging can be used to quantify resting state regional and global cerebral metabolic activity. Functional neuroimaging with FDG PET is abnormal in patients with MSA, DLB, PSP, and CBD, even in early-stage patients (Poston and Eidelberg 2009; Mosconi et al. 2008) (Table 1). In MSA patients, FDG PET revealed reduced glucose metabolism in the putamen, thalamus, pons, and cerebellum (Antonini et al. 1998; De Volder et al. 1989; Eidelberg et al. 1993; Otsuka et al. 1996). This is in contrast to IPD patients,

TABLE 1: CHARACTERISTIC FDG PET ABNORMALITIES IN NEURODEGENERATIVE DISEASES

Neurodegenerative disease	Regional FDG PET abnormalities	Reference
Parkinson's disease	Hypermetabolism of the putamen and thalamus Hypometabolism of the lateral frontal, inferior parietal, and parieto-occipital cortex	(Eidelberg et al. 1994; Eidelberg et al. 1995; Fukuda et al. 2001; Berding et al. 2001; Eidelberg et al. 1990)
Multiple system atrophy	Hypometabolism of the putamen, cerebellum, and pons	(Antonini et al. 1998; De Volder et al. 1989; Eidelberg et al. 1993; Otsuka et al. 1996; Ghaemi et al. 2002; Taniwaki et al. 2002)
Progressive supranuclear palsy	Hypometabolism of the midbrain, midline frontal cortex, and striatum	(Foster et al. 1988; Park et al. 2009; Hosaka et al. 2002; Blin et al. 1990)
Corticobasal degeneration	Asymmetric hypometabolism in the hemispheric cortex and striatum contralateral to the more affected limbs	(Hosaka et al. 2002; Nagahama et al. 1997; Eidelberg et al. 1991)
Dementia with Lewy bodies	Hypometabolism of the parieto-occipital cortex	(Mosconi et al. 2008; Ishii et al. 1998b; Yong et al. 2007)
Alzheimer's dementia	Hypometabolism of the parietotemporal cortex and posterior cingulate	(Mosconi et al. 2008; Ishii et al. 1998b; Minoshima et al. 1997; Herholz 1995)
Frontotemporal dementia	Hypometabolism of the frontal and anterior temporal cortex	(Poston and Eidelberg 2009; Ishii et al. 1998a)

who show increased basal ganglia activity, even in the early stages of disease (Eidelberg et al. 1994; Ghaemi et al. 2002; Ma et al. 2009; Spetsieris and Eidelberg 2011). Several studies have demonstrated that striatal FDG PET values discriminate individual MSA patients from those with IPD, (Eidelberg et al. 1993; Eidelberg et al. 1994; Antonini et al. 1997), although an overlap with healthy control subjects has been noted (Otsuka et al. 1997). Using a voxel-based comparison with a statistical parametric mapping technique, Juh et al. (2005a) reported that glucose metabolism in the pons, cerebellum, and putamen can be used as the variable factor for differentiating between individual IPD and MSA patients. Using perfusion SPECT, Van Laere and colleagues have shown similar results with reduced putaminal blood flow in MSA patients compared to those with IPD (Van Laere et al. 2004; Eckert et al. 2007). Therefore, visualization of decreased striatal, pontine, and cerebellar metabolism with FDG PET or reduced striatal blood flow with ECD SPECT can be used to diagnose MSA in a parkinsonian patient (Figure 3). Specifically, cerebellar hypometabolism on FDG PET can help distinguish MSA-P from IPD in patients without clinically evident ataxia (Gilman 2005). Likewise, putamen hypometabolism can help diagnose MSA-C in ataxic patients without clinically evident parkinsonism. Indeed, the most recent consensus statement for the diagnosis of MSA includes putamen, brainstem, or cerebellar hypometabolism on FDG PET as an additional feature of possible MSA-P and putamen hypometabolism as an additional feature of possible MSA-C (Gilman et al. 2008). FDG PET can also be useful in distinguishing MSA

patients with minimal parkinsonian or ataxic features from patients with pure autonomic failure (PAF). Fulham et al. (Fulham et al. 1991) have shown prominent reduction in cerebellum, brainstem, striatum, frontal, and motor cerebral metabolic rates in patients with MSA compared to those with PAF.

A few studies have examined the use of FDG PET in patients with parkinsonism and dementia. In particular, patients with DLB have characteristic parieto-occipital hypometabolism on FDG PET imaging, as opposed to parieto-temporal and posterior cingulate hypometabolism in Alzheimer's dementia or prominent frontal and anterior temporal hypometabolism in frontotemporal dementia (Mosconi et al. 2008). In one study using FDG PET in parkinsonian patients with dementia, patients with clinically diagnosed DLB were found to have reduced metabolism of the anterior cingulate when compared to patients with IPD-related dementia (Yong et al. 2007). Further investigations in early patients with parkinsonism and dementia are needed to determine the utility of FDG PET in the clinical diagnosis of this patient subgroup.

FDG PET is also abnormal in patients with PSP and CBD and can be used to assist in distinguishing between these two tauopathies. Patients with PSP have characteristic hypometabolism of the midbrain and midline frontal cortex in addition to striatal hypometabolism (Foster et al. 1988; Park et al. 2009; Hosaka et al. 2002). By contrast, CBD patients show characteristic asymmetric cortical glucose metabolism with more pronounced hypometabolism in the hemispheric cortex and striatum contralateral to the more

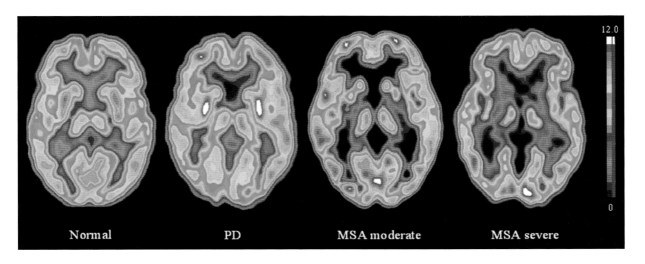

Figure 3 FDG PET in a healthy, normal subject, an IPD patient, and a moderately and severely affected MSA patient (parkinsonian subtype). Note the increased glucose metabolism in the IPD patient and the decreased glucose metabolism in the MSA patients in the lentiform nucleus compared to healthy subjects (Eckert & Eidelberg 2004). [Metabolic increases are color-coded from red to yellow; metabolic decreases are color-coded from blue to purple]. [Reprinted from *Clin Auton Res* 14, 2004 p. 84–91, The role of functional neuroimaging in the differential diagnosis of idiopathic Parkinson's disease and multiple system atrophy, Eckert, T., and Eidelberg, D., Figure 1 with permission of Springer Science+Business Media.]

affected limbs (Hosaka et al. 2002; Nagahama et al. 1997). Coulier et al. (2003) have shown that patients with a final diagnosis of CBD have an asymmetric pattern of reduced glucose metabolism, specifically in the peri-rolandic cortex, striatum, and thalamus, which in two patients was evident prior to clinical diagnosis. Using voxel-based analysis with statistical parametric mapping, Juh et al. (2005b) have shown a similar distinction with additional asymmetric reduction of glucose metabolism in the parietal, frontal, and cingulate region in CBD patients, while in PSP patients glucose metabolism is lower in the orbitofrontal, middle frontal, thalamic, and midbrain regions. A similar method was used to distinguish individual patients with moderate disease severity (Hoehn and Yahr Stage 2–3) and a clinical diagnosis of PSP, MSA and IPD (Juh et al. 2004). The results of these FDG PET studies suggest that this imaging approach in conjunction with voxel-based analysis can improve diagnosis in atypical parkinsonian disorders; however, this method has not been verified in larger patient cohorts prior to clinical diagnosis.

More sophisticated analysis techniques have been applied to FDG PET to further improve diagnostic accuracy in parkinsonian patients. Eckert et al. (2005) have developed a computer-assisted technique with FDG PET to differentiate IPD, MSA, PSP, and CBD patients prior to clinical diagnosis. In this study, non-expert readers visually compared 135 individual patient scans to characteristic disease templates and correctly categorized 92.4% of patients when compared to clinical follow-up on average two years later. This method was later used to accurately categorize four pathology-confirmed patients with CBD, with accurate imaging diagnosis prior to clinical diagnosis in two cases (Poston et al. 2009b). Although this technique still relies on user visual interpretation, the computer-assisted analysis of individual PET scans with disease-specific templates can improve diagnostic accuracy compared to standard visual PET reading.

The recent application of a spatial covariance approach based on principal component analysis (PCA) to FDG PET imaging has allowed for the identification of several disease-specific metabolic patterns (Eidelberg 2009; Habeck and Stern 2010; Spetsieris and Eidelberg 2011). These disease-specific patterns can then be prospectively applied to individual subjects to further improve diagnostic accuracy in patients with parkinsonian symptoms (Poston and Eidelberg 2009; Spetsieres et al. 2009). In addition to the Parkinson's disease-related metabolic pattern (PDRP; see Chapter 3 for a detailed description), MSA and PSP have also been associated with specific and highly stable metabolic brain networks by applying strictly defined statistical criteria to imaging data (Eckert et al. 2008 ; Spetsieris

et al. 2009); a novel asymmetrical CBD-related metabolic pattern has recently been identified (Niethammer et al. 2011). The MSA-related pattern (MSARP) is characterized by bilateral metabolic decreases in the putamen and cerebellum (Figure 4, top). By contrast, the PSP-related pattern (PSPRP) is characterized by metabolic decreases predominantly in the upper brainstem and medial prefrontal cortex as well as in the medial thalamus, the caudate nuclei, the anterior cingulate area, the ventrolateral prefrontal cortex, and the frontal eye fields (Figure 4, bottom). In both diseases, pattern expression has been shown to be significantly elevated in patients relative to age-matched healthy subjects (Eckert et al. 2008). In addition, pattern expression has also been shown to be elevated in two independent prospectively scanned patient groups when compared to a healthy control group. Achieving a high sensitivity in separating individual patients from normal subjects suggests potential application of these patterns as functional imaging biomarkers for MSA and PSP.

In an interesting study, Varrone et al. (2007) used [99mTc] ECD SPECT with PCA to identify abnormal patterns associated with PSP; these patterns are characterized by relative blood flow reduction in the cingulate cortex, prefrontal cortex, and caudate with relative increases in parietal cortical blood flow. The patterns in this study were then used to distinguish PSP patients from controls and those with IPD. These findings suggest that disease-specific patterns identified using spatial covariance analysis are not imaging modality specific. Rather, the spatial patterns represent abnormal brain networks reflecting the underlying disease-related pathology in the resting state (Eckert et al. 2007).

Recent evidence suggests that multiple disease-specific patterns used in concert can increase the diagnostic accuracy of FDG PET in patients with uncertain clinical parkinsonism (Spetsieris et al. 2009). Tang and colleagues (2010) have developed an automated imaged-based classification procedure using FDG PET to differentiate individual patients with IPD, MSA, and PSP prior to clinical diagnosis. Using multiple disease-related patterns with logistic regression, 167 patients with an uncertain parkinsonian clinical diagnosis were categorized by an automated algorithm. Final clinical diagnosis was determined by blinded movement disorders specialists on average 2.6 years later; the initial image-based classification was then compared to the final clinical diagnosis. Image-based classification for IPD had 84% sensitivity, 97% specificity, 98% positive predictive value (PPV), and 82% negative predictive value (NPV). Imaging classification was also highly accurate for MSA (85% sensitivity, 96% specificity, 97% PPV, and 83% NPV) and PSP (88% sensitivity, 94% specificity,

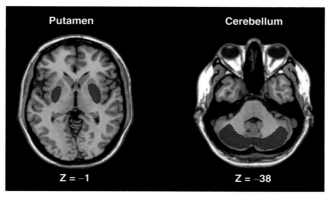

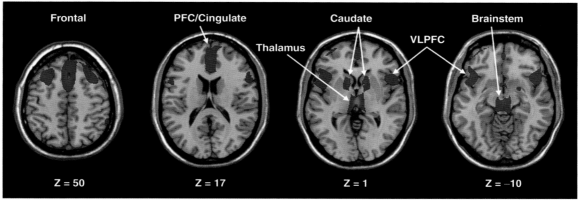

Figure 4 Spatial covariance patterns associated with multiple system atrophy and progressive supranuclear palsy. Top: Metabolic pattern associated with multiple system atrophy (MSARP) characterized by covarying metabolic decreases in the putamen and cerebellum (Eckert et al. 2008). Bottom: Metabolic pattern associated with progressive supranuclear palsy-related spatial covariance pattern (PSPRP) characterized by covarying metabolic decreases in the medial prefrontal cortex (PFC), frontal eye fields, ventrolateral prefrontal cortex (VLPFC), caudate nuclei, medial thalamus, and the upper brainstem. (Eckert et al. 2008) [The covariance patterns were overlaid on T1-weighted MR-template images. The displays represent regions that contributed significantly to the network and that were demonstrated to be reliable by bootstrap resampling. Voxels with negative region weights (metabolic decreases) are color-coded blue.] [Reprinted from *Mov Disord*; 23:727–733, Figures 1 and 3, Copyright © 2008 with permission of John Wiley and Sons.]

91% PPV, and 92% NPV). The sensitivity of imaging classification remained high (>88%) in patients with less than two years of symptoms at the time of imaging, which is in contrast to the relatively low sensitivity (<60%) of an initial clinical diagnosis of MSA and PSP (Osaki et al. 2004; Osaki et al. 2002). The results of this study were further validated in a cohort of 22 subjects with accurate classification on repeat FDG PET imaging 3.1±2.2 years after initial imaging classification and in nine patients with confirmed diagnosis at autopsy. These results indicate that disease-specific patterns with FDG PET can be used to accurately diagnose clinically uncertain parkinsonian patients. Further prospective studies in early patients with long-term follow-up and autopsy confirmation will be needed to determine the utility of this approach in clinical practice.

In addition to aiding in the diagnosis of atypical parkinsonian syndromes, FDG PET abnormalities can be used as a biomarker for disease progression. Lyoo et al. (2008) have studied FDG PET in a cross-sectional study with 37 MSA patients with parkinsonian or cerebellar symptoms for less than three years. In this study, patients with less than one year of symptoms showed hypometabolism in the frontal cortex, and in the anterior cerebellar hemisphere and vermis, whereas patients with 2–3 years of symptoms showed hypometabolism in the frontal and parieto-temporal cortices, bilateral caudate, and posterolateral putamen. Based on neuropsychological testing at the time of PET, they postulated that the spreading pattern of hypometabolism coincided with progressive cognitive decline and that early caudate hypometabolism may contribute to cognitive impairment. In this patient cohort, parkinsonian motor deficits preceded the putaminal hypometabolism, whereas cerebellar hypometabolism occurred early in the clinical course. Network analysis of FDG PET has also been used in MSA patients, with increases in MSARP activity observed in longitudinally assessed patients (Poston et al. 2009a). These studies suggest that FDG PET could be a sensitive biomarker for disease severity in patients with MSA.

NEUROTRANSMITTER IMAGING

Several neuroimaging techniques use radioligands to determine the synthesis, binding, and reuptake of specific neurotransmitters within various brain regions. In parkinsonian and other tremor disorders, the density and activity of these specific neurotransmitters can vary according to the different pathological processes. Understanding the underlying pathology is important for considering how these imaging modalities can be used to differentiate and shed light on these disorders. For instance, IPD is characterized by the loss of dopaminergic neurons projecting from the substantia nigra pars compacta in the midbrain to the putamen and caudate nucleus (Braak and Braak 2000). Thus, the nerve terminals from these nigrostriatal dopaminergic neurons reside in the striatum. Imaging techniques that show degeneration of this nigrostriatal pathway, either by cell body loss in the midbrain or nerve terminal loss in the striatum, can differentiate IPD from other parkinsonian and tremor disorders that do not cause nigrostriatal degeneration, such as vascular parkinsonism, essential tremor (ET), and drug-induced parkinsonism. However, the neurodegenerative atypical parkinsonian syndromes, such as MSA, DLB, PSP, and CBD, share with IPD a common pathological neuronal loss in the nigrostriatal pathway. Therefore, similar to IPD, abnormal striatal imaging can help differentiate atypical parkinsonian disorders from normal. However, more complex imaging techniques of the nigrostriatal pathway are required to differentiate MSA, DLB, PSP, and CBD from IPD or from each other. By contrast, there is a substantial loss of striatal postsynaptic spiny interneurons in both MSA and PSP compared to IPD; therefore the postsynaptic neuron density is more likely to differentiate IPD from these atypical parkinsonian syndromes.

Dopamine cell loss can be assessed by binding biological compounds tagged with PET and SPECT isotopes to different regions of the presynaptic nerve terminal. The regions of the dopamine nerve terminal used in imaging studies include the (1) enzyme aromatic-amino-acid decarboxylase (AADC), located inside the presynaptic neuron; (2) dopamine transporter (DAT), located on the axonal plasma membrane of the presynaptic neuron; and (3) vesicular monoamine transporter 2 (VMAT2), which allows for packaging of dopamine into synaptic vesicles and is located on the vesicular membrane (Table 2). By contrast, striatal postsynaptic neuronal integrity can be assessed by biological compounds tagged with radioisotopes that reversibly bind to the dopamine (D_2) receptors in the putamen.

The tracer ^{18}F-6-fluorodopa (FDOPA) provides a measure of AADC activity and is used with PET as a marker of the accumulation and metabolism of levodopa at the dopamine nerve terminal. In patients with IPD, an asymmetric loss of tracer accumulation is seen in the putamen using three-dimensional PET, which can be used to distinguish IPD from normal (Morrish, Sawle, and Brooks 1995). The distinction between IPD and atypical parkinsonian syndromes is more challenging since there is also loss of nigrostriatal nerve terminals in MSA, PSP, CBD, and DLB; however, the pattern of nigrostriatal loss in these disorders may be informative (Table 3). In IPD, the nigral projections

TABLE 2: COMMON PRE- AND POST SYNAPTIC DOPAMINE RADIOLIGANDS WITH PET AND SPECT

	PET	SPECT	Both
AADC	^{18}F-6-fluorodopa		
DAT	^{11}C-nomifensine ^{11}C or ^{18}F-ß-CFT (-2-beta-carbomethoxy-3beta-[4-fluorophenyl]tropane) ^{11}C-RTI-32 (methyl [1R-2-exo-3-exo]-8-methyl-3-[4-methylphenyl]-8-azabicyclo[3.2.1] octane-2-carboxylate)	^{123}I-ß-CIT (carbomethoxy-3-[4-iodophenyl]tropane) ^{99m}Tc-TRODAT ^{99m}Tc-technepine	ß-FP CIT (N-omega-fluoropropyl-2 beta-carbomethoxy-3 beta-[4-iodophenyl]nortropane); ^{18}F for PET, ^{123}I for SPECT Altropane; ^{11}C for PET, ^{123}I for SPECT ß-CIT-FE (N-[2-fluoroethyl]-2beta-carbomethoxy-3beta-[4-iodophenyl]tropane); ^{11}C for PET, ^{123}I for SPECT PE21 (N-[3-iodoprop-2-enyl]-2beta-carbomethoxy-3beta-[4'-methy lphenyl] nortropane); ^{11}C for PET, ^{123}I for SPECT
VMAT2	^{11}C-dihydrotetrabenazine		
D2- receptor	^{11}C-raclopride ^{18}F-desmethoxyfallypride ^{18}F-fallypride	^{123}I-iodobenzamide ^{123}I-iodobenzofuran ^{123}I-epidepride	

to the caudal putamen are earliest affected with relative sparing of the projections to the caudate (Fearnley and Lees 1991). By contrast, in PSP and MSA the loss of nigral cells is more uniform and extensive, with early loss of nigral projections to the caudate. Therefore, on FDOPA PET the caudal putamen-caudate nucleus ratio can be used to help differentiate IPD from atypical parkinsonian syndromes (Brooks et al. 1990a; Brooks et al. 1990b; Sawle et al. 1991; Nagasawa et al. 1996). However, significant overlap still exists, and most studies have found that individual parkinsonian patients with IPD, MSA, PSP, CBD, and DLB cannot be distinguished using visualization of FDOPA uptake alone (Ghaemi et al. 2002; Antonini et al. 1997; Eidelberg et al. 1995; Laureys et al. 1999; Otsuka et al. 1991; Hu et al. 2000).

Radiotracers have also been developed for PET and SPECT to assess the transport of dopamine across the presynaptic neuronal cell membrane and the presynaptic vesicular membrane by binding to DAT and VMAT2, respectively (Table 2). Like FDOPA, these tracers assess the integrity of the presynaptic dopamine neuron in the striatum and provide a sensitive means of distinguishing normal individuals from those with nigrostriatal cell loss, such as patients with IPD, MSA, PSP, CBD, and DLB (Klaffke et al. 2006; Walker and Walker 2009; Vlaar et al. 2007; Kim et al. 2002). In MSA patients S-^{11}C-nomifensine, a PET ligand for DAT, has been shown to have reduced uptake in the striatum, with a similar reduction in IPD patients (Brooks et al. 1990a). By contrast, caudate uptake is also reduced in MSA, whereas in IPD caudate uptake is

TABLE 3: COMMON ABNORMALITIES ON DOPAMINE IMAGING IN PARKINSONIAN DISORDERS

Reference	Imaging Modality	IPD	MSA	PSP	CBD	DLB	Comments
(Ghaemi et al. 2002; Antonini et al. 1997; Brooks et al. 1990a; Brooks et al 1990b; Sawle et al. 1991; Nagasawa et al. 1996; Burn, Sawle, and Brooks 1994; Laureys et al. 1999; Otsuka et al. 1991; Hu et al. 2000)	FDOPA PET	Asymmetric reduced (putamen > caudate) binding	Symmetric reduced (putamen = caudate) binding	Symmetric reduced (putamen = caudate) binding	Asymmetric reduced (putamen = caudate) binding	Symmetric reduced (putamen = caudate binding	PET and SPECT presynaptic striatal imaging is not sensitive for discriminating between individual patients with these disorders (Vlaar et al. 2007; Vlaar et al. 2008a; Ransmayr et al. 2001)
(Brooks et al. 1990b; Klaffke et al. 2006; Walker and Walker 2009; Vlaar et al. 2007; Kim et al. 2002; Pirker et al. 2000; Seppi et al. 2006)	DAT PET and SPECT	Asymmetric reduced (putamen > caudate) binding	Symmetric reduced (putamen = caudate), and reduced midbrain binding	Symmetric reduced (putamen = caudate) and reduced midbrain binding	Asymmetric reduced (putamen = caudate) binding	Symmetric reduced (putamen = caudate binding	
(Martin et al. 2008; Gilman et al. 1996; Gilman et al. 1999; Albin and Koeppe 2006)	VMAT2 PET	Reduced bilateral caudate and asymmetric ✓ putamen binding	Reduced caudate and putamen binding			Reduced caudate and putamen binding	Studies limited to small patient groups
(Antonini et al. 1997; Klaffke et al. 2006; Kim et al. 2002; Vlaar et al. 2008a; Knudsen et al. 2004; Wenning et al. 1998; Schwarz et al. 1993; Kaasinen et al. 2000)	D_2- receptors with PET and SPECT	Increased putamen binding in early untreated patients, normal binding in treated patients	Reduced putamen binding	Reduced putamen binding	Normal or reduced putamen binding		Studies limited to small patient groups

relatively preserved. However, this observation is limited by poor discriminatory power due to overlap between syndromes. Using [^{123}I]β-CIT SPECT, Pirker et al. (2000) reported reduced striatal binding in MSA, PSP, CBD, and IPD, without overlap between patients and normals. Reduced putamen-caudate nucleus ratio is more pronounced in IPD than PSP, CBD, or MSA using group-wise analysis, but there is individual overlap in patients from all groups. Similarly, IPD and CBD patients have increased right–left asymmetry of [^{123}I]β-CIT binding compared to controls, MSA, and PSP patients, but these differences are not statistically significant. Indeed, it has been shown in multiple studies that presynaptic striatal imaging, either by PET or SPECT, cannot accurately discriminate between individual patients with IPD, MSA, PSP, CBD, and DLB (Vlaar et al. 2007; Vlaar et al. 2008a; Ransmayr et al. 2001). Despite these findings, PET and SPECT DAT imaging can provide valuable information in some patients with neurodegenerative disorders. For instance, in patients whose primary symptom is dementia, not parkinsonism, it has been shown that striatal FPCIT uptake with SPECT provides greater than 75% sensitivity for detecting clinically probable DLB and greater than 90% specificity for excluding non-DLB with overall good accuracy in discriminating patients with pathologically confirmed DLB from those with Alzheimer's disease, but not from those with IPD dementia (Walker et al. 2007; Walker and Walker 2009; McKeith et al. 2007; Walker et al. 2004). By contrast, in patients whose primary symptom is parkinsonism, using DAT PET or SPECT ligands to distinguish between syndromes requires analysis of regions outside of the striatum (Scherfler et al. 2005). Voxel-wise statistical parametric mapping analysis with [^{123}I]β-CIT SPECT in patients with MSA-P and PSP has shown a reduction in midbrain binding compared with controls and IPD patients, allowing for discrimination between these atypical parkinsonian syndromes and IPD in 91.3% of patients; however, this method fails to discriminate between MSA-P and PSP patients (Seppi et al. 2006). DAT ligands have also been used to study longitudinal changes in nigrostriatal cell density over time in patients with atypical parkinsonism. Pirker et al. (2002) have shown that β-CIT binding declines 14.9% over almost two years in patients with MSA, PSP, and CBD, compared to a 7.1% decline in early IPD patients.

The VMAT2 PET ligand (+)-[^{11}C]dihydrotetrabenazine ([^{11}C]DTBZ) has been used in patients with IPD, MSA, and sporadic olivopontocerebellar atrophy to understand changes in nigrostriatal function associated with each of these diseases (Martin et al. 2008). Gilman et al. (1996) has shown reduced putamen-specific binding of [^{11}C]DTBZ

in MSA compared to sporadic olivopontocerebellar atrophy or normals. In addition, a normalized binding potential is further reduced in patients with MSA-P compared to those with MSA-C (Gilman et al. 1999). In this study, a negative correlation between striatal binding and severity of parkinsonian symptoms provides further evidence that the degree of clinical parkinsonism in MSA is due to degeneration in the nigrostriatal pathway.

Pathologic studies of atypical parkinsonian disorders revealed postsynaptic striatal cell loss in addition to that found in the presynaptic nigrostriatal pathway. Radioligands that bind to striatal dopamine D_2 receptors, such as ^{11}C-raclopride in PET, can therefore estimate the density of postsynaptic neuronal loss in these disorders. It has been shown in several studies that in MSA and PSP there is a significant reduction in D_2 radiotracer binding (Antonini et al. 1997; Kim et al. 2002; Knudsen et al. 2004), whereas in CBD, D_2 binding is sometimes preserved (Klaffke et al. 2006; Plotkin et al. 2005). By contrast, D_2 binding is often increased in early untreated IPD, likely due to receptor upregulation (Wenning et al. 1998; Schwarz et al. 1993; Kaasinen et al. 2000), and is within normal range in treated IPD, ET, and DLB (Plotkin et al. 2005). Although these studies suggest that D_2 receptor ligands, such as ^{11}C-raclopride, show some discrimination capacity between MSA and IPD, this tracer is available only at limited centers, and synthesis requires an in-house cyclotron. Furthermore, in contrast to these earlier studies, Vlaar et al. have shown in a study of 248 parkinsonian patients minimal discriminatory value between IPD, MSA, PSP, and DLB with the SPECT D_2 receptor ligand ^{123}I-iodobenzamide (Vlaar et al. 2008a).

MIBG SCINTIGRAPHY

Metaiodobenzylguanidine (MIBG) is an inactive physiologic analog of norepinephrine that is taken up and stored in sympathetic nerve endings. Functional imaging studies using [^{123}I]MIBG scintigraphy have demonstrated myocardial postganglionic sympathetic dysfunction in patient with IPD, particularly in those with autonomic failure (Goldstein et al. 2000; Orimo et al. 1999), whereas postganglionic sympathetic fibers remain intact in MSA (Druschky et al. 2000; Braune 2001). Despite early reports using [^{123}I] MIBG scintigraphy to differentiate MSA from IPD in parkinsonian patients (Orimo et al. 2002), there are several limiting features of this technique (Brooks and Seppi 2009). First, although MIBG SPECT can discriminate established MSA-P and IPD, MIBG uptake can be normal in early IPD and in genetic PD (Orimo et al. 2005; Suzuki et al. 2005;

Nagayama et al. 2005). Therefore, a normal MIBG SPECT scan is less reliable for definitively diagnosing MSA-P in early parkinsonian patients with autonomic dysfunction (Satoh et al. 1999). Second, the optimal testing parameter and cut-off value for use in differential diagnosis is unclear (Frohlich et al. 2010). In a recent study, Chung et al. (2009) have shown that the washout ratio, rather than the early or late heart-to-mediastinal ratio, is more specific for differentiating MSA-P from IPD with autonomic dysfunction. By contrast, the heart-to-mediastinal ratio was superior in the diagnosis of IPD and DLB in other studies (Estorch et al. 2008). Third, [123I]MIBG scintigraphy has limited utility in distinguishing MSA from other forms of parkinsonism, as uptake is also normal in most patients with PSP, vascular parkinsonism, and ET (Brooks and Seppi 2009; Raffel et al. 2006). In addition, several studies have shown that cardiac sympathetic denervation can occur in some patients with MSA, PSP, and CBD (Nagayama et al. 2005; Frohlich et al. 2010). Indeed, in a study of 50 parkinsonian patients where initial [123I]MIBG-based diagnosis was compared to final clinical diagnosis after 9.5±1.3 months of follow-up, Frohlich et al. (2010) have found accurate diagnosis with [123I]MIBG in only two-thirds of patients. In a larger series, Nagayama et al. (2005) have shown an 87.7% sensitivity but only 37.4% specificity for accurately detecting IPD using [123I]MIBG. Indeed, in this study of 391 patients, 21.4% of MSA patients, 85.7% of PSP patients, and 80% of vascular parkinsonism patients exhibited low [123I]MIBG uptake. However, all final diagnoses were based on clinical assessment. Further studies with autopsy-confirmed diagnoses will be valuable in determining the utility of this technique in the diagnosis of parkinsonism.

Similar to other Lewy body disorders, [123I]MIBG scintigraphy is decreased in patients with DLB and may be helpful when diagnosing patients with a primary dementia (Kashihara et al. 2006; Yoshita, Taki, and Yamada 2001; Novellino et al. 2010). Indeed, reduced [123I]MIBG is now included as a "supportive feature" of the diagnostic criteria for DLB by the Consortium on Dementia with Lewy Bodies (McKeith et al. 2005). In a study of 65 patients with dementia who underwent [123I]MIBG at the first clinical appointment, Estorch et al. (2008) showed accurate differentiation of DLB from other dementias (PSP, MSA, Alzheimer's dementia, frontotemporal dementia, vascular parkinsonism) with 94% sensitivity and 95% specificity compared to final clinical diagnosis after four-year follow-up. In contrast to prior studies, heart-to-mediastinal ratio was more accurate than washout ratio. In this study, however, 32% of initial patients were not included in the final evaluation due to inability to determine a final clinical diagnosis

after four years of follow-up. By contrast, in patients who present with parkinsonism and mild cognitive dysfunction, [123I]MIBG scintigraphy is not able to distinguish between patients with IPD and DLB (Taki et al. 2004).

TCS

Transcranial sonography (TCS) is an imaging technique that has recently been studied in patients with parkinsonism. This approach, described in detail in Chapter 5, has been applied to aid in the diagnosis of IPD and also atypical parkinsonian syndromes. Becker et al. (2005) originally reported IPD-related hyperechogenicity of the substantia nigra (SN), which is found in 90% of IPD patients, but less than 10% of healthy subjects (Berg, Siefker, and Becker 2001; Berg et al. 2002; Walter et al. 2003). By contrast, hyperechogenicity of the lentiform nucleus (LN, i.e. the putamen and globus pallidus) is found in patients with MSA, PSP, CBD, and DLB (Walter et al. 2003; Walter et al. 2006; Walter et al. 2004). In the past decade, several studies have examined the discriminatory power of TCS in patients with atypical parkinsonism, with mixed results (Vlaar et al. 2009; Vlaar et al. 2008b). Walter et al. (2003) have studied atypical patients with a clinically probable diagnosis of MSA and PSP and found that only 2% of MSA and PSP patients have SN hyperechogenicity compared to 96% of IPD. Later studies suggest that normal SN echogenicity indicates MSA rather than IPD with 90% sensitivity and 98% specificity, whereas third ventricle dilation in combination with LN hyperechogenicity indicates PSP rather than IPD with 84% sensitivity and 98% specificity (Walter et al. 2007). In this study, however, moderate or marked SN echogenicity was also found in 47% of PSP patients and LN hyperechogenicity was found in up to 30% of IPD patients. By contrast, SN hyperechogenicity is found in 88% of CBD patients and 80% of DLB patients (Walter et al. 2006; Walter et al. 2004). In most DLB patients SN echogenicity is bilateral, compared to only a third of IPD patients with dementia.

In a prospective study of 60 parkinsonian patients, of whom only 37% had a definitive clinical diagnosis at the time of TCS, SN hyperechogenicity yielded 90.7% sensitivity and 82.4% specificity for the diagnosis of IPD, whereas LN hyperechogenicity yielded only 66.7% sensitivity and 68.6% specificity for a diagnosis of atypical parkinsonism (Gaenslen et al. 2008). In this study, no patients with MSA or PSP had SN hyperechogenicity. However, only 10 atypical patients were included, and the diagnosis was not confirmed by autopsy. Other studies, however, indicate a lower predictive power of SN hyperechogenicity in the diagnosis of IPD due to false positive results (i.e., the presence of SN hyperechogenicity in non-IPD), specifically in patients with MSA, PSP, DLB, and vascular parkinsonism (Vlaar et al. 2008b). Therefore, larger studies in atypical patients, which include pathology, are needed to determine the diagnostic power of TCS in early parkinsonian patients with a final diagnosis of MSA, PSP, CBD, and DLB.

TCS has several advantages over other imaging techniques in that it is widely available, easy to use in patients who have tremor, does not require radioactive tracers, and is less expensive than MRI, PET, or SPECT. However, there are several technical issues that can limit the usefulness of TCS, which include the inability to acquire a two-dimensional view of intracranial structures in 5%–25% of subjects due to an inappropriate temporal bone window. In addition, there is a considerable level of technical expertise required to correctly perform and interpret TCS, which is likely contributing to the inconsistent outcomes reported in the literature (Vlaar et al. 2009).

CONCLUSION

Recent advances in imaging technology provide new means of assessing patients with atypical forms of parkinsonism and offer both clinicians and researchers more accurate differential diagnoses than history and exam alone. The optimal technique is one that provides high discriminatory power between atypical syndromes in individual patients presenting with early symptoms, ideally without requiring significant technical expertise. Such techniques are invaluable to researchers, and eventually clinicians, as new treatments are developed, tested, and ultimately made available for patients with atypical parkinsonian syndromes.

REFERENCES

Abe, K., T. Hikita, M. Yokoe et al. 2006. The "cross" signs in patients with multiple system atrophy: A quantitative study. *J Neuroimaging* 16:73–77.

Albin, R., and R. Koeppe. 2006. Rapid loss of striatal VMAT2 binding associated with onset of Lewy body dementia. *Movement Disorders* 21:287–288.

Antonini, A., K. Kazumata, A. Feigin et al. 1998. Differential diagnosis of parkinsonism with [18F]fluorodeoxyglucose and PET. *Mov Disord* 13:268–274.

Antonini, A., K. L. Leenders, P. Vontobel et al. 1997. Complementary PET studies of striatal neuronal function in the differential diagnosis between multiple system atrophy and Parkinson's disease. *Brain* 120:2187–2195.

Becker, G., J. Seufert, U. Bogdahn et al. 1995. Degeneration of substantia nigra in chronic Parkinson's disease visualized by transcranial color-coded real-time sonography. *Neurology* 45:182–184.

Berding, G., P. Odin, D. J. Brooks et al. 2001. Resting regional cerebral glucose metabolism in advanced Parkinson's disease studied in the off and on conditions with [(18)F]FDG-PET. *Mov Disord* 16:1014–1022.

Berg, D., C. Siefker, and G. Becker. 2001. Echogenicity of the substantia nigra in Parkinson's disease and its relation to clinical findings. *J Neurol* 248:684–689.

Berg, D., W. Roggendorf, U. Schroder et al. 2002. Echogenicity of the substantia nigra: Association with increased iron content and marker for susceptibility to nigrostriatal injury. *Arch Neurol* 59:999–1005.

Bhattacharya, K., D. Saadia, B. Eisenkraft et al. 2002. Brain magnetic resonance imaging in multiple-system atrophy and Parkinson disease: A diagnostic algorithm. *Arch Neurol* 59:835–842.

Blin, J., J. C. Baron, B. Dubois et al. 1990. Positron emission tomography study in progressive supranuclear palsy. Brain hypometabolic pattern and clinicometabolic correlations. *Arch Neurol* 47:747–752.

Boeve, B. F., A. E. Lang, and I. Litvan. 2003. Corticobasal degeneration and its relationship to progressive supranuclear palsy and frontotemporal dementia. *Annals of Neurology* 54:S15–S19.

Boxer, A. L., M. D. Geschwind, N. Belfor et al. 2006. Patterns of brain atrophy that differentiate corticobasal degeneration syndrome from progressive supranuclear palsy. *Arch Neurol* 63:81–86.

Braak, H., and E. Braak. 2000. Pathoanatomy of Parkinson's disease. *J Neurol* 247 (Suppl 2): II3–10.

Braune, S. 2001. The role of cardiac metaiodobenzylguanidine uptake in the differential diagnosis of parkinsonian syndromes. *Clin Auton Res* 11:351–355.

Brooks, D. J., and J. Seppi. 2009. Proposed neuroimaging criteria for the diagnosis of multiple system atrophy. *Mov Disord* 24:949–964.

Brooks, D. J., E. P. Salmon, C. J. Mathias et al. 1990a. The relationship between locomotor disability, autonomic dysfunction, and the integrity of the striatal dopaminergic system in patients with multiple system atrophy, pure autonomic failure, and Parkinson's disease, studied with PET. *Brain* 113 (Pt 5):1539–1552.

Brooks, D. J., V. Ibanez, G. V. Sawle et al. 1990b. Differing patterns of striatal 18F-dopa uptake in Parkinson's disease, multiple system atrophy, and progressive supranuclear palsy. *Ann Neurol* 28:547–555.

Burn, D. J., G. V. Sawle, and D. J. Brooks. 1994. Differential diagnosis of Parkinson's disease, multiple system atrophy, and Steele-Richardson-Olszewski syndrome: Discriminant analysis of striatal 18F-dopa PET data. *J Neurol Neurosurg Psychiatry* 57:278–284.

Chung, E. J., W. Y. Lee, W. T. Yoon et al. 2009. MIBG scintigraphy for differentiating Parkinson's disease with autonomic dysfunction from Parkinsonism-predominant multiple system atrophy. *Mov Disord* 24:1650–1655.

Coulier, I. M., J. J. de Vries, K. L. Leenders. 2003. Is FDG-PET a useful tool in clinical practice for diagnosing corticobasal ganglionic degeneration? *Mov Disord* 18:1175–1178.

De Volder, A. G., J. Francart, C. Laterre et al. 1989. Decreased glucose utilization in the striatum and frontal lobe in probable striatonigral degeneration. *Ann Neurol* 26:239–247.

Druschky, A., M. J. Hilz, G. Platsch et al. 2000. Differentiation of Parkinson's disease and multiple system atrophy in early disease stages by means of I-123-MIBG-SPECT. *J Neurol Sci* 175:3–12.

Eckert, T., A. Barnes, V. Dhawan et al. 2005. FDG PET in the differential diagnosis of parkinsonian disorders. *Neuroimage,* 26:912–921.

Eckert, T., and D. Eidelberg. 2004. The role of functional neuroimaging in the differential diagnosis of idiopathic Parkinson's disease and multiple system atrophy. *Clin Auton Res* 14:84–91.

Eckert, T., C. Tang, Y. Ma et al. 2008. Abnormal metabolic networks in atypical parkinsonism. *Movement Disorders* 23:727–733.

Eckert, T., K. Van Laere, C. Tang et al. 2007. Quantification of Parkinson's disease-related network expression with ECD SPECT. *Eur J Nucl Med Mol Imaging* 34:496–501.

Eidelberg, D. 2009. Metabolic brain networks in neurodegenerative disorders: A functional imaging approach. *Trends Neurosci* 32:548–557.

(Jahanshahi et al. 1995; Playford et al. 1992; Samuel et al. 1997a; Samuel et al. 1997b). The most common tests include the uni-manual task, involving either repeated thumb to other finger opposition movements or manipulation of a joystick in different directions. For example, when normal subjects performed repetitive right-hand joystick movements in freely selected directions while undergoing [^{15}O] H$_2$O PET, an increase in regional cerebral blood flow (rCBF) was found in the contralateral primary sensorimotor cortex and lentiform nucleus. Activation was also seen bilaterally in the anterior cingulate gyrus, supplementary motor area (SMA), lateral premotor cortex, and dorsolateral prefrontal cortex (Playford et al. 1992). In contrast, PD patients presented a more complicated activation pattern, showing impaired rCBF changes in the lentiform nucleus, anterior cingulate gyrus, SMA, and dorsolateral prefrontal cortex and normal activation at the level of sensorimotor cortex, lateral, and parietal premotor cortex compared with the healthy controls (Jahanshahi et al. 1995; Playford et al. 1992). It has been observed that the pattern of activation in PD varies depending upon the stage of the disease, exposure to medication, and the type of motor task. Samuel et al. (1997a) hypothesized that nigrostriatal dopaminergic degeneration results in hypoactivation of a mesial premotor system (SMA, anterior cingulate gyrus, and dorsolateral prefrontal cortex), prevalently involved in self-paced movements. A different network, engaging the lateral premotor cortex and primary motor cortex, and heavily connected with parietal cortex and cerebellum (prevalently involved in externally cued movements), is relatively preserved in PD and may compensate for the failure in generating self-paced movements (Jahanshahi et al. 1995). The same group was also able to demonstrate that activation of the SMA significantly improved when akinesia was reversed with apomorphine (Jenkins et al. 1992). In particular, rCBF was measured in PD patients at rest and when performing paced joystick movements with the right hand in one of four freely chosen directions. All patients were studied before treatment, in an off state, and when "on" with apomorphine. Under resting conditions apomorphine had no effect on CBF, while significant activation of the SMA was observed while using the joystick with apomorphine. The authors concluded that the concomitant supplementary motor area activation and motor function improvement in apomorphine-treated patients with PD provided further evidence for the role of this structure in generating motor programs. Recent studies have generated more controversial findings. Haslinger et al. (2001), in an fMRI study, measured blood oxygen level dependent (BOLD) cortical signal changes in PD patients associated with volitional

limb movements while off and on levodopa. Compared to the control group, patients both off and on levodopa showed movement-related impaired activation in the rostral supplementary motor area and increased activation in the primary motor cortex (M1) and the lateral premotor cortex bilaterally. However, levodopa led to a relative normalization of the impaired activation in the mesial premotor cortex, M1, lateral premotor, and superior parietal cortex. They concluded that levodopa may improve impaired motor initiation in the supplementary motor area and decrease hyperfunction of the lateral premotor and primary motor cortex during simple volitional movements. Another interesting fMRI study by Eckert et al. (2006) reported a relatively increased BOLD response of the pre-SMA in patients with early, drug-naïve PD before and after initiation of dopaminergic medication compared with healthy age-matched controls while performing simple temporally self-initiated hand movements.

These apparently contradicting studies provide some insights into the role of chronic medication effects and disease progression on different activation patterns.

Other studies have also attempted to investigate the pattern of activation associated with levodopa-induced dyskinesias. Rascol et al. (1998) carried out a [133Xe]SPECT rCBF measurement at rest and during a sequential finger opposition motor task in two groups of PD patients with and without dyskinesias. Hyperactivation of SMA and ipsi- and contralateral primary motor cortex was found in dyskinetic PD patients but not in non-dyskinetic patients and healthy subjects. This hyperactivation favored the view that dyskinesias could be the consequence of a disinhibition of primary motor cortex and accessory motor areas as a result of an excessive drive of the pallido-thalamocortical motor pathway. More recent studies with [^{15}O]H$_2$O PET in PD patients with focal limb dyskinesias have confirmed that resting levels of rCBF after oral levodopa are increased during dyskinesias in lentiform nuclei, motor, premotor, and dorsal prefrontal cortex (Brooks et al. 2000).

Several PET activation studies have tested the effect of surgical therapies on motor activation. Electrophysiological experiments in non-human primate models of nigrostriatal dopamine degeneration have reported a significant increase in the firing rate of neurons in the subthalamic nucleus (glutamatergic) and in the internal globus pallidus (GABAergic). In turn there was a marked inhibition of thalamocortical projections (Alexander et al. 1990; Feger et al. 1997). Thus, improvement of the akinetic-rigid syndrome by pallidotomy, internal globus pallidus, or subthalamic electrical stimulation should be associated with a reversibility of the impaired cortical activation. This hypothesis has been confirmed by a number of PET studies. In fact, in PD patients performing a motor task, unilateral pallidotomy was associated with an increased activation of SMA, lateral premotor cortex, and dorsolateral prefrontal cortex (Samuel et al. 1997b). In another PET study performed in PD patients with an electrode surgically implanted in either the internal globus pallidus or the subthalamic nucleus (Limousin et al. 1997), high-frequency deep brain stimulation (DBS) was associated with rCBF decrement in motor and premotor regions during rest, and with an increment in rCBF in SMA, anterior cingulate gyrus and dorsolateral prefrontal cortex during a uni-manual motor task. Similarly, Strafella et al. (2003), using $[^{15}O]H_2O$ PET in Parkinsonian patients with bilateral electrical stimulators implanted in the STN, determined the effect of unilateral and bilateral STN stimulation delivered at different frequencies on rCBF activation during paced self-selected joystick movements. Five different stimulation settings were used: stimulation OFF, unilateral low- (60 Hz) and high- (185 Hz) frequency stimulation contralateral to hand movement, unilateral high-frequency stimulation ipsilateral to hand movement, and bilateral high-frequency stimulation. Both unilateral low- and high-frequency stimulation of the STN contralateral to hand movement restored activation of the supplementary motor area and anterior cingulate cortex and improved motor performance. Bilateral high-frequency stimulation of the STN produced the most pronounced improvement in motor performance and the greatest extent of activation in cortical areas with additional bilateral activation of the globus pallidus. They concluded that STN stimulation produces its clinical effects by normalizing the pattern of brain activity during movement.

In the past few years, studies have suggested that chronic electrical stimulation of the primary motor cortex (MCS) may also relieve motor symptoms of PD (Canavero et al. 2002; Canavero et al. 2003; Pagni et al. 2003). This novel approach may be considered as an alternative for PD patients who are not good candidates for DBS of the STN. In order to understand the cortical and subcortical effects of MCS, Strafella et al. (2007) used $[^{15}O]H_2O$ PET to investigate changes in rCBF while testing motor performance with a joystick motor task. Interestingly, they found that MCS at 50 and 130 Hz did not produce significant changes in joystick motor performance or rCBF at cortical or subcortical levels. They concluded that while MCS was probably a simpler and safer surgical procedure than DBS of the STN, it failed to modify the pattern of movement-related rCBF activation in PD patients.

It is well known that patients with advanced PD may develop disabling axial symptoms, including gait disturbances,

freezing, and postural instability, that are poorly responsive to levodopa replacement therapy. Recently, a new surgical target in the brainstem, i.e., the pedunculopontine nucleus (PPN), has been identified as a potential new treatment for PD. The PPN is involved in locomotion, control of posture, and behavioral states [i.e., wakefulness, rapid eye movement (REM) sleep] (Lim et al. 2007; Pahapill and Lozano 2000). Recent reports suggested that PPN modulation with DBS may be beneficial in the treatment of axial symptoms. However, the mechanisms underlying these effects are still unknown. Ballanger et al. (2009a) (Figure 1) used $[^{15}O]$ H_2O PET to investigate rCBF in patients with advanced PD who underwent implantation of unilateral PPN-DBS. Patients were studied off-medication with stimulator off and on, both at rest and during a self-paced alternating motor task of the lower limbs. Stimulation induced significant rCBF increases in subcortical regions such as the thalamus ($p < 0.006$), cerebellum ($p < 0.001$), and midbrain ($p < 0.001$), as well as different cortical areas involving medial sensorimotor cortex extending into caudal SMA (BA 4/6; $p < 0.001$). PPN-DBS in advanced PD resulted in blood flow and presumably neuronal activity changes in subcortical and cortical areas involved in balance and motor control, including the mesencephalic locomotor region (e.g., PPN) and closely interconnected structures within the cerebello-(rubro)-thalamocortical circuit. Whether these findings are associated with PPN-DBS, the clinical effect remains to be proven. However, they suggest that PPN modulation may induce functional changes in neural networks associated with the control of lower limb movements.

ACTIVATION STUDIES OF COGNITIVE FUNCTIONS

PD is traditionally associated with motor symptoms; however, neuropsychological studies have also revealed deficits across a range of cognitive functions (Dubois and Pillon 1997; Taylor and Saint-Cyr 1995; Taylor et al.1986). Cognitive disabilities include deficits of executive function, language, visuospatial/visuoconstructive abilities, memory, attention, and skill learning (Monchi et al. 2004; Monchi et al. 2007; Owen 2004; Taylor and Saint-Cyr 1995; Zgaljardic et al. 2004). Several studies have documented that in PD, dopamine depletion is restricted in the earlier stages to the putamen and the dorsal caudate nucleus and only later progresses to the more ventral parts of the striatum and the mesocorticolimbic dopaminergic system (Cools et al. 2001; Kish et al. 1988; Rosvold 1972; Swainson et al. 2000). Thus, the evolving pattern of cognitive impairments

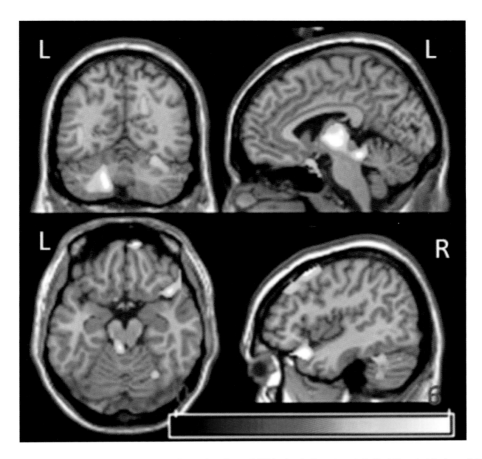

Figure 1 Statistical parametric maps of brain regions showing the main effect of PPN stimulation at a statistical threshold of p < 0.001 (uncorrected) at the single voxel level and p < 0.05 (corrected) at the cluster level. Areas of increased rCBF involve mainly the subcortical structures. These areas are superimposed on sagittal, coronal, and transverse sections of a single subject brain MRI from SPM2. rCBF = regional cerebral blood flow; PPN = pedunculopontine nucleus; R = right; L = left. From Ballanger et al., *Hum Brain Mapp.* 2009; 30(12):3901–9. Reprinted with permission from John Wiley & Sons.

observed in these patients is explained in terms of the spatiotemporal progression of dopamine depletion within the striatum and the terminal distribution of its cortical afferents. Neurochemical studies have revealed an uneven pattern of striatal dopamine loss in patients with PD (Kish et al. 1988). This uneven dopaminergic loss explains why dopaminergic therapy, while improving motor symptoms, may not necessarily have the same effects on various cognitive functions (Cools et al. 2001; Swainson et al. 2000). In fact, there is evidence that different cognitive disabilities may be differentially affected by dopaminergic replacement therapy depending on the underlying neural pathways (Gotham et al. 1988).

Several neuroimaging studies in PD patients have documented the involvement of the frontostriatal networks in executive dysfunctions, in particular those that engage the nigrostriatal and mesocortical pathways (Cools et al. 2002; Dagher et al. 2001; Mattay et al. 2002; Owen et al. 1998). Monchi et al. (2004) measured performance of the Wisconsin Card Sorting Task (WCST) in PD patients and healthy

controls during fMRI. PD patients showed a decreased activation in both the ventrolateral prefrontal cortex (VLPFC) (when receiving negative feedback) and the posterior prefrontal cortex (PFC) (when matching after negative feedback). In the healthy controls, these prefrontal regions specifically co-activated with the striatum during those stages of task performance. In contrast, when receiving positive or negative feedback, greater activation was found in the PD patients in prefrontal areas that were not co-activated with the striatum in healthy control subjects. These findings suggest that both decreased and increased activation can occur in prefrontal areas during cognitive performance, and that the pattern of activity observed in a specific area of the PFC depends on its specific relationship with the striatum for the task at hand. Later, these observations were confirmed in another fMRI study using a different set-shifting task (i.e., Montreal Card Sorting Task [MCST]) (Monchi et al. 2007), where a pattern of cortical activation was characterized by either reduced or increased activation depending on whether the caudate nucleus was involved or not in the task. These findings do not agree with the traditional model, which proposes that nigrostriatal dopamine depletion results in decreased cortical activity. Rather, the data support the hypothesis that not only nigrostriatal but also mesocortical dopaminergic pathways play a significant role in the cognitive deficits observed in PD. A H_2 [15] O-PET study in healthy subjects as well as mildly affected PD patients (Dagher et al. 2001) showed no behavioral differences on the Tower of London (TOL) test, although there were differences in neuronal activation pattern. In the two groups, overlapping areas of the PFC were activated but, whereas the right caudate nucleus was activated in the control group, this was not evident in the PD patients. The authors suggested that normal frontal lobe activation can occur in PD despite abnormal processing within the basal ganglia. Moreover, they found that right hippocampal activity was suppressed in the controls and enhanced in the PD patients. This could represent a shift during performance of the TOL task, possibly resulting from insufficient working memory capacity within the frontostriatal system. In another study, Owen and colleagues (Owen et al. 1998) examined the effects of striatal dopamine depletion on cortical and subcortical blood flow changes with the same task (i.e., TOL) in patients with moderate PD and age-matched controls. Relative to control conditions, the planning task was associated with an increase in cerebral blood flow in the internal segment of the right globus pallidus in the age-matched control subjects and a decrease in the same region in the patients with PD. They concluded that striatal dopamine depletion disrupts the normal pattern of basal ganglia outflow in PD and consequently affects the expression of frontal-lobe functions by interrupting normal transmission of information through frontostriatal circuitry.

To date, there is some interesting imaging evidence that dopamine replacement therapy may not have the same effect on the identified motor and cognitive frontostriatal networks. In fact, previous FDG-PET studies have shown that unlike the PD-related motor pattern (PDRP), the PD-related cognitive pattern (PDCP) expression is not significantly altered by antiparkinsonian treatment with either intravenous levodopa or deep brain stimulation (Huang et al. 2007; also see Chapter 9).

Recently, it has been proposed that in PD, the dysfunction in dopaminergic frontostriatal networks may be influenced by a common functional polymorphism (val [158] met) within the catechol O-methyltransferase (COMT) gene. COMT is an enzyme that regulates dopamine levels in cortical areas. A polymorphism in COMT resulting in a substitution of valine for methionine at codon 158 (val [158] met) may affect PD cognitive performance (Williams-Gray et al. 2008). A low

activity COMT genotype (met/met), for example, causes higher dopamine levels in the PFC, decreases performance on the TOL test, and decreases frontoparietal activity (Williams-Gray et al. 2007). Williams-Gray et al. (2008) compared PD patients with high (val/val) to low (met/met) activity COMT genotypes using an attentional control task. Genotype had a critical impact on task strategy: while patients with high activity COMT genotypes (val/val) adopted a typical approach of preferentially shifting attention, those with low activity genotypes (met/met) failed to adopt such a strategy, suggesting an inability to form an attentional "set." Moreover, this behavior was associated with significant underactivation across the frontoparietal attentional network. Furthermore, they demonstrated an interactive effect of COMT genotype and dopaminergic medication on task performance and BOLD response. Exogenous levodopa caused a larger decrease of prefrontal functions in val/val compared to met/met PD patients (Williams-Gray et al. 2008).

To date, the bulk of functional neuroimaging experiments have studied executive deficits in PD patients with regard to task-related brain activation. However, recent reports suggest that executive performance also relies on the integrity of the default mode network (i.e., medial prefrontal cortex, mPFC; posterior cingulate, PCC; precuneus) characterized by a deactivation of these cortical areas during the performance of executive tasks. In a recent study designed to examine the integrity of the default mode network in PD patients using fMRI (van Eimeren et al. 2009b) (Figure 2), during a card-sorting task compared to a simple sensory-motor matching task, the authors found that PD patients and matched controls showed comparable deactivation of the medial PFC but different deactivation in the posterior parietal cortex (PPC) and precuneus. Compared to controls, PD patients not only showed less deactivation of the PCC and the precuneus, they even demonstrated a reversed pattern of activation and deactivation. Connectivity analysis yielded that in contrast to healthy individuals, the medial PFC and rostral ventromedial caudate nucleus were functionally disconnected in PD. These findings suggest a specific malfunctioning of the default mode network in PD in relation to executive processing. However, other important cognitive processes such as sequence learning are also closely linked with deactivation of the default mode network (Argyelan et al. 2008). In this study, the authors used PET to measure rCBF in 15 PD patients while they performed a motor sequence learning task. Scanning was conducted before and during intravenous levodopa infusion; the pace and extent of movement was controlled across tasks and treatment conditions. In unmedicated PD patients, learning-related deactivation was present in the

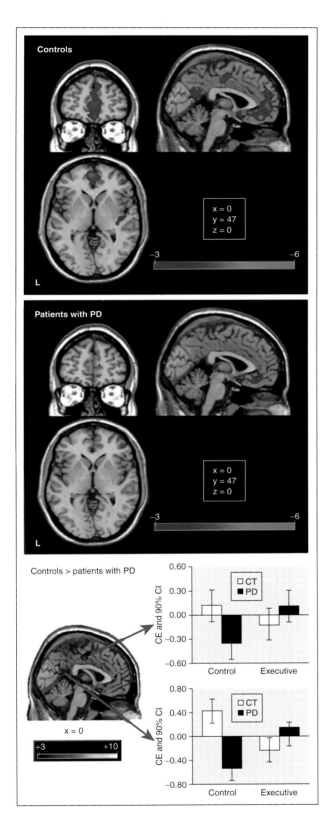

ventromedial prefrontal cortex. This response was absent in the treated condition. Treatment-mediated changes in deactivation correlated with baseline performance and with the $val^{158}met$ catechol O-methyltransferase genotype. These findings suggest that dopamine can influence prefrontal deactivation during learning and that these changes are linked to baseline performance and genotype. Similar observations were reported in another study showing that dopamine modulates default mode network deactivation in PD patients during the Tower of London task (Nagano-Saito et al. 2009).

ACTIVATION STUDIES OF BEHAVIORAL SYMPTOMS

In the last few years there have been increasing reports of PD patients experiencing severe behavioral symptoms in response to medication. In fact, while dopamine replacement treatment is titrated to compensate for the deficiencies in the motor basal ganglia network and to alleviate motor symptoms, this may result in a dopaminergic "overdosing effect" in corticobasal ganglia pathways mediating cognitive and behavioral functions (Rowe et al., 2008). As a result, dopamine agents can worsen non-motor symptoms (Cools 2006; Park and Stacy 2009), cause compulsive medication use (Evans et al. 2009), and trigger certain forms of behavioral addiction. In particular, dopamine agonists have been implicated in the development of impulse control disorders (ICDs), including hypersexuality (Voon et al. 2006; Voon et al. 2007; Voon and Fox 2007; Weintraub et al. 2006; Weintraub 2008; Weintraub et al., 2008), compulsive shopping (Voon et al. 2006; Weintraub 2008; Weintraub et al. 2008), compulsive eating (Nirenberg and Waters 2006; Weintraub 2008; Weintraub et al. 2008), and, more commonly, pathological gambling (Grosset et al. 2007; Lu et al. 2006; Voon et al. 2006; Weintraub et al. 2006; Weintraub 2008; Weintraub et al. 2008). Recent functional imaging studies that have compared PD patients on agonists with and without ICDs have revealed specific differences in frontostriatal function during tasks that mimic—or tap some of

Figure 2 Cerebral deactivations as indexed by blood oxygen level dependent decreases during executive relative to control trials. The statistical T maps are superimposed on sections (corresponding stereotactic coordinates are stated in millimeters) of the T1-weighted magnetic resonance imaging template implemented in MRIcro. Controls (CT) show deactivation of the medial prefrontal cortex, posterior cingulate cortex, and precuneus. Patients with Parkinson's disease (PD) show deactivation of the medial prefrontal cortex only. Controls show more deactivation of the posterior cingulate cortex and precuneus. The bar graphs plot the contrast estimates (CEs) and 90% confidence intervals (CIs) per group and condition for the respective peak voxels within the posterior cingulate cortex and precuneus. From Van Emeiren et al., *Arch Neuro* 2009; 66(7):877–83. Reprinted with permission from American Medical Association.

the underlying constructs of—the pathological behavior in question (Riba et al. 2008; Steeves et al. 2009; van Eimeren et al. 2009a; van Eimeren et al. 2009b). What is emerging from these studies is evidence that the tonic stimulation of dopamine receptors via agonists may impair reward processing in ways that promote pathological repetition of behaviors. Dopaminergic medications could potentially stimulate compulsive behaviors at multiple levels. Proposed mechanisms have included (1) differential DA receptor stimulation preferentially affecting limbic circuits regulating reward, reinforcing effects of excessive or continuous DA receptor stimulation conferring excessive salience, or

impairing its eventual withdrawal; and (2) a more specific priming effect of dopamine agonists inducing excess release of DA in ventral striatal circuits that could increase salience and thus trigger craving for the relevant stimulus. Given the involvement of the ventral striatum in drug and behavioral addictions described above, it is sensible to predict that excessive limbic dopaminergic stimulation plays a role in the development of ICDs in PD patients treated with agonists. Limbic regions of the striatum are relatively unimpaired in PD (Kish et al. 1988), which is proposed to account for the deficits in particular cognitive tasks when patients are on medication (Cools 2006). Thus, PD patients

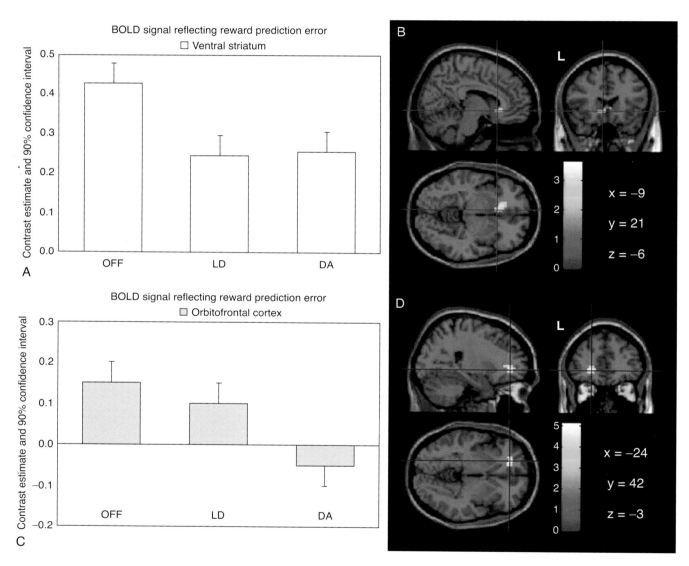

Figure 3 Effect of dopaminergic medication on reward processing. (a) Contrast estimates and 90% confidence interval of regression with trial-by-trial reward prediction values (RPE) in the ventral striatum (x:9, y:21, z:6 mm). OFF, without dopaminergic medication; LD, on levodopa; DA, on pramipexole. (b) Both medications (LD/DA) significantly diminished local reward processing (compared to OFF). L, left hemisphere. (c) Contrast estimates and 90% confidence interval of regression with trial-by-trial reward prediction values (RPE) in the orbitofrontal cortex (x:24, y:42, z:3 mm). OFF, without dopaminergic medication; LD, on levodopa; DA, on pramipexole. (d) Only pramipexole greatly diminished local reward processing. L, left hemisphere. From Van Emeiren et al., *NPP* 2009; 34(13):2758–66. Reprinted with from Nature Publishing Group.

with preserved ventral striatal dopamine projections at the time of initial treatment may be particularly at risk of developing ICDs. One fMRI study comparing agonist vs. placebo found decreased striatal BOLD responses to rewards when subjects (without a history of gambling) were on pramipexole (Riba et al. 2008), suggesting that the activation of presynaptic autoreceptors had decreased the sensitivity of the reward circuit. Similarly, in another fMRI study, in a group of PD patients without any ICD, van Eimeren et al. (2009a) (Figure 3) found that both agonists and levodopa diminished ventral striatal reward processing and that agonists, but not levodopa, increased activity in the orbitofrontal cortex during the receipt of reward. This increase was found to be due to a relatively increased orbitofrontal response to negative feedback compared with the healthy controls. The authors suggested that agonists prevent pauses in dopamine transmission and thus impair the processing of negative reinforcement. Those findings were confirmed in a more recent [^{15}O]H$_2$O PET study (van Eimeren et al. 2009c). In this study, the authors investigated dopamine agonist-induced changes in brain activity that may differentiate PD patients with agonist-induced pathological gambling from PD patients who remained free of the disorder. Patients were scanned before and after administration of dopamine agonists to measure changes in rCBF

during a card selection game with feedback. The authors found that dopamine agonists increased activity in brain areas associated with impulse control in patients without pathological gambling. The gamblers on the other hand showed a significant dopamine agonist-induced reduction of activity.

In the last couple years, there has also been growing evidence suggesting that in PD patients, DBS of the STN may also contribute to certain impulsive behavior under high-conflict conditions (Ballanger et al. 2009b; Frank et al. 2007). A neurocomputational model of the basal ganglia has proposed that this behavioral aspect may be related to the role played by the STN in relaying a "hold your horses" signal intended to allow more time to settle on the best option (Frank et al. 2007). Recently, Ballanger et al. (2009b) (Figure 4) used [^{15}O]H$_2$O PET to measure rCBF during a Go/No-Go paradigm to study the motor improvement and response-inhibition deficits associated with STN-DBS in patients with PD. They found that while improving UPDRS motor ratings and inducing a global decrease in reaction time during task performance, STN-DBS impaired response inhibition as revealed by an increase in commission errors in No-Go trials. These behavioral effects were accompanied by changes in synaptic activity consisting in a reduced activation in the cortical networks responsible for

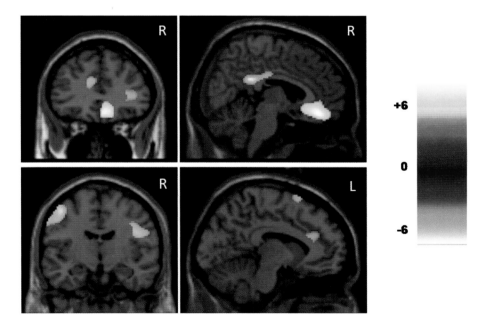

Figure 4 Statistical parametric maps of brain regions showing common significant changes with subthalamic nucleus (STN) stimulation during both Go and Go/NoGo tasks at a statistical threshold of p < 0.001 (uncorrected) at the single-voxel level. Areas of increased regional cerebral blood flow (rCBF) with STN stimulation involving the ventral anterior cingulate cortex (ACC) are in yellow. Areas of decreased rCBF during STN stimulation involving the left motor and premotor areas, the medial dorsal ACC, posterior cingulate cortex, and pre-supplementary motor area are in blue. These areas are superimposed on sagittal (right column) and coronal (left column) sections of a single subject's brain magnetic resonance imaging from SPM2. R = right; L = left. From Ballanger et al. 2009 *Ann Neurol.* 66(6): 817–824. Reprinted with from John Wiley & Sons.

reactive and proactive response inhibition. They suggested that, while improving motor functions in PD patients, modulation of STN hyperactivity with DBS may tend at the same time to favor the appearance of impulsive behavior by acting on the gating mechanism involved in response initiation.

In conclusion, activation studies have been able to shed new light into the pathophysiology of PD and the neurobiological underpinnings of its motor, cognitive, and behavioral manifestations. They have been able to provide a large bulk of information on the role of current dopaminergic and surgical therapies in normalizing cortical and subcortical abnormalities and have set the ground for testing potential novel surgical targets and medical treatment for the management of Parkinson's disease.

REFERENCES

Alexander, G. E., M. D. Crutcher, and M. R. DeLong. 1990. Basal ganglia-thalamocortical circuits: Parallel substrates for motor, oculomotor, 'prefrontal' and 'limbic' functions. *Progress in Brain Research* 85:119–146.

Alexander, G. E., M. R. DeLong, and P. L. Strick. 1986. Parallel organization of functionally segregated circuits linking basal ganglia and cortex. *Annual Review of Neuroscience* 9:357–381.

Argyelan, M., M. Carbon, M. F. Ghilardi, A. Feigin, P. Mattis, C. Tang, V. Dhawan, and D. Eidelberg. 2008. Dopaminergic suppression of brain deactivation responses during sequence learning. *Journal of Neuroscience* 28 (no. 42): 10687–10695.

Ballanger, B., A. M. Lozano, E. Moro,T. van Eimeren, C. Hamani, R. Chen, R. Cilia, S. Houle, Y. Y. Poon, A. E. Lang, and A. P. Strafella. 2009a. Cerebral blood flow changes induced by pedunculopontine nucleus stimulation in patients with advanced Parkinson's disease: A [(15)O] H2O PET study. *Human Brain Mapping* 30 (no. 12): 3901–3909.

Ballanger, B., T. van Eimeren, E. Moro, A. M. Lozano, C. Hamani, P. Boulinguez, G. Pellecchia, S. Houle, Y. Y. Poon, A. E. Lang, and A. P. Strafella. 2009b. Stimulation of the subthalamic nucleus and impulsivity: Release your horses. *Annals of Neurology* 66 (no. 6): 817–824.

Braak, H., J. R. Bohl, C. M. Muller, U. Rub, R. A. de Vos, and K. Del Tredici. 2006. Stanley Fahn Lecture (2005): The staging procedure for the inclusion body pathology associated with sporadic Parkinson's disease reconsidered. *Mov Disord* 21 (no. 12): 2042–2051.

Brooks, D. J., P. Piccini, N. Turjanski, and M. Samuel. 2000. Neuroimaging of dyskinesia. *Annals of Neurology* 47 (no. 4, Suppl 1): S154–S158.

Calzavara, R., P. Mailly, and S. N. Haber. 2007. Relationship between the corticostriatal terminals from areas 9 and 46, and those from area 8A, dorsal and rostral premotor cortex and area 24c: An anatomical substrate for cognition to action. *European Journal of Neuroscience* 26 (no. 7): 2005–2024.

Canavero, S., V. Bonicalzi, R. Paolotti, G. Castellano, S. Greco-Crasto, L. Rizzo, O. Davini, and R. Maina. 2003. Therapeutic extradural cortical stimulation for movement disorders: A review. *Neurological Research* 25 (no. 2): 118–122.

Canavero, S., R. Paolotti, V. Bonicalzi, G. Castellano, S. Greco-Crasto, L. Rizzo, O. Davini, F. Zenga, and P. Ragazzi. 2002. Extradural motor cortex stimulation for advanced Parkinson disease. Report of two cases. *Journal of Neurosurgery* 97 (no. 5): 1208–1211.

Cools, R. 2006. Dopaminergic modulation of cognitive function-implications for L-DOPA treatment in Parkinson's disease. *Neuroscience and Biobehavioral Reviews* 30 (no. 1): 1–23.

Cools, R., R. A. Barker, B. J. Sahakian, and T. W. Robbins. 2001. Mechanisms of cognitive set flexibility in Parkinson's disease. *Brain* 124 (no. Pt 12): 2503–2512.

Cools, R., E. Stefanova, R. A. Barker, T. W. Robbins, and A. M. Owen. 2002. Dopaminergic modulation of high-level cognition in Parkinson's disease: The role of the prefrontal cortex revealed by PET. *Brain* 125 (no. Pt 3): 584–594.

Dagher, A., A. M. Owen, H. Boecker, and D. J. Brooks. 2001. The role of the striatum and hippocampus in planning: A PET activation study in Parkinson's disease. *Brain* 124 (no. Pt 5): 1020–1032.

Dubois, B. and B. Pillon. 1997. Cognitive deficits in Parkinson's disease. *Journal of Neurology* 244 (no. 1): 2–8.

Eckert, T., T. Peschel, H. J. Heinze, and M. Rotte. 2006. Increased pre-SMA activation in early PD patients during simple self-initiated hand movements. *Journal of Neurology* 253 (no. 2): 199–207.

Evans, A. H., A. D. Lawrence, and A. J. Lees. 2009. Changes in psychomotor effects of L-dopa and methylphenidate after sustained dopaminergic therapy in Parkinson's disease. *Journal of Neurology, Neurosurgery and Psychiatry* 80 (no. 3): 267–272.

Feger, J., O. K. Hassani, and M. Mouroux. 1997. The subthalamic nucleus and its connections. New electrophysiological and pharmacological data. *Advances in Neurology* 74:31–43.

Frank, M. J., J. Samanta, A. A. Moustafa, and S. J. Sherman. 2007. Hold your horses: Impulsivity, deep brain stimulation, and medication in parkinsonism. *Science* 318 (no. 5854): 1309–1312.

Gotham, A. M., R. G. Brown, and C. D. Marsden. 1988. 'Frontal' cognitive function in patients with Parkinson's disease 'on' and 'off' levodopa. *Brain* 111 (Pt 2): 299–321.

Grabli, D., K. McCairn, E. C. Hirsch, Y. Agid, J. Feger, C. Francois, and L. Tremblay. 2004. Behavioural disorders induced by external globus pallidus dysfunction in primates: I. Behavioural study. *Brain* 127 (no. Pt 9): 2039–2054.

Grosset, K. A., D. G. Grosset, G. Macphee, G. Pal, D. Stewart, A. Watt, and J. Davie. 2007. Dopamine agonists and pathological gambling. *Parkinsonism Relat Disord* 13 (no. 4): 259.

Haber, S. N., K. S. Kim, P. Mailly, and R. Calzavara. 2006. Reward-related cortical inputs define a large striatal region in primates that interface with associative cortical connections, providing a substrate for incentive-based learning. *Journal of Neuroscience* 26 (no. 32): 8368–8376.

Haber, S. N., K. Kunishio, M. Mizobuchi, and E. Lynd-Balta. 1995. The orbital and medial prefrontal circuit through the primate basal ganglia. *Journal of Neuroscience* 15 (no. 7, Pt 1): 4851–4867.

Haslinger, B., P. Erhard, N. Kampfe, H. Boecker, E. Rummeny, M. Schwaiger, B. Conrad, and A. O. Ceballos-Baumann. 2001. Event-related functional magnetic resonance imaging in Parkinson's disease before and after levodopa. *Brain* 124 (Pt 3): 558–570.

Huang, C., C. Tang, A. Feigin, M. Lesser, Y. Ma, M. Pourfar, V. Dhawan, and D. Eidelberg. 2007. Changes in network activity with the progression of Parkinson's disease. *Brain* 130 (Pt 7): 1834–1846.

Jahanshahi, M., I. H. Jenkins, R. G. Brown, C. D. Marsden, R. E. Passingham, and D. J. Brooks. 1995. Self-initiated versus externally triggered movements. I. An investigation using measurement of regional cerebral blood flow with PET and movement-related potentials in normal and Parkinson's disease subjects. *Brain* 118 (Pt 4): 913–933.

Jenkins, I. H., W. Fernandez, E. D. Playford, A. J. Lees, R. S. Frackowiak, R. E. Passingham, and D. J. Brooks. 1992. Impaired activation of the supplementary motor area in Parkinson's disease is reversed when akinesia is treated with apomorphine. *Annals of Neurology* 32 (no. 6): 749–757.

Kish, S. J., K. Shannak, and O. Hornykiewicz. 1988. Uneven pattern of dopamine loss in the striatum of patients with idiopathic Parkinson's disease. Pathophysiologic and clinical implications. *New England Journal of Medicine* 318 (no. 14): 876–880.

Kostopoulos, P. and M. Petrides. 2003. The mid-ventrolateral prefrontal cortex: Insights into its role in memory retrieval. *European Journal of Neuroscience* 17 (no. 7): 1489–1497.

Levy, R. and P. S. Goldman-Rakic. 2000. Segregation of working memory functions within the dorsolateral prefrontal cortex. *Experimental Brain Research* 133 (no. 1): 23–32.

Lim, A. S., A. M. Lozano, E. Moro, C. Hamani, W. D. Hutchison, J. O. Dostrovsky, A. E. Lang, R. A. Wennberg, and B. J. Murray. 2007. Characterization of REM-sleep associated ponto-geniculo-occipital waves in the human pons. *Sleep* 30 (no. 7): 823–827.

Limousin, P., J. Greene, P. Pollak, J. Rothwell, A. L. Benabid, and R. Frackowiak. 1997. Changes in cerebral activity pattern due to subthalamic nucleus or internal pallidum stimulation in Parkinson's disease. *Annals of Neurology* 42 (no. 3): 283–291.

Lu, C., A. Bharmal, and O. Suchowersky. 2006. Gambling and Parkinson disease. *Archives of Neurology* 63 (no. 2): 298.

Mattay, V. S., A. Tessitore, J. H. Callicott, A. Bertolino, T. E. Goldberg, T. N. Chase, T. M. Hyde, and D. R. Weinberger. 2002. Dopaminergic modulation of cortical function in patients with Parkinson's disease. *Annals of Neurology* 51 (no. 2): 156–164.

Monchi, O., M. Petrides, J. Doyon, R. B. Postuma, K. Worsley, and A. Dagher. 2004. Neural bases of set-shifting deficits in Parkinson's disease. *Journal of Neuroscience* 24 (no. 3): 702–710.

Monchi, O., M. Petrides, B. Mejia-Constain, and A. P. Strafella. 2007. Cortical activity in Parkinson's disease during executive processing depends on striatal involvement. *Brain* 130 (Pt 1): 233–244.

Nagano-Saito, A., J. Liu, J. Doyon, and A. Dagher. 2009. Dopamine modulates default mode network deactivation in elderly individuals during the Tower of London task. *Neuroscience Letters* 458 (no. 1): 1–5.

Nirenberg, M. J., and C. Waters. 2006. Compulsive eating and weight gain related to dopamine agonist use. *Mov Disord* 21 (no. 4): 524–529.

Owen, A. M. 2004. Cognitive dysfunction in Parkinson's disease: The role of frontostriatal circuitry. *Neuroscientist* 10 (no. 6): 525–537.

Owen, A. M., J. Doyon, A. Dagher, A. Sadikot, and A. C. Evans. 1998. Abnormal basal ganglia outflow in Parkinson's disease identified with PET. Implications for higher cortical functions. *Brain* 121 (Pt 5): 949–965.

Pagni, C. A., S. Zeme, and F. Zenga. 2003. Further experience with extra-dural motor cortex stimulation for treatment of advanced Parkinson's disease. Report of 3 new cases. *Journal of Neurosurgical Sciences* 47 (no. 4): 189–193.

Pahapill, P. A., and A. M. Lozano. 2000. The pedunculopontine nucleus and Parkinson's disease. *Brain* 123 (Pt 9): 1767–1783.

Parent, A. 1990. Extrinsic connections of the basal ganglia. *Trends in Neurosciences* 13 (no. 7): 254–258.

Parent, A., and L. N. Hazrati. 1995a. Functional anatomy of the basal ganglia. I. The cortico-basal ganglia-thalamo-cortical loop. *Brain Research Brain Research Reviews* 20 (no. 1): 91–127.

Parent, A., and L. N. Hazrati. 1995b. Functional anatomy of the basal ganglia. II. The place of subthalamic nucleus and external pallidum in basal ganglia circuitry. *Brain Research Brain Research Reviews* 20 (no. 1): 128–154.

Park, A., and M. Stacy. 2009. Non-motor symptoms in Parkinson's disease. *Journal of Neurology* 256 (Suppl 3): 293–298.

Petrides, M. 2002. The mid-ventrolateral prefrontal cortex and active mnemonic retrieval. *Neurobiology of Learning and Memory* 78 (no. 3): 528–538.

Petrides, M. 2005. Lateral prefrontal cortex: Architectonic and functional organization. *Philos Trans R Soc Lond B Biol Sci* 360 (no. 1456): 781–795.

Petrides, M., and D. N. Pandya. 2002. Comparative cytoarchitectonic analysis of the human and the macaque ventrolateral prefrontal cortex and corticocortical connection patterns in the monkey. *European Journal of Neuroscience* 16 (no. 2): 291–310.

Playford, E. D., I. H. Jenkins, R. E. Passingham, J. Nutt, R. S. Frackowiak, and D. J. Brooks. 1992. Impaired mesial frontal and putamen activation in Parkinson's disease: A positron emission tomography study. *Annals of Neurology* 32 (no. 2): 151–161.

Rascol, O., U. Sabatini, C. Brefel, N. Fabre, S. Rai, J. M. Senard, P. Celsis, G. Viallard, J. L. Montastruc, and F. Chollet. 1998. Cortical motor overactivation in parkinsonian patients with L-dopa-induced peak-dose dyskinesia. *Brain* 121 (Pt 3): 527–533.

Riba, J., U. M. Kramer, M. Heldmann, S. Richter, and T. F. Munte. 2008. Dopamine agonist increases risk taking but blunts reward-related brain activity. *PLoS One* 3 (no. 6): e2479.

Rizzuto, D. S., A. N. Mamelak, W. W. Sutherling, I. Fineman, and R. A. Andersen. 2005. Spatial selectivity in human ventrolateral prefrontal cortex. *Nature Neuroscience* 8 (no. 4): 415–417.

Rosvold, H. E. 1972. The frontal lobe system: Cortical-subcortical inter-relationships. *Acta Neurobiol Exp (Wars)* 32 (no. 2): 439–460.

Rowe, J. B., L. Hughes, B. C. Ghosh, D. Eckstein, C. H. Williams-Gray, S. Fallon, R. A. Barker, and A. M. Owen. 2008. Parkinson's disease and dopaminergic therapy—differential effects on movement, reward and cognition," *Brain* 131 (no. Pt 8): 2094–2105.

Samuel, M., A. O. Ceballos-Baumann, J. Blin, T. Uema, H. Boecker, R. E. Passingham, and D. J. Brooks. 1997a. Evidence for lateral premotor and parietal overactivity in Parkinson's disease during sequential and bimanual movements. A PET study. *Brain* 120 (Pt 6): 963–976.

Samuel, M., A. O. Ceballos-Baumann, N. Turjanski, H. Boecker, A. Gorospe, G. Linazasoro, A. P. Holmes, M. R. DeLong, J. L. Vitek, D. G. Thomas, N. P. Quinn, J. A. Obeso, and D. J. Brooks. 1997b. Pallidotomy in Parkinson's disease increases supplementary motor area and prefrontal activation during performance of volitional movements an H2(15)O PET study. *Brain* 120 (Pt 8): 1301–1313.

Steeves, T. D., J. Miyasaki, M. Zurowski, A. E. Lang, G. Pellecchia, T. van Eimeren, P. Rusjan, S. Houle, and A. P. Strafella. 2009. Increased striatal dopamine release in Parkinsonian patients with pathological gambling: A [11C] raclopride PET study. *Brain* 132 (no. Pt 5): 1376–1385.

Strafella, A. P., A. Dagher, and A. F. Sadikot. 2003. Cerebral blood flow changes induced by subthalamic stimulation in Parkinson's disease. *Neurology* 60 (no. 6): 1039–1042.

Strafella, A. P., A. M. Lozano, A. E. Lang, J. H. Ko, Y. Y. Poon, and E. Moro. 2007. Subdural motor cortex stimulation in Parkinson's disease does not modify movement-related rCBF pattern. *Mov Disord* 22 (no. 14): 2113–2116.

Strafella, A. P., A. F. Sadikot, and A. Dagher. 2003. Subthalamic deep brain stimulation does not induce striatal dopamine release in Parkinson's disease. *Neuroreport* 14 (no. 9): 1287–1289.

Swainson, R., R. D. Rogers, B. J. Sahakian, B. A. Summers, C. E. Polkey, and T. W. Robbins. 2000. Probabilistic learning and reversal deficits in patients with Parkinson's disease or frontal or temporal lobe lesions: Possible adverse effects of dopaminergic medication. *Neuropsychologia* 38 (no. 5): 596–612.

Taylor, A. E., and J. A. Saint-Cyr. 1995. The neuropsychology of Parkinson's disease. *Brain Cogn* 28 (no. 3): 281–296.

Taylor, A. E., J. A. Saint-Cyr, and A. E. Lang. 1986. Frontal lobe dysfunction in Parkinson's disease. The cortical focus of neostriatal outflow. *Brain* 109 (Pt 5): 845–883.

van Eimeren, T., B. Ballanger, G. Pellecchia, J. M. Miyasaki, A. E. Lang, and A. P. Strafella. 2009a. Dopamine agonists diminish value sensitivity of the orbitofrontal cortex: A trigger for pathological gambling in Parkinson's disease? *Neuropsychopharmacology* 34 (no. 13): 2758–2766.

van Eimeren, T., O. Monchi, B. Ballanger, and A. P. Strafella. 2009b. Dysfunction of the default mode network in Parkinson disease: A functional magnetic resonance imaging study. *Archives of Neurology* 66 (no. 7): 877–883.

van Eimeren T., G. Pellecchia, J. Miyasaki, B. Ballanger, T. Steeves, S. Houle, A. E. Lang, and A. Strafella. 2009c. Tonic stimulation of the orbitofrontal cortex by dopamine agonists in PD wipes out reward processing and increases risk taking behaviour: Are they at risk of gambling? *Movement Disorders* 24: Abstract S217.

Voon, V., and S. H. Fox. 2007. Medication-related impulse control and repetitive behaviors in Parkinson disease. *Archives of Neurology* 64 (no. 8): 1089–1096.

Voon, V., K. Hassan, M. Zurowski, M. de Souza, T. Thomsen, S. Fox, A. E. Lang, and J. Miyasaki. 2006. Prevalence of repetitive and reward-seeking behaviors in Parkinson disease. *Neurology* 67 (no. 7): 1254–1257.

Voon, V., T. Thomsen, J. M. Miyasaki, M. de Souza, A. Shafro, S. H. Fox, S. Duff-Canning, A. E. Lang, and M. Zurowski. 2007. Factors associated with dopaminergic drug-related pathological gambling in Parkinson disease. *Archives of Neurology* 64 (no. 2): 212–216.

Weintraub, D. 2008. Dopamine and impulse control disorders in Parkinson's disease. *Annals of Neurology* 64 (Suppl 2): S93–100.

Weintraub, D., C. L. Comella, and S. Horn. 2008. Parkinson's disease— Part 3: Neuropsychiatric symptoms. *American Journal of Managed Care* 14 (no. 2 Suppl): S59–S69.

Weintraub, D., A. D. Siderowf, M. N. Potenza, J. Goveas, K. H. Morales, J. E. Duda, P. J. Moberg, and M. B. Stern. 2006. Association of dopamine agonist use with impulse control disorders in Parkinson disease. *Archives of Neurology* 63 (no. 7): 969–973.

Williams-Gray, C. H., T. Foltynie, C. E. Brayne, T. W. Robbins, and R. A. Barker. 2007. Evolution of cognitive dysfunction in an incident Parkinson's disease cohort. *Brain* 130 (no. Pt 7): 1787–1798.

Williams-Gray, C. H., A. Hampshire, R. A. Barker, and A. M. Owen. 2008. Attentional control in Parkinson's disease is dependent on COMT val 158 met genotype. *Brain* 131 (no. Pt 2): 397–408.

Zgaljardic, D. J., N. S. Foldi, and J. C. Borod. 2004. Cognitive and behavioral dysfunction in Parkinson's disease: Neurochemical and clinicopathological contributions. *Journal of Neural Transmission* 111 (no. 10–11): 1287–1301.

9

FUNCTIONAL MARKERS OF COGNITION IN PARKINSON'S DISEASE

^{18}F-FDG AND H_2 ^{15}O POSITRON EMISSION TOMOGRAPHY STUDIES

Paul J. Mattis and Maren Carbon

Parkinson's disease (PD) is characterized by motor symptoms including resting tremor, rigidity, and bradykinesia. However, cognitive and behavioral problems in PD are common (Emre et al. 2007) and have a significant relationship to quality of life (Aarsland et al. 1999; Martinez-Martin et al. 2009). The prevalence of dementia in patients with PD has conservatively been estimated to range between 24% and 31% (Aarsland et al. 2005). The cognitive profile observed in PD patients with dementia (PDD) is substantially different than that of the primarily cortical dementia of Alzheimer's disease (AD). Patients with PDD typically exhibit difficulties with executive functions, the retrieval aspects of memory, and visuospatial skills (Aarsland et al. 2005). This pattern of cognitive decline is often characterized as subcortical dementia to differentiate it from disorders such as AD that affect cortical areas early in the disease process and often include clear aphasia, apraxia, or agnosia (see Table 1). The onset of dementia in PD is insidious, typically occurring years after the onset of motor symptoms. However, cognitive difficulties have been observed even in early PD (Foltynie et al. 2004). The pattern of early cognitive dysfunction in PD is believed to be generally similar to that of PDD (Huang et al. 2007b; Green et al. 2002).

The pathophysiology of cognitive symptoms in PD likely differs from the pathophysiology of motor symptoms (Mentis et al. 2002; Lozza et al. 2004; Huang et al. 2007a). In vivo imaging data and postmortem studies suggest multiple, potentially interrelated mechanisms of disease, including dopamine depletion in the striatum and, to a far lesser degree, in the prefrontal cortex. Disruption of dopamine levels at either site may lead to frontal-like deficits either directly or via downstream effects in striato-pallidal-thalamocortical loops (CSPTC) (Scatton et al. 1982;

Monchi et al. 2007; Jokinen et al. 2009). In this vein, the heterogeneity of cognitive deficits prior to the development of PDD could result from a differential involvement of segregated dorsolateral, orbitofrontal, and medial prefrontal CSPTC loops (Wichmann and DeLong 1996; Goldman-Rakic 1998; Swainson et al. 2000). Importantly, additional evidence points to widespread cortical cholinergic dysfunction as a factor of cognitive decline in PD (Hilker et al. 2005; Shimada et al. 2009; Klein et al. 2010; for review see Bohnen and Albin 2010). Adrenergic (Scatton et al. 1983; Pavese et al. 2010) and serotonergic (Scatton et al. 1983; Guttman et al. 2007; Boileau et al. 2008) deficits have also been described in PD but are associated with behavioral rather than cognitive function. Moreover, other pathological processes, such as regional cortical Lewy body formation, are also likely to contribute to cognitive decline in PD (Kovari et al. 2003; Lyoo et al. 2010).

The functional effects of these pathologies can be assessed in vivo with resting state metabolic imaging using radio-labeled glucose (^{18}F-FDG) and positron emission tomography (PET) as well as during the performance of cognitive tasks using radiolabeled water (H_2 ^{15}O) and PET. Local measurements of FDG uptake reflect mainly afferent synaptic activity (Sibson et al. 1998). By contrast, H_2 ^{15}O PET measurements of regional cerebral blood flow reflect changes in local field potentials, i.e., afferent synaptic input and local processing subsequent to the input (Lauritzen 2001). Since the advent of functional magnetic resonance imaging (fMRI), one may question the reasons for continued use of radiolabeled tracers. However, resting state studies with fMRI have only recently been found informative through the use of novel analytical techniques. More importantly, in the case of movement disorders, fMRI is not suited to examine the effects of deep brain stimulation (DBS), an

TABLE 1: PATTERN OF NEUROPSYCHOLOGICAL IMPAIRMENT IN PARKINSON'S DISEASE, DIFFUSE LEWY BODY DISEASE AND ALZHEIMER'S DISEASE

	PD	DLB	AD
Orientation	Ø	Ø	↓
Immediate recall	↓	↓	↓
Delayed recall	↓	↓↓	↓↓↓
Recognition memory	Ø	↓	↓
Executive functioning	↓↓	↓↓↓	↓
Naming	↓	↓↓	↓↓↓
Verbal Fluency	↓↓	↓↓↓	↓
Visuospatial	↓↓	↓↓	↓

increasingly used but still incompletely understood anti-parkinsonian intervention (Poewe 2009).

METABOLIC MARKERS OF COGNITIVE DECLINE: RESTING STATE STUDIES

Although PD has traditionally been conceptualized as a subcortical dementia, resting state FDG PET has consistently revealed cortical prefrontal and lateral parietal hypometabolism in early non-demented PD patients (Mentis et al. 2002; Huang et al. 2007a; Huang et al. 2008). There is also evidence to support the idea that over the course of the disease, these metabolic reductions extend spatially to include occipital and medial frontal regions at moderately advanced disease stages (Mohr et al. 1992; Hilker et al. 2004; Hosokai et al. 2009; Borghammer et al. 2010). In fact, in patients with PDD, more widespread hypometabolism has been observed in parietal, occipital, and frontal cortex, as well as anterior cingulate, suggesting a progression of cortical hypometabolism in parallel to cognitive decline (Peppard et al. 1990; Hilker et al. 2004; Yong et al. 2007; Hosokai et al. 2009). It is currently unclear whether or not this extension of hypometabolism relates to local cortical pathology or to deficient subcortical modulation. Consistent with the shared characteristic of widespread cortical cholinergic deficits found in Alzheimer's disease (AD) and PDD (for review see Bohnen and Albin 2010), cortical hypometabolism in advanced PDD shows similarities with AD (Peppard et al. 1990), and Diffuse Lewy Body Disease (DLBD) (Yong et al. 2007).

Nevertheless, metabolic reductions are more pronounced and widespread in AD and DLBD than in PDD. Interestingly, the regional distribution of hypometabolism in vivo has been suggested (Yong et al. 2007) to parallel the distribution of Lewy body formation as documented in postmortem histological studies of PDD and DLBD (Harding et al. 2002).

Although dementia is common in advanced PD, circumscribed cognitive deficits, such as deficits in executive strategies, attentional set-shifting, working memory, and temporal sequencing, can be present in the early stages of the disease (Rodriguez-Oroz et al. 2009). The presence of cognitive deficits upon assessment, but without significant decline in daily functioning, is termed "mild cognitive impairment (MCI)." Comparisons of PD patients with and without MCI suggest that the extent and intensity of abnormal cortical hypometabolism reflects the severity of cognitive impairment (Peppard et al. 1990; Yong et al. 2007; Hosokai et al. 2009). PD patients without cognitive dysfunction exhibited only very circumscribed frontal hypometabolism (Hosokai et al. 2009), whereas those with MCI exhibited greater metabolic reductions in temporal and parietal cortices, and premotor areas. Furthermore, PD subjects with deficient performance in more than one cognitive area (multiple domain MCI) have been found to exhibit reduced metabolism in the inferior parietal lobule and middle frontal gyrus compared to those patients with impairment in a single cognitive area (single domain MCI). Surprisingly, PD patients with single-domain or multiple-domain MCI showed increased cingulate metabolism compared to PD patients without MCI and normal controls (Huang et al. 2008).

Abnormal prefrontal metabolism has been specifically linked to working memory deficits in PD (Lozza et al. 2004; Nagano-Saito et al. 2004). Using network analysis, Marié and colleagues (1995) observed a positive correlation between prefrontal glucose metabolism and working memory deficit in PD, whereas an inverse correlation was observed with the mediodorsal thalamic nucleus, suggesting a relationship between working memory dysfunction and subcortico-frontal networks. While informative with regard to mechanisms of cognitive decline in PD, these relationships are not necessarily disease-specific, and their prospective value remains to be demonstrated.

To identify PD-specific metabolic brain networks, Eidelberg et al. have applied a voxel-based spatial covariance approach to the analysis of resting state FDG PET data (Eidelberg 2009). This approach has allowed for the identification of abnormal disease-related metabolic patterns

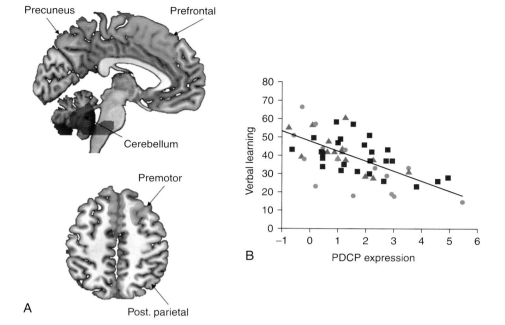

A

B

Figure 1 The Parkinson's Disease Cognition-Related Pattern (PDCP). **A.** Spatial covariance analysis of FDG PET scans during the resting state in Parkinson's disease (PD) identified significant covarying metabolism associated with measures of cognitive performance (Huang et al. 2007a). This pattern was characterized by relative metabolic decreases in the medial prefrontal cortex, premotor cortex, and posterior parietal cortex associated with metabolic increases in the cerebellum. The pattern was superimposed on a single-subject MRI T1 template. The color scale represents voxels that contribute significantly to the network at P = 0.001 and that were demonstrated to be reliable (p < 0.001) on bootstrap estimation. Voxels with positive region weights (metabolic increases) are color-coded red; those with negative region weights (metabolic decreases) are color-coded blue. [Reproduced with permission from Elsevier, Huang 2007 34:714–723]. **B.** PDCP expression correlates with performance on neuropsychological tests of memory and executive functioning in non-demented PD patients. For the California Verbal Learning Test: Sum 1 to 5 (CVLT sum), this correlation was significant for the entire cohort (n = 56, r = –0.67, p < 0.001), as well as for the original group used for pattern derivation (*circles*: n = 15, r = –0.71, p = 0.003) and in two prospective validation groups (*squares*: n = 25, r = –0.53, p = 0.007; *triangles*: n = 16: r = –0.80, p < 0.001) (Huang et al. 2007a). [Reproduced with permission from Elsevier, Eidelberg 2009 32:548–557].

(i.e., brain networks) and the quantification of the expression of these patterns (i.e., network activity) in individual subjects. In addition to the Parkinson's disease-related motor pattern (see Chapters 3 and 12), Huang et al. (2007a) identified and validated a distinct cognition-related metabolic pattern (PDCP) in non-demented PD patients (Figure 1A). This pattern is characterized by metabolic reductions in frontal and parietal association areas, with relative metabolic increases in the cerebellum. The PDCP has been demonstrated to correlate with neuropsychological measures commonly associated with the subcortical dementia syndrome, with network expression most strongly associated with performance on tests of memory and executive functioning (Figure 1B); a less robust relationship with visuospatial and perceptual-motor speed has been observed (Huang et al. 2007b). PDCP subject scores exhibited a stepwise increase in PD patients without MCI, with MCI, and with dementia (Figure 2). Furthermore, recent data (Tang et al. 2011) showed that abnormally elevated PDCP expression is associated with

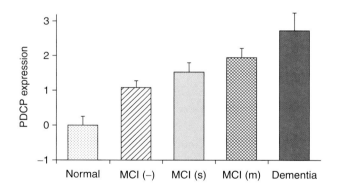

Figure 2 PDCP Expression Increases with Cognitive Decline. Prospective calculation of PDCP network expression (*bar graph*) in healthy controls and PD patients with varying degrees of cognitive impairment showed a significant stepwise increase of PDCP expression with increasing loss of cognitive function (Eidelberg 2009). PD groups included all stages of cognitive impairment from patients without cognitive impairment (*far left*) to PD-related dementia (*far right*); transitioning through minimal cognitive impairment in a single domain (MCI-s) and minimal cognitive impairment in multiple domains (MCI-m). [Reproduced with permission from Elsevier, Eidelberg 2009 32:548–557].

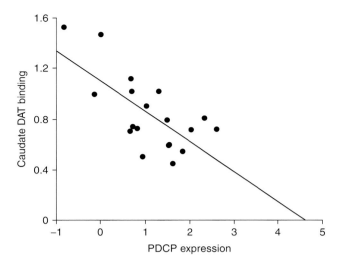

Figure 3 Relationship between PDCP expression and caudate binding. In 19 PD patients who underwent both FDG PET and FPCIT PET imaging, PDCP expression was found to have a significant inverse correlation (r = –0.67, p < 0.0003) with DAT binding in the caudate nucleus. (Courtesy of Dr. M. Niethammer).

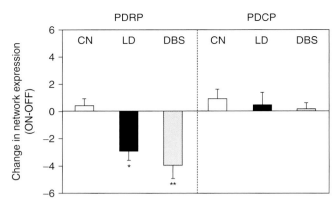

Figure 4 Effect of treatment on PDRP and PDCP expression. Bar graph illustrating mean (±SE) treatment-mediated changes in the expression of the PDRP (*left*) and PDCP (*right*) (Huang et al. 2007a). ON-OFF differences in network activity with levodopa infusion (LD: *black*) and subthalamic nucleus deep brain stimulation (DBS; *gray*) compared with changes in network activity without intervention (CN; *white*). Significant treatment-mediated changes were observed only for the motor-related PDRP network. [*p < 0.05, **p < 0.01] [Reproduced with permission from Elsevier, Huang 2007 34:714–723].

reduced dopaminergic function in the caudate nucleus in individual patients with PD (Figure 3).

The PDCP has some regional overlap with the PDRP. However, these network biomarkers are dissociable in multiple ways (Huang et al. 2007a, b; Feigin et al. 2007; Lin et al. 2008). PDRP is closely related to scores on the motor UPDRS (Eidelberg 2009). In a longitudinal study (Huang et al. 2007b), PDRP expression was found to be only slightly elevated in early disease, and a significantly abnormal degree of PDCP expression can be discerned approximately six years after symptom onset. In other words, network expression parallels symptom onset, with the motor manifestations preceding the development of cognitive dysfunction.

While PDRP expression is sensitive to pharmacologic and surgical therapies directed at the motor manifestations of the disease (Asanuma et al. 2006; Trost et al. 2006), PDCP expression is generally unaffected by these interventions (Huang et al. 2007a). Studies examining the effect of levodopa (LD) infusion and pallidal (GPi) or subthalamic (STN) DBS have demonstrated significant PDRP suppression with successful suppression of motor symptoms (Asanuma et al. 2006). By contrast, while showing highly heterogeneous effects on cognitive performance, these interventions did not robustly alter PDCP expression (Figure 4). However, LD-mediated changes in cognitive functioning, specifically verbal learning, were recently found to be associated with altered PDCP expression at the individual subject level (Mattis et al. in press). Of note, the treatment-mediated

PDCP changes were found to be independent of concurrent changes in motor functioning and/or PDRP expression. Interestingly, when stratified based on reliable change index (RCI) analysis of performance measures (Maassen 2004), those patients with a positive cognitive response to LD exhibited a significant concomitant suppression of PDCP activity. By contrast, there were no treatment-induced changes in PDCP activity in those patients who did not experience an improvement in verbal learning with LD. Further, in a cohort of PD subjects receiving placebo in expectation of a treatment improving cognition, a subgroup exhibited an improvement in verbal learning. However, in these patients, considered to have a significant placebo effect, there was no associated change in PDCP expression. Moreover, we found that the catechol O-methyltransferase (COMT; 22q11.2) genotype was a significant predictor of the degree of change in PDCP activity experienced with LD treatment. Importantly, while meaningful for LD-mediated cognitive changes, the COMT genotype was not associated with baseline descriptors (motor UPDRS score, baseline verbal learning, and PDCP, PDRP) or LD-mediated PDRP changes (Mattis et al. 2011).

ACTIVATION DEFICITS IN COGNITIVE TASKS

The basal ganglia have been shown to mediate specific aspects of motor learning, especially the process of combining individual movements into sequences (Beauchamp et al. 2008). Thus, given resting state functional abnormalities in this region in PD patients, motor sequence learning was chosen as a behavioral paradigm for the study of brain-performance relationships in PD (Carbon and Eidelberg 2006; Doyon 2008). In a series of experiments conducted with $H_2^{15}O$ PET, participants performed an explicit, externally paced motor sequence learning task (MSEQ) while in the PET scanner. Performance was recorded in all subjects during the scan. Although cognitively less challenging than more complex paradigms (see below), motor sequence learning is particularly suited to study learning mechanisms during imaging, as behavioral changes can be measured during the short duration time of single scans.

Network analysis has been used to identify brain activation patterns that correlated with measures of retrieval and acquisition during MSEQ in healthy subjects (Nakamura et al. 2001; Carbon et al. 2003). The retrieval pattern comprised bilateral activation of the dorsolateral and inferior prefrontal cortex, the rostrocaudal premotor cortex, and the occipital association cortices, as well as activation of the anterior cingulate area. The acquisition pattern importantly included caudate nucleus activation in conjunction with the cerebellar dentate nucleus, and left ventral prefrontal as well as inferior parietal activation. Early- and advanced-stage PD patients exhibited activation of the retrieval-related motor sequence learning pattern but did not express the normal acquisition-related pattern (Nakamura et al. 2001; Carbon et al. 2002). By contrast, acquisition in PD was related to bilateral dorso-lateral prefrontal cortex (DLPFC) activation (Nakamura et al. 2001; Carbon et al. 2002). It has been demonstrated that the dopaminergic modulation of cortical activation serves to improve the signal-to-noise ratio and to subsequently focus prefrontal activation. The observed bilateralization can thus be understood to reflect the loss of dopaminergic modulation in early PD. In fact, Carbon et al. (2004) subsequently showed that increased prefrontal activation partly reflects a loss of dopaminergic mesocortical focusing function in the DLPFC. Alternatively, this bilateralization may be indicative of a compensatory effort of homologous brain areas. Utilizing a cognitively more challenging trial-and-error guided sequence learning task, Mentis et al. (2003) supported the latter alternative. In order to achieve a comparable level of performance as controls, early PD patients showed a significant bilateralization of dorsolateral prefrontal, premotor, and parietal activation. Interestingly, a similar compensatory mechanism was found during a verbal working memory task (Grossman et al. 2003).

In addition to resting state experiments, activation studies have been employed to assess cognitive decline in PD patients over time. Carbon et al. (2010) studied sequence learning and related brain activation responses in a group of early-stage PD patients over the course of two years. The authors utilized the MSEQ paradigm along with an observational sequence learning task to control for motor-related changes. Surprisingly, there was only a marginal, non-significant decline in sequence learning performance at the group level, with a wide range of variance in the longitudinal development of learning measures. Despite this behavioral variability, a significant decline in sequence-learning related brain activation responses was found in the DLPFC, precuneus, and parietal association cortex (Figure 5). Longitudinal activation increases were localized to the dorsal anterior cingulate. In order to identify compensatory brain activation responses, the authors made use of the behavioral variability and studied those subjects who maintained stable performance levels throughout the two-year observation period. These high-performing PD subjects exhibited increased activation of the right hippocampus. A similar shift from striatal to hippocampus activation has been found previously and is thought to represent increased use of declarative memory strategies in the presence of deficient implicit learning (see below).

The presence of frontal-like deficits in PD prompted a series of imaging studies using frontal activation paradigms (Jagust et al. 1992; Jenkins et al. 1992). Using the Tower of London (TOL) task as a paradigm for higher executive functioning, Owen et al. (Dagher et al. 1999; Owen and Doyon 1999) reported significantly reduced pallidal activation concomitant to normal prefrontal activation in moderately advanced PD patients. However, with increasing difficulty during the TOL task, impaired activation of the cingulate cortex and caudate nucleus was identified (Dagher et al. 2001). Moreover, PD patients shifted from striatal to abnormal hippocampal processing, possibly indicating the inappropriate use of declarative memory strategies in the presence of impaired implicit striatum-mediated learning (Dagher et al. 2001). This hypothesis was recently further substantiated in a recent study (Beauchamp et al. 2008) in which PD patients in a two-hour learning session were able to improve their performance on the TOL task. This was attributed to enhanced activation of the DLPFC and hippocampus. Moreover, frontopolar and posterior cingulate activation were abnormally sustained throughout the learning period.

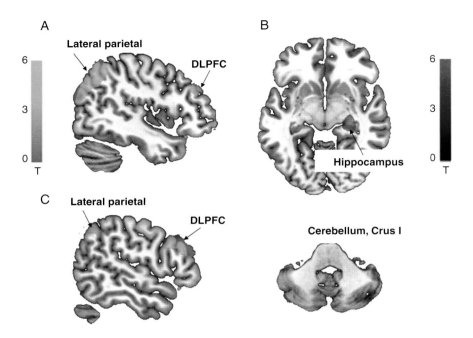

Figure 5 Longitudinal changes in brain activation during sequence learning. Reduced brain activation in the dorsolateral prefrontal cortex (DLPFC) and in the lateral parietal cortex during motor and visual sequence learning (**A**), as well as trial-and-error guided sequence learning (**C**). Additional decreases during the more challenging trial-and-error guided sequence learning were present in the cerebellar cortex (**C**, *right*). The subgroup of subjects who maintained high performance throughout the two-year observation exhibited increased hippocampal activation at follow-up (**B**), indicating a shift from deficient striatal to compensatory hippocampal activation. [SPM{t} maps were superimposed on a single-subject MRI T1 template. The color scale represents T-values thresholded at 3.0 corresponding to p < 0.001 uncorrected.]

TREATMENT-INDUCED CHANGES IN ACTIVATION DURING THE PERFORMANCE OF COGNITIVE TASKS

The effects of medical or surgical antiparkinsonian therapy on cognitive functioning have been found to be highly heterogeneous (Carbon et al. 2003; Cools 2006; Hirano et al. 2009; Jahanshahi et al. 2010). Behavioral and neuroimaging studies in PD patients and experimental models have associated this heterogeneity to (i) task-specific differences in regional activation responses, (ii) differences in the degree/location of dopaminergic denervation depending on the stage of disease progression, (iii) baseline genetic features such as the COMT genotype, and (iv) individual treatment status (Cools 2006).

In a series of studies, the motor sequence learning paradigm was used to assess performance modulation and related brain activation responses during medical and surgical antiparkinsonian treatment (Fukuda et al. 2002; Feigin et al. 2003; Carbon et al. 2003; Argyelan et al. 2007, 2008). On a group level, GPi and STN stimulation was associated with improved sequence learning performance, whereas LD was not (Argyelan et al. 2008). Changes in task performance during LD infusion depended on baseline performance. Bad learners profited from LD, whereas

performance in good learners declined with treatment (Argyelan et al. 2008). Concomitantly, the activity of normal sequence learning-related networks was reduced with LD. Additional changes were characterized by a loss of the normal sequence learning response in the ventromedial prefrontal cortex and in the posterior insula. The loss of ventromedial prefrontal cortex deactivation points to a deficient modulation of the default mode network in PD. Levodopa also induced an abnormally increased response in the pre-supplementary motor cortex, while a recovery to the normal level of response was present in the premotor cortex (Argyelan et al. 2008).

Treatment-mediated normalization of prefrontal activation has also been suggested by other studies using the TOL paradigm and a variant of the n-back task (Cools et al. 2002; Mattay et al. 2002). Although deficits in accuracy of task performance were related to abnormally increased prefrontal activation, this normalization was not accompanied by clear performance improvement. The authors interpreted their findings as a support for the specific, beneficial effect of LD on mesocortical dopaminergic pathways. This interpretation is in keeping with animal models (Goldman-Rakic 1998; for review see Kulisevsky 2000), which have shown that dopaminergic input to the prefrontal cortex leads to a reduction of memory receptive fields in parallel to

TABLE 1: FUNCTIONAL CONSEQUENCES OF REGIONAL LEWY BODY PATHOLOGY IN PD AND DEMENTIA. NEURONAL DEGENERATION RESULTING IN THE DYSFUNCTION OF MULTIPLE SUBCORTICAL NEUROMODULATOR PROJECTIONS ALONG WITH REGIONAL LEWY BODY PATHOLOGY IN SUBCORTICAL AND CORTICAL REGIONS HAS BEEN DESCRIBED (KALAITZAKIS AND PEARCE 2009)

Cortex	Local neuronal degeneration and/or disruption of local neural circuits
Limbic System	Local neuronal degeneration and/or disruption of local neural circuits
Substantia Nigra/Ventral Tegmental Area	Degeneration of striatal, limbic, and ascending mesofrontal cortical dopaminergic projections
Nucleus Basalis of Meynert	Degeneration of limbic and ascending cortical cholinergic projections
Pedunculopontine Nucleus & Laterodorsal Tegmental Nucleus	Degeneration of ascending subcortical cholinergic projections
Locus Ceruleus	Degeneration of noradrenergic subcortical and cortical projections
Raphe Nucleus	Degeneration of serotonergic subcortical and cortical projections

PD patients is found to improve functions of working memory and cognitive sequencing, more pure measures of executive functioning do not show significant benefit with dopaminergic agents (Cooper et al. 1992; Gotham, Brown, and Marsden 1988). In addition to the well-known dopaminergic reductions, cholinergic system degeneration is also an early feature of PD and worsens with the appearance of dementia (Ruberg et al. 1986; Shimada et al. 2009). For example, significant loss of cholinergic forebrain neurons has been reported in PD brains (Whitehouse et al. 1983), and a postmortem study found greater reductions of acetylcholinesterase (AChE) in the frontal cortex of demented (−68%) compared to non-demented (−35%) patients with PD (Ruberg et al. 1986). Lewy first identified the eponymous Lewy body in neurons of the nbM (Lewy 1913), the source of cholinergic innervation of the cerebral cortex. Cholinergic denervation may occur early in PD. For example, nigral and magnocellular basal forebrain pathologies occur simultaneously in the Braak et al. staging schema of PD pathology (Braak et al. 2003).

CHOLINERGIC MARKERS

There are two major sources of cholinergic projections in the brain. First, magnocellular neurons of the basal forebrain provide widespread cholinergic input to the telencephalon (Mesulam and Geula 1988; Mesulam 1996). Cholinergic neurons of the medial septal nucleus (also known as the Ch1 cell group) and the vertical limb nucleus of the diagonal band (Ch2) provide the major cholinergic input of the hippocampus; cholinergic neurons of the horizontal limb nucleus of the diagonal band (Ch3) provide the major cholinergic input of the olfactory bulb; and cholinergic neurons of the nbM (or Ch4) provide the principal cholinergic input of the remaining cerebral cortex and amygdala (Mesulam, Mufson, Levy et al. 1983; Everitt et al. 1988). Trajectories of cholinergic pathways containing AChE within the cerebral hemispheres of the human brain have been identified (Selden et al. 1998).

Second, the pedunculopontine nucleus-laterodorsal tegmental complex (PPN-LDTC; hereafter referred to as the PPN), a brainstem center, provides cholinergic inputs to the thalamus, cerebellum, several brainstem nuclei, some striatal fibers, and the spinal cord (Mesulam, Mufson, Wainer et al. 1983; Heckers, Geula, and Mesulam 1992). The striatum contains a population of cholinergic interneurons, and small populations of cholinergic neurons are present in the cortex, the medial habenula, and parts of the reticular formation (de Lacalle, Hersh, and Saper 1993; Fibiger 1982; Mesulam et al. 1992; Lecourtier and Kelly 2007). Figure 1 illustrates the two major cholinergic projection systems in the brain: a cortical system originating from the nbM and a subcortical system originating mainly from the brainstem PPN and laterodorsal tegmental nucleus.

Neurochemical, histochemical, immunohistochemical, and radiotracer imaging identification of cholinergic neurons and pathways depends on cholinergic neuron expression of proteins dedicated to acetylcholine synthesis, storage, and degradation (Table 2). Choline acetyltransferase (ChAT) and AChE are the two ubiquitous constituents of cholinergic pathways of the human brain (Mesulam and Geula 1992). Acetylcholine is synthesized via acetylation of choline by the cytosolic enzyme ChAT and then pumped into

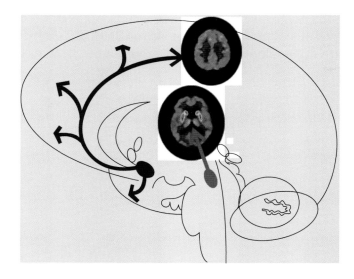

Figure 1 Schematic overview of the major cholinergic cerebral projections. The major cortical input originates from cholinergic forebrain neurons (in blue), whereas thalamic inputs have significant origination from brainstem cholinergic nuclei (pedunculopontine nucleus and laterodorsal tegmental nucleus; in red). Representative transaxial slices of [C-11]PMP AChE PET images (summed radioactivity images 0–25 minutes post-injection) illustrate the utility of this imaging technique to assess the integrity of the two major ascending cholinergic systems in the brain.

synaptic vesicles by the vesicular acetylcholine transporter (VAChT). After exocytosis, acetylcholine is degraded within the synapse by cholinesterase enzymes located on both pre- and postsynaptic membranes. There are two principal cholinesterases in the human brain: AChE and butyrylcholinesterase (BuChE). AChE has a neuronal and BuChE a neuroglial distribution (Wright, Geula, and Mesulam 1993). Acetylcholine is hydrolyzed by both AChE and BuChE, but AChE catalyzes the hydrolysis of acetylcholine much more efficiently than BuChE. The physiological role of BuChE is poorly understood, but studies from AChE knockout mice show that this enzyme may have the potential to substitute

TABLE 2: CHOLINERGIC MARKERS IN PATHOLOGY AND IN VIVO LIGAND IMAGING

	Pathology marker	Radioligand
Acetyltransferase (ChAT)	√	None
Vesicular acetylcholine transporter (VAChT)	√	√
Acetylcholinesterase (AChE)	√	√
Butyrylcholinesterase (BuChE)	√	√
Nicotinic cholinergic receptors (nAChR)	√	√
Muscarinic cholinergic receptors (mAChR)	√	√

for AChE (Mesulam et al. 2002). AChE has been recognized since 1966 as a reliable marker for brain cholinergic pathways, including in the human brain (Shute and Lewis 1966). The distribution of AChE enzyme activity is highest in the basal ganglia and the basal forebrain nucleus, intermediate in the cerebellum, and lower in the cortex (Atack et al. 1986).

EX VIVO PATHOLOGY FINDINGS OF THE CHOLINERGIC SYSTEM IN PD AND PARKINSONIAN DEMENTIA

ALZHEIMER'S DISEASE IS ASSOCIATED WITH CORTICAL BUT NO SIGNIFICANT SUBCORTICAL CHOLINERGIC DEFICITS

Substantial loss of the cholinergic innervation of the cerebral cortex is accepted as a major pathological feature of advanced AD (Geula and Mesulam 1989). This is most severe in the temporal lobes, including the entorhinal cortex, in which up to 80% of cholinergic axons can be depleted (Mesulam and Geula 1988; Geula and Mesulam 1996, 1999). In contrast to the degeneration of the basal forebrain complex, the cholinergic innervation of the striatum (mainly originating from striatal interneurons) and of the thalamus (mainly originating from the brainstem PPN) remain relatively intact. Therefore, there is no general cholinergic lesion in AD (Mesulam 2004).

PARKINSON'S DISEASE AND DEMENTIA

A key pathologic event of PD is loss of midbrain neurons in the substantia nigra, pars compacta, and their terminals in the striatum. In addition to the well-known reductions in dopamine, there is convergent evidence for alterations in cholinergic neurotransmission in PD. For example, muscarinic binding and ChAT activity are reduced in the pars compacta of the substantia nigra (Ruberg et al. 1982), hippocampus, and especially in the neocortex (Lange et al. 1993). A postmortem autoradiographic study of the nicotinic cholinergic receptor ligand 5-[I-125]-A-85380 demonstrated loss of striatal binding that closely paralleled the loss of nigrostriatal dopaminergic markers (Pimlott et al. 2004). At postmortem losses of nicotinic receptors of up to 30% have been reported in the striatum and thalamus of PD subjects (Schmaljohann et al. 2006). The reduction in cortical nicotinic cholinergic receptor numbers in PD patients appears also to parallel the degree of dementia observed with progression of the disease (Whitehouse et al. 1988; Aubert et al. 1992). Loss of cholinergic neurons in the nbM has been reported in PD brains, as it also has in AD (Arendt et al. 1983; Whitehouse et al. 1983; Candy et al. 1983; Nakano and Hirano 1984; Tagliavini et al. 1984; Rogers, Brogan, and Mirra 1985). Arendt et al. found even greater forebrain neuronal loss in PD than in AD (Arendt et al. 1983), suggesting that cholinergic deficits may be at least as prominent in PD as in AD. Similarly, a postmortem study found greater reductions of AChE in the frontal cortex of demented (−68%) compared to non-demented (−35%) patients with PD (Ruberg et al. 1986). Therefore, degeneration of the cholinergic system may play a significant role in the cognitive decline in PD. Although dementia in PD has often been attributed to co−existent AD pathology (Mahler and Cummings 1990), cognitive impairment has been found to correlate with cortical ChAT levels but not with the extent of plaque or tangle formation in PD (Mattila et al. 2001; Perry et al. 1985).

Unlike relatively preserved subcortical cholinergic innervation in AD, there is postmortem evidence of decreased brainstem cholinergic functions in at least a subset of PD. For example, there are reports that about 50% of the large cholinergic neurons of the lateral part of the PPN, pars compacta, degenerate in PD (Hirsch et al. 1987; Jellinger 1988; Zweig et al. 1989; Gai et al. 1991). The PPN is a brainstem locomotor center (Lee, Rinne, and Marsden 2000), and PPN dysfunction has been associated with dopamine-resistant akinesia in PD (Stein 2009).

IN VIVO IMAGING FINDINGS OF THE CHOLINERGIC SYSTEM IN PD AND PARKINSONIAN DEMENTIA

Neurochemical PET (positron emission tomography) or SPECT (single photon emission computed tomography) imaging studies complement neuropathology studies by allowing in vivo assessment of the regional distribution and quantitative measurement of cholinergic neurotransmitter, enzymes, or receptors in the brain of patients with PD or related dementias. The ability to measure cholinergic synapses in the living brain offers also the opportunity to study cholinergic neurotransmission at early stages of PD before the development of dementia. Cholinergic neurons and their synaptic connections provide molecular targets suitable for radiolabeling (Figure 2). These include ligands of acetylcholine neuronal integrity and cholinergic receptors (see also Table 2).

A traditional presynaptic marker of cholinergic neurons, ChAT, has not been imaged successfully in vivo. Although there are no radioligands for ChAT, there are radiotracers

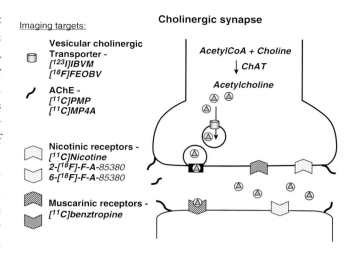

Figure 2 Schematic overview of a cholinergic nerve terminal with listing of different classes of and examples of cholinergic neurotransmission ligands.

for AChE, or the acetylcholine vesicular transporter, that have been shown to map acetylcholine cells in the brain and to have a good correspondence with ChAT (Mesulam and Geula 1992; Weihe et al. 1996).

CHOLINESTERASE SUBSTRATE TRACERS

Radioligand imaging of AChE is a suitable tool to study the integrity of neocortical cholinergic afferents in vivo. AChE is localized predominantly in cholinergic cell bodies and axons. In the cortex, AChE is present in axons innervating it from the basal forebrain (Mesulam and Geula 1991). There also is AChE in intrinsic cortical neurons, and low levels of AChE are probably present in the non-cholinergic structures postsynaptic to the nucleus basalis innervation (Heckers, Geula, and Mesulam 1992). Though AChE is anchored in presynaptic membranes in the acetylcholine neuron as well as in postsynaptic membranes and in the intersynaptic space, it has a very good correspondence with ChAT. Therefore, AChE PET imaging measures the pre- and postsynaptic functional integrity of cortical cholinergic transmission in general.

The most commonly applied AChE PET imaging technique utilizes a radiolabeled lipophilic acetylcholine analog that diffuses into the brain, where it is metabolized by AChE to produce a hydrophilic metabolite that is trapped at the site of its production (Irie et al. 1994). Rats with a unilateral nbM lesion demonstrated reduced cortical AChE activity (−30% to −50%) when studied by autoradiography using [C-14] acetylcholine analogs (Irie et al. 1996). Kilbourn et al. studied in vivo AChE activity in mice using the labeled substrates methyl-4-piperidyl acetate (MP4A) and methyl-4-piperidinyl propionate (PMP) (Kilbourn et al. 1996). After peripheral injection in mice, each ester showed rapid penetration into the brain and a regional retention of radioactivity reflecting known levels of AChE activity in the brain (Atack et al. 1986). PMP studies showed better discrimination between regions of high, intermediate, and low AChE activities compared to MP4A. MP4A has the relative advantage that it is slightly more specific for AChE (94%) compared to PMP (85%–88%). However, the PMP ester has a slower rate of hydrolysis (k3) compared to MP4A and is less flow limited than MP4A. Enzyme hydrolysis estimates are close to optimal for PMP in cortex and less optimal for MP4A. Striatal PMP estimates are only fair, and striatal MP4A estimates are quite flow limited. Kuhl and colleagues using [C-11]PMP found a distribution of AChE activity in normal volunteers that closely correlated with postmortem histochemical distribution (Kuhl, Koeppe et al. 1996).

The Chiba group reported reduced AChE activity in the cerebral cortex in PD that was greater in patients with dementia (Shinotoh et al. 1999). Hilker et al. reported significant reductions of cortical AChE in PD without dementia (10.7%) but severe reductions in PDD (29.7%) (Hilker et al. 2005). We previously reported that cortical AChE deficits were greatest and more extensive in PDD when compared to AD of approximately equal degree of dementia severity (Bohnen et al. 2003), and Herholz et al. reported more significant in vivo cortical losses of AChE activity in a patient with DLB compared to AD (Herholz et al. 2000). We found that cortical AChE activity was also significantly reduced in the PD without dementia group when compared to the control subjects (Bohnen et al. 2003). We did not find significant differences in cortical AChE activity between PDD and DLB subjects. PD without dementia had less severe but significant reductions in cortical AChE activity that were most prominent in the temporal lobe (Bohnen et al. 2003).

Recently, Shimada et al. specifically evaluated whether brain cholinergic deficits occur in early PD, antedating the occurrence of dementia (Shimada et al. 2009). First, the authors replicated our findings of more prominent and widespread reductions in cortical AChE in the demented subject groups that were similar in the DLB and PDD groups. Interestingly, the authors found a significant reduction of cortical AChE activity in early drug naïve patients with PD. The most prominent AChE reductions in PD subjects with early disease occurred in the medial occipital secondary visual cortex (Brodmann area 18). These results correlate well with prior postmortem data indicating that this region (the cuneus) experiences the greatest degree of cholinergic denervation (Perry et al. 1985). Thus, these findings confirm postmortem evidence suggesting that basal forebrain cholinergic system degeneration appears early in PD and then worsens with the appearance of dementia (Ruberg et al. 1986). The in vivo AChE imaging studies in PD, PDD, and DLB are summarized in Table 3.

Radioligands have also been developed to study BuChE by radiolabeling 1-methyl-4-piperidinyl esters, such as 1-[C-11]methyl-4-piperidinyl n-butyrate (BMP) (Snyder et al. 2001) but have not yet been studied in the PD population.

TABLE 3: IN VIVO IMAGING FINDINGS OF CORTICAL AChE ACTIVITY IN PD AND PARKINSONIAN DEMENTIA. MILD CORTICAL REDUCTIONS ARE PRESENT IN PD WITHOUT DEMENTIA WITH MORE EXTENSIVE AND GREATER LOSSES IN DLB AND PDD GROUPS. HOWEVER, THERE DO NOT APPEAR TO BE GROSS DIFFERENCES IN AVERAGE CORTICAL AChE BETWEEN PDD AND DLB GROUPS

Radioligand	Study subjects	Cortical AChE activity	Reference
[C-11]PMP	PD	−12.9%	(Bohnen et al. 2003)
[C-11]MP4A	PD	−10.7%	(Hilker et al. 2005)
[C-11]MP4A	PD	−11.8%	(Shimada et al. 2009)
[C-11]PMP	PD	−10.2%	(Bohnen et al. 2009)
[C-11]MP4A	PD/PDD	−17.0%	(Shinotoh et al. 1999)
[C-11]PMP	PDD	−19.8%	(Bohnen et al. 2003)
[C-11]PMP	DLB	−20.2%	(Bohnen et al. 2003)
[C-11]MP4A	PDD	−29.7%	(Hilker et al. 2005)
[C-11]MP4A	PDD/DLB	−26.8%	(Shimada et al. 2009)

ACETYLCHOLINE VESICULAR TRANSPORTER AND IMAGING

The vesicular ACh transporters (VAChT) are localized in the acetylcholine terminals and carry acetylcholine from the cytoplasm into the vesicles. Radiolabeling of these vesicular transporters would provide a presynaptic marker of cholinergic innervation. Several radioligands that target the ACh vesicular transporter have been labeled (Kuhl et al. 1994). Of these, only (−)-5-[I-123]iodobenzovesamicol ([I-123] IBVM), a SPECT radiotracer, has been used to image the living human brain (Kuhl et al. 1994). [I-123]IBVM is an analog of vesamicol that binds to the acetylcholine vesicular transporter. The relative distributions of [I-123]IBVM in the human brain correspond well with postmortem values reported for ChAT (Kuhl et al. 1994). A structurally similar F-18 label of benzovesamicol has been synthesized (5-[F-18] fluoroethoxybenzovesamicol (FEOBV) and studied in the rat (Mulholland et al. 1998). A potentially clinical advantage of a VAChT ligand is that it may allow in vivo assessment of integrity of cholinergic nerve terminals despite patients taking cholinesterase inhibitor drugs.

Previous VAChT imaging studies have reported cholinergic deficits in PD and PDD patients (Kuhl, Minoshima et al. 1996). In PD without dementia, [I-123]-IBVM binding was reduced modestly in the average cortex (−9%) but significantly only in the parietal (−19%) and occipital (−21%) cortices in PD subjects without dementia, but demented PD subjects had extensive cortical binding decreases most prominently in the occipital (−39%) and posterior cingulate (−45%) cortices (Table 4). Furthermore, cortical VAChT losses were greater in PDD compared to AD of the late onset type and comparable to AD of early onset (Kuhl, Minoshima et al. 1996).

CHOLINERGIC RECEPTOR IMAGING

Radioligands have also been developed to measure cholinergic receptors (see also Figure 2). These receptors

are localized in both presynaptic and postsynaptic targets. Cholinergic ligands are selective for either muscarinic (mAChR) or nicotinic (nAChR) receptors.

NICOTINIC RECEPTORS

Nicotinic (nAChR) receptors belong to the ligand-gated ion channels. The nAChRs have a pentameric structure composed of five membrane-spanning subunits that provide the basis for the heterogeneity of structure and function observed in the nAChR subtypes. It appears that the majority of high-affinity nAChRs in the brain comprise the $\alpha_4\beta_2$ subtype (Flores et al. 1992). Neuronal nAChRs are involved in cognitive processes in the brain where both α_4 and α_7 subunits are suggested to play an important role in cognitive function (Nordberg 2001).

There have been three general classes of compounds developed as radiotracers for nAChR: nicotine and its derivatives, epibatidine or azetidine and its derivatives, and 3-pyridyl ether derivatives, including A-85380 and A-84543 (Sihver, Langstrom, and Nordberg 2000). The first PET ligand applied in monkeys and humans for visualizing nAChRs in the brain was [C-11]nicotine. Because [C-11]nicotine is an agonist of nicotinic receptors, it is not an ideal PET ligand, owing to a relatively high level of nonspecific binding, short receptor interaction, and strong dependence on cerebral blood flow (Maziere and Delforge 1995). Quantitative assessment of [C-11]nicotine binding, therefore, requires a dual tracer model with administration of [O-15]H_2O for regional cerebral blood flow to calculate a flow-compensated measure of [C-11]nicotine binding (Kadir et al. 2006). The discovery of the potent high-affinity nicotinic receptor agonist epibatidine has provided a new venue for the in vivo imaging of nAChRs. Epibatidine was labeled with fluorine-18, where fluorine is substituted for the chlorine atom that is present in the natural product to produce [F-18]norchlorofluoroepibatidine ([F-18]NFEP) (Ding et al. 1996). Human use of [F-18]NFEP is limited by its toxicity (Volkow et al. 2001). It is evident from in vitro binding studies that various 3-pyridyl ether derived PET ligands—such as [Br-76]Br-A-85380 (Sihver et al. 1999), 6-[F-18]fluoro-A-85380 (Gundisch et al. 2005), and 2-[F-18]fluoro-A-85380 (Chefer et al. 1999)—also show a very high affinity for α_4 nAChR subunits, whereas [C-11]nicotine also shows a high affinity for non-α_4 nAChR subtypes (Mogg et al. 2004). A-85380 displays an affinity for $\alpha_4\beta_2$ receptors equal to that of epibatidine, but significantly lower affinity for α_7 receptors than epibatidine. A-85380 may also bind to the $\alpha_6\beta_2$ nAChR subtype. A relative drawback of 2-[F-18]fluoro-A-85380 and 6-[F-18]fluoro-A-85380 as PET ligands is the very long scanning time (hours) that

TABLE 4: IN VIVO IMAGING FINDINGS OF CEREBRAL VAChT ACTIVITY IN PD AND PDD COMPARED TO NON-PD CONTROL SUBJECTS

Radioligand	Study subjects	Cortical VAChT activity	Reference
[I-123]IBVM	PD	−9%	(Kuhl, Minoshima et al. 1996)
[I-123]IBVM	PDD	−34%	(Kuhl, Minoshima et al. 1996)

is needed. The derivative 2-fluoro-3-[2-(*S*)-3-pyrrolinyl) methoxy]pyridine ([F-18]-nifene) is a PET $\alpha_4\beta_2$ nicotinic ligand, which has faster binding kinetics, allowing shorter imaging time (Pichika et al. 2006). More recently, analogs of [^{11}C]CH$_3$-PVC, a radiolabeled derivative of A-84543, have been synthesized that show promising kinetics in animal studies (Gao et al. 2009).

nAChR SPECT ligands have also been developed, including radioiodinated 5-I-A-85380 (Musachio et al. 1999). For example, a [I-123]-5-I-A-85380 SPECT study found widespread significant decrease (10%) in not only cortical but also subcortical regions in PD patients without dementia (Fujita et al. 2006). A 5-[I-123]-iodo-3-(2(S)-azetidinylmethoxy)pyridine ([I-123]I-5IA), a derivative of A-85380, SPECT study also found widespread reductions (–15% to –25%) in the cortex, especially the frontal cortex, and subcortical regions (thalamus, striatum, cerebellum, and brainstem) in PD subjects (Oishi et al. 2007). A recent 2-[F-18]fluoro-A-85380 PET study found evidence of more widespread reduction of $\alpha_4\beta_2$ nicotinic receptors in PD in the cortex and subcortical regions, including the midbrain, putamen, hippocampus, amygdala, pons, and cerebellum (Meyer et al. 2009). Kas et al., also using the PET 2-[F-18]fluoro-A-85380 ligand and a simplified imaging acquisition, found reduced $\alpha_4\beta_2$ nicotinic receptors in the striatum (–10%) and substantia nigra (–14.9%) in PD (Kas et al. 2009). There was no left-to-right asymmetry in $\alpha_4\beta_2$ nAChR binding despite the clinical asymmetry in motor symptoms in these patients.

Cortical reductions, however, were not significantly lower from control subjects.

A [I-123]-5-I-A-85380 SPECT study found evidence of reduced binding in striatal, frontal, temporal, and cingulate regions (O'Brien et al. 2008). However, there was a relative increase in occipital binding that was more prominent in subjects with a recent history of visual hallucinations. These findings suggest a link between cholinergic changes in the occipital lobe and visual hallucinations in parkinsonian dementia. However, the authors did not find evidence of a correlation between [I-123]-5-I-A-85380 binding and cognitive functions in these subjects. A follow-up study of the same group found that reduced normalized regional cortical [I-123]-5-I-A-85380 activity in a combined group of DLB and AD patients significantly correlated with a decline in executive cognitive functions (Colloby et al. 2010). Table 5 provides an overview of nAChR imaging studies in PD and dementia.

MUSCARINIC RECEPTOR IMAGING

Muscarinic receptors mediate the metabotropic actions of acetylcholine in the nervous system (Eglen 2006), and include pharmacologically defined M1–M3 subtypes. On a molecular level, there are 5 distinct receptor subtype gene products designated m1–m5. There is a complex and overlapping relationship of the molecular to the pharmacologically defined subtypes, owing to the similarity of the proteins and the ligand recognition site structures. The M1

TABLE 5: IN VIVO IMAGING FINDINGS OF CEREBRAL nAChR ACTIVITY IN PD AND PARKINSONIAN DEMENTIA COMPARED TO NON-PD CONTROL SUBJECTS. ALL OF THESE STUDIES SHOW DECREASED SUBCORTICAL BINDING, WITH THE MAJORITY OF THE STUDIES ALSO SHOWING DECREASED CORTICAL nAChR ACTIVITY. A DLB STUDY SUGGESTS WIDESPREAD CORTICAL AND SUBCORTICAL nAChE REDUCTIONS EXCEPT FOR INCREASED OCCIPITAL LOBE ACTIVITY THAT MAY RELATE TO RECENT VISUAL HALLUCINATIONS

Ligand	Study subjects	Findings	Reference
[I-123]-5-I-A-85380	PD	Widespread cortical and subcortical losses, including the thalamus, striatum, pons, and cerebellum	(Fujita et al. 2006)
[I-123]I-5IA	PD	Widespread cortical and subcortical reductions; most significant reductions in the frontal cortex and brainstem	(Oishi et al. 2007)
2-[F-18]fluoro-A-85380	PD	Widespread cortical and subcortical losses, including the thalamus, putamen, amygdala hippocampus, and cerebellum	(Meyer et al. 2009)
2-[F-18]fluoro-A-85380	PD	Reduced binding in the striatum and substantia nigra; no significant cortical reductions	(Kas et al. 2009)
[I-123]-5-I-A-85380	DLB	Reduced binding in striatal, frontal, temporal, and cingulate regions; however, there was relative increase in occipital binding	(O'Brien et al. 2008)

subtype (including the m1 and m4 molecular subtypes) is postsynaptic and accounts for 80% of cortical muscarinic receptors, occurring in high concentration in limbic and paralimbic areas including the cingulate gyrus (Mash, White, and Mesulam 1988).

Imaging muscarinic receptors, which are the dominant post-synaptic cholinergic receptors in the brain, has been pursued by many tracers for SPECT ([I-123]quinuclidinyl-benzylate [QNB], and PET ([C-11]QNB, [C-11]2-tropanyl-benzylate [TRB], [C-11]-N-methylpiperidyl-benzylate [NMPB], [C-11] scopolamine, and [C-11]benztropine) (Eckelman et al. 1984; Dewey et al. 1990; Zubieta et al. 2001). For the most part these radiotracers are limited by the lack of selectivity for the muscarinic receptor subtypes (M1–M3/ m1–m5), except for [F-18]3-(3-(3-fluoropropylthio)-1,2,5-thiadiazol-4-yl)-1,2,5,6-tetrahydro-1-methylpyridine ([F-18]FP-TZTP), which appears to bind predominantly to M2 (including m2 and possibly also m4 receptors) (Carson et al. 1998; Volkow et al. 2001).

Muscarinic receptor PET studies using the radioligand [C-11]NMPB demonstrated increased mAChR binding in the frontal cortex in non-demented PD patients (Asahina et al. 1995; Asahina et al. 1998). This finding may reflect denervation hypersensitivity caused by loss of the ascending cholinergic input to that region from the basal forebrain. Colloby et al. found evidence of increased mAChR in the occipital lobe in PDD and DLB subjects using [I-123] QNB and SPECT (Colloby et al. 2006). Findings were independent of regional cerebral blood flow changes. The authors hypothesize that these occipital mAChR upregulations may be related to visual disturbances that are prevalent in these patients. However, the authors did not find evidence of cognitive or neuropsychiatric correlates of altered mAChR expression in these subjects (Colloby et al. 2006). Table 6 provides an overview of mAChR imaging studies in PD and dementia.

IN VIVO COGNITIVE CORRELATES OF CHOLINERGIC DENERVATION IN PD

Previous in vivo imaging studies have shown reduced cortical AChE and VAChT activity in PDD or DLB compared to PD without dementia (Kuhl, Minoshima et al. 1996; Bohnen et al. 2003; Hilker et al. 2005; Shimada et al. 2009). Several studies have correlated performance on cognitive tests with cortical cholinergic activity. For example, Shinotoh et al. did not find a significant correlation between cortical AChE activity and scores on the Mini-Mental State Examination (MMSE) or the Wisconsin Card Sorting Test in a predominant non-demented PD population (Shinotoh et al. 1999). However, they noticed significantly lower cortical AChE activity in PD subjects with visual hallucinations compared to those without hallucinations. We recently reported a modest correlation between cortical AChE activity and scores on the MMSE in a larger series of PD subjects without dementia (*P = 0.02*) (Bohnen et al. 2009). Shimada et al. did find a significant correlation between cortical AChE activity and scores on the MMSE in the combined PD, PDD, and DLB groups (*P < 0.005*) (Shimada et al. 2009). Furthermore, a subgroup analysis revealed a more robust inverse correlation between AChE activity in the posterior cingulate gyrus and the MMSE scores in the DLB subjects (Shimada et al. 2009).

Cognitive impairment in PD has been attributed to a subcortico-cortical syndrome that is characterized mainly by attentional and executive dysfunction (Lees and Smith 1983; Stern et al. 1983; Dubois et al. 1990). We previously determined in vivo cortical AChE levels were greater and more extensive in parkinsonian dementia compared to AD of similar dementia severity (Bohnen et al. 2003). The degree of cognitive impairment correlated with cortical AChE activity (Bohnen et al. 2006). Analysis of the cognitive data within the patient groups demonstrated that scores

TABLE 6: IN VIVO IMAGING FINDINGS OF mAChR ACTIVITY IN PD AND PARKINSONIAN DEMENTIA COMPARED TO NON-PD CONTROL SUBJECTS

Ligand	Study subjects	Findings	Reference
[C-11]NMPB	PD/PDD	Increased frontal receptor activity (22%). Frontal increase was more prominent in a single PDD subject. There were non-significant increases in the parietotemporal cortices (16%) and striatum (16%).	(Asahina et al. 1998)
C-11]NMPB	PD	Increased frontal receptor activity (20%)	(Asahina et al. 1995)
[I-123]QNB	PDD	Increased binding in right and left occipital lobes	(Colloby et al. 2006)
[I-123]QNB	DLB	Increased binding in right occipital lobe	(Colloby et al. 2006)

on the WAIS-III Digit Span, a test of working memory and attention, had the most robust correlation with cortical AChE activity ($P < 0.005$). There were also significant correlations between cortical AChE activity and other tests of attentional and executive functions, such as the Trail Making Test and Stroop Color Word Test (Bohnen et al. 2006). In contrast, there were no significant correlations with tests of delayed verbal learning. The data are consistent with pharmacological observations that anti-cholinergic drugs have disproportionately adverse effects on attentional and executive processes (Cooper et al. 1992; Bedard et al. 1999). For example, Dubois et al. reported that the use of anti-cholinergic medications in patients with PD led to severe impairment on attentional and executive tests, such as the Digit Span test and the Wisconsin Card Sorting Task (Dubois et al. 1987; Dubois et al. 1990). In addition, anti-cholinergic drug administration caused a transient dysexecutive syndrome in PD patients, but not in normal controls, indicating specific anti-cholinergic vulnerability in PD (Bedard et al. 1998; Bedard et al. 1999). These findings indicate that the behavioral correlates of cholinergic denervation better predict the cognitive profile of PD compared to typical AD (Dubois et al. 1987) and support a cholinergic model of dementia that may be more applicable to parkinsonian dementia than prototypical AD.

It should be noted that PD is a multisystem neurodegeneration syndrome and that cognitive impairment in PD is likely the result of an interplay of deficiencies in multiple neurotransmitters, including dopamine. For example, effects of dopaminergic denervation, especially of the caudate nucleus (Dahlstrom and Fuxe 1964), and dopaminergic mesolimbic and mesocortical pathways that innervate parts of the limbic system and the mesiofrontal neocortex (Bjorklund and Lindvall 1984), may in part affect cognitive functions mediated by the frontal lobe, and early, more posterior cortical activity may reflect cholinergic denervation of the nbM (Williams-Gray et al. 2009). However, Hilker et al. did not observe any difference in striatal FDOPA reductions between PD and PDD groups, whereas the PDD had significantly reduced cortical AChE compared to the PD subjects (Hilker et al. 2005). The cuneus is thought to be the most vulnerable region to cholinergic deafferentation, as there is more severe loss of cholinergic projections to the cuneus than to any other cortical region (Candy et al. 1983; Perry et al. 1983; Hilker et al. 2005). Although cholinergic denervation may cause early posterior cortical denervation, progression of dementia is associated with more diffuse and severe frontal cholinergic deficits (Shimada et al. 2009). Mixed effects of dopaminergic and cholinergic denervation contribute to the cognitive phenotype PD.

However, unlike early stage PD, where there is evidence of uniform and severe dopaminergic denervation, convergent evidence from in vivo imaging and postmortem studies shows that cholinergic denervation worsens with the appearance of dementia in patients with this disorder.

MOTOR PHENOTYPE AND RISK OF DEMENTIA IN PD: IS THE CHOLINERGIC SYSTEM IMPLICATED?

The rate of disease progression is quite variable among PD patients. Patients with tremor-predominant disease, for example, tend to progress more slowly than patients with postural instability and gait disturbances (PIGD). Some studies have shown an association between the PIGD motor phenotype in PD and increased risk of dementia (Taylor et al. 2008). An association between the PIGD phenotype and a greater degree of cholinergic cortical denervation is plausible. For example, we recently reported lower cortical and in particular subcortical (thalamic) AChE activity in subjects with PD and a history of falls compared to PD subjects without a fall history (Bohnen et al. 2009). In contrast, there was no significant difference in the degree of nigrostriatal denervation between these groups. Thalamic AChE activity in part represents cholinergic output of the PPN, a key node for gait control (Lee, Rinne, and Marsden 2000), and PPN dysfunction may relate to the presence of dopamine nonresponsive gait and balance impairments, including falls in PD (Stein 2009). Further studies are needed to determine the relationship between specific motor phenotypes in PD and degree of subcortical cholinergic denervation. PD can be viewed as a multisystem disease, so differences in the degree or rate of degeneration in different neural systems may account for differences in phenotypic features.

EX VIVO EVIDENCE OF COMORBID ALZHEIMER PATHOLOGY IN PD AND PARKINSONIAN DEMENTIA

Although the pathological hallmark of parkinsonian dementia is the presence of extra-nigral Lewy bodies (Mattila et al. 1998; Aarsland et al. 2005), there may be a spectrum of neuropathological changes of dementia in parkinsonism leading to overlapping and neuropathologically heterogeneous syndromes, including comorbid AD (Mahler and Cummings 1990). Although different studies cannot be directly compared because of differences in defining AD pathology, use

SUMMARY ASSESSMENT OF PROTEIN AGGREGATION BINDING CHARACTERISTICS OF PIB AND FDDNP LIGANDS. THE PRELIMINARY INFORMATION IS BASED ON LIMITED AVAILABLE DATA

	Soluble amyloid	Amyloid angiopathy	Fibrillary amyloid		Neurofibrillary tangle	Lewy body
			Neuritic plaques	Diffuse plaques		
PIB	–	+	+	+	–	–
FDDNP	–	+	+	+	+	?

ACKNOWLEDGEMENTS

The authors gratefully acknowledge research support from the NIH-NINDS, the Department of Veterans Affairs, and the Michael J. Fox Foundation.

REFERENCES

Aarsland, D., and M. W. Kurz. 2010. The epidemiology of dementia associated with Parkinson disease. *J Neurol Sci* 289:18–22.

Aarsland, D., R. Perry, A. Brown, J. P. Larsen, and C. Ballard. 2005. Neuropathology of dementia in Parkinson's disease: a prospective, community-based study. *Ann Neurol* 58 (5):773–6.

Apaydin, H., J. E. Ahlskog, J. E. Parisi, B. F. Boeve, and D. W. Dickson. 2002. Parkinson disease neuropathology: Later-developing dementia and loss of the levodopa response. *Arch Neurol* 59:102–112.

Arendt, T., V. Bigl, A. Arendt, and A. Tennstedt. 1983. Loss of neurons in the nucleus basalis of Meynert in Alzheimer's disease, paralysis agitans and Korsakoff's Disease. *Acta Neuropathol (Berl)* 61:101–108.

Asahina, M., H. Shinotoh, K. Hirayama, T. Suhara, F. Shishido, O. Inoue, and Y. Tateno. 1995. Hypersensitivity of cortical muscarinic receptors in Parkinson's disease demonstrated by PET. *Acta Neurol Scand* 91 (6):437–43.

Asahina, M., T. Suhara, H. Shinotoh, O. Inoue, K. Suzuki, and T. Hattori. 1998. Brain muscarinic receptors in progressive supranuclear palsy and Parkinson's disease: A positron emission tomographic study. *J Neurol Neurosurg Psychiatry* 65 (2):155–63.

Atack, J. R., E. K. Perry, J. R. Bonham, J. M. Candy, and R. H. Perry. 1986. Molecular forms of acetylcholinesterase and butyrylcholinesterase in the aged human central nervous system. *J Neurochem* 47: 263–277.

Aubert, I., D. M. Araujo, D. Cecyre, Y. Robitaille, S. Gauthier, and R. Quirion. 1992. Comparative alterations of nicotinic and muscarinic binding sites in Alzheimer's and Parkinson's diseases. *J Neurochem* 58:529–541.

Bacskai, B. J., M. P. Frosch, S. H. Freeman, S. B. Raymond, J. C. Augustinack, K. A. Johnson, M. C. Irizarry, W. E. Klunk, C. A. Mathis, S. T. Dekosky, S. M. Greenberg, B. T. Hyman, and J. H. Growdon. 2007. Molecular imaging with Pittsburgh Compound B confirmed at autopsy: A case report. *Arch Neurol* 64 (3):431–4.

Ballard, C., I. Ziabreva, R. Perry, J. P. Larsen, J. O'Brien, I. McKeith, E. Perry, and D. Aarsland. 2006. Differences in neuropathologic characteristics across the Lewy body dementia spectrum. *Neurology* 67 (11):1931–4.

Bedard, M. A., S. Lemay, J.F. Gagnon, H. Masson, and F. Paquet. 1998. Induction of a transient dysexecutive syndrome in Parkinson's disease using a subclinical dose of scopolamine. *Behav Neurol* 11: 187–195.

Bedard, M. A., B. Pillon, B. Dubois, N. Duchesne, H. Masson, and Y. Agid. 1999. Acute and long-term administration of anticholinergics in Parkinson's disease: Specific effects on the subcortico-frontal syndrome. *Brain Cogn* 40:289–313.

Bjorklund, A., and O. Lindvall. 1984. Dopamine-containing systems in the CNS. In *Handbook of chemical neuroanatomy*, ed. A. Bjorklund and T. Hokfelt. Amsterdam: Elsevier, pp. 55–122.

Bohnen, N. I., D. I. Kaufer, R. Hendrickson, L. S. Ivanco, B. J. Lopresti, G. M. Constantine, A. Mathis Ch, J. G. Davis, R. Y. Moore, and S. T. Dekosky. 2006. Cognitive correlates of cortical cholinergic denervation in Parkinson's disease and parkinsonian dementia. *J Neurol* 253 (2):242–7.

Bohnen, N. I., D. I. Kaufer, L. S. Ivanco, B. Lopresti, R. A. Koeppe, J. G. Davis, C. A. Mathis, R. Y. Moore, and S. T. DeKosky. 2003. Cortical cholinergic function is more severely affected in parkinsonian dementia than in Alzheimer disease: An in vivo positron emission tomographic study. *Arch Neurol* 60 (12):1745–8.

Bohnen, N. I., M. L. Muller, R. A. Koeppe, S. A. Studenski, M. A. Kilbourn, K. A. Frey, and R. L. Albin. 2009. History of falls in Parkinson disease is associated with reduced cholinergic activity. *Neurology* 73 (20):1670–6.

Boller, F., T. Mizutani, U. Roessmann, and P. Gambetti. 1980. Parkinson's disease, dementia and Alzheimer's disease: Clinicopathologic correlations. *Ann Neurol* 7:329–335.

Braak, H., K. Del Tredici, U. Rub, R. A. de Vos, E. N. Jansen Steur, and E. Braak. 2003. Staging of brain pathology related to sporadic Parkinson's disease. *Neurobiol Aging* 24 (2):197–211.

Bresjanac, M., L. M. Smid, T. D. Vovko, A. Petric, J. R. Barrio, and M. Popovic. 2003. Molecular-imaging probe 2-(1-[6-[(2-fluoroethyl) (methyl) amino]-2-naphthyl]ethylidene) malononitrile labels prion plaques in vitro. *J Neurosci* 23 (22):8029–33.

Brown, D. F., R. C. Risser, E. H. Bigio, P. Tripp, A. Stiegler, E. Welch, K. P. Eagan, C. L. Hladik, and C. L. White. 1998. Neocortical synapse density and Braak stage in the Lewy body variant of Alzheimer's disease: A comparison with classic Alzheimer disease and normal aging. *J Neuropathol Exp Neurol* 57:955–960.

Burack, M. A., J. Hartlein, H. P. Flores, L. Taylor-Reinwald, J. S. Perlmutter, and N. J. Cairns. 2010. In vivo amyloid imaging in autopsy-confirmed Parkinson disease with dementia. *Neurology* 74 (1):77–84.

Candy, J. M., R. H. Perry, E. K. Perry, D. Irving, G. Blessed, A. F. Fairbairn, and B. E. Tomlinson. 1983. Pathological changes in the nucleus of Meynert in Alzheimer's and Parkinson's diseases. *J Neurol Sci* 59:277–289.

Carson, R. E., D. O. Kiesewetter, E. Jagoda, M. G. Der, P. Herscovitch, and W. C. Eckelman. 1998. Muscarinic cholinergic receptor measurements with [18F]FP-TZTP: control and competition studies. *J Cereb Blood Flow Metab* 18 (10):1130–42.

Chefer, S. I., A. G. Horti, A. O. Koren, D. Gundisch, J. M. Links, V. Kurian, R. F. Dannals, A. G. Mukhin, and E. D. London. 1999. 2-[18F]F-A-85380: A PET radioligand for alpha4beta2 nicotinic acetylcholine receptors. *Neuroreport*, 10 (13):2715–21.

Chui, H. C., J. A. Mortimer, U. Slager, C. Zarow, W. Bondareff, and D. D. Webster. 1986. Pathologic correlates of dementia in Parkinson's disease. *Arch Neurol* 43:991–995.

Churchyard, A., and A. J. Lees. 1997. The relationship between dementia and direct involvement of the hippocampus and amygdala in Parkinson's disease. *Neurology* 49:1570–1576.

Colloby, S. J., S. Pakrasi, M. J. Firbank, E. K. Perry, M. A. Piggott, J. Owens, D. J. Wyper, I. G. McKeith, D. J. Burn, E. D. Williams, and J. T. O'Brien. 2006. In vivo SPECT imaging of muscarinic acetylcholine receptors using (R,R) 123I-QNB in dementia with Lewy bodies and Parkinson's disease dementia. *Neuroimage* 33 (2):423–9.

Colloby, S. J., E. K. Perry, S. Pakrasi, S. L. Pimlott, D. J. Wyper, I. G. McKeith, E. D. Williams, and J. T. O'Brien. 2010. Nicotinic ^{123}I-5IA-85380 single photon emission computed tomography as a predictor of cognitive progression in Alzheimer's disease and dementia with Lewy bodies. *Am J Geriatr Psychiatry* 18 (1):86–90.

Cooper, J. A., H. J. Sagar, S. M. Doherty, N. Jordan, P. Tidswell, and E. V. Sullivan. 1992. Different effects of dopaminergic and anticholinergic therapies on cognitive and motor function in Parkinson's disease. A follow-up study of untreated patients. *Brain* 115:1701–1725.

Dahlstrom, A., and K. Fuxe. 1964. Evidence for the existence of monoamine-containing neurons in the central nervous system. I. Demonstration of monoamines in the cell bodies of brain stem neurons. *Acta Physiol Scand* 62 [Suppl 232]:231–255.

de Lacalle, S., L. B. Hersh, and C. B. Saper. 1993. Cholinergic innervation of the human cerebellum. *J Comp Neurol* 328:364–376.

Del Ser, T., V. Hachinski, H. Merskey, and D. G. Munoz. 2001. Clinical and pathologic features of two groups of patients with dementia with Lewy bodies: Effect of coexisting Alzheimer-type lesion load. *Alzheimer Dis Assoc Disord* 15:31–44.

Dewey, S. L., N. D. Volkow, J. Logan, R. R. MacGregor, J. S. Fowler, D. J. Schlyer, and B. Bendriem. 1990. Age-related decreases in muscarinic cholinergic receptor binding in the human brain measured with positron emission tomography (PET. *J Neurosci Res* 27 (4):569–75.

Ding, Y. S., S. J. Gatley, J. S. Fowler, N. D. Volkow, D. Aggarwal, J. Logan, S. L. Dewey, F. Liang, F. I. Carroll, and M. J. Kuhar. 1996. Mapping nicotinic acetylcholine receptors with PET. *Synapse* 24 (4):403–7.

Dubois, B., F. Danze, B. Pillon, G. Cusimano, F. Lhermitte, and Y. Agid. 1987. Cholinergic-dependent cognitive deficits in Parkinson's disease. *Ann Neurol* 22:26–30.

Dubois, B., B. Pillon, F. Lhermitte, and Y. Agid. 1990. Cholinergic deficiency and frontal dysfunction in Parkinson's disease. *Ann Neurol* 28:117–121.

Eckelman, W. C., R. C. Reba, W. J. Rzeszotarski, R. E. Gibson, T. Hill, B. L. Holman, T. Budinger, J. J. Conklin, R. Eng, and M. P. Grissom. 1984. External imaging of cerebral muscarinic acetylcholine receptors. *Science* 223 (4633):291–3.

Edison, P., C. C. Rowe, J. O. Rinne, S. Ng, I. Ahmed, N. Kemppainen, V. L. Villemagne, G. O'Keefe, K. Nagren, K. R. Chaudhury, C. L. Masters, and D. J. Brooks. 2008. Amyloid load in Parkinson's disease dementia and Lewy body dementia measured with [^{11}C]PIB positron emission tomography. *J Neurol Neurosurg Psychiatry* 79 (12):1331–8.

Eglen, R. M. 2006. Muscarinic receptor subtypes in neuronal and non-neuronal cholinergic function. *Auton Autacoid Pharmacol* 26 (3):219–33.

Everitt, B. J., T. E. Sirkia, A. C. Roberts, G. H. Jones, and T. W. Robbins. 1988. Distribution and some projections of cholinergic neurons in the brain of the common marmoset, Callithrix jacchus. *J Comp Neurol* 271 (4):533–58.

Fibiger, H. C. 1982. The organization and some projections of cholinergic neurons of the mammalian forebrain. *Brain Res Rev* 4:327–388.

Flores, C. M., S. W. Rogers, L. A. Pabreza, B. B. Wolfe, and K. J. Kellar. 1992. A subtype of nicotinic cholinergic receptor in rat brain is composed of alpha 4 and beta 2 subunits and is up-regulated by chronic nicotine treatment. *Mol Pharmacol* 41 (1):31–7.

Fodero-Tavoletti, M. T., D. P. Smith, C. A. McLean, P. A. Adlard, K. J. Barnham, L. E. Foster, L. Leone, K. Perez, M. Cortes, J. G. Culvenor, Q. X. Li, K. M. Laughton, C. C. Rowe, C. L. Masters, R. Cappai, and V. L. Villemagne. 2007. In vitro characterization of Pittsburgh compound-B binding to Lewy bodies. *J Neurosci* 27 (39): 10365–71.

Friedland, R. P., R. Kalaria, M. Berridge, F. Miraldi, P. Hedera, J. Reno, L. Lyle, and C. A. Marotta. 1997. Neuroimaging of vessel amyloid in Alzheimer's disease. *Ann N Y Acad Sci* 826:242–7.

Fujita, M., M. Ichise, S. S. Zoghbi, J. S. Liow, S. Ghose, D. C. Vines, J. Sangare, J. Q. Lu, V. L. Cropley, H. Iida, K. M. Kim, R. M. Cohen, W. Bara-Jimenez, B. Ravina, and R. B. Innis. 2006. Widespread decrease of nicotinic acetylcholine receptors in Parkinson's disease. *Ann Neurol* 59 (1):174–7.

Gai, W. P., G. M. Halliday, P. C. Blumbergs, L. B. Geffen, and W. W. Blessing. 1991. Substance P-containing neurons in the mesopontine tegmentum are severely affected in Parkinson's disease. *Brain* 114 (Pt 5): 2253–67.

Galpern, W. R., and A. E. Lang. 2006. Interface between tauopathies and synucleinopathies: A tale of two proteins. *Ann Neurol* 59 (3):449–58.

Gandy, S. 2005. The role of cerebral amyloid beta accumulation in common forms of Alzheimer disease. *J Clin Invest* 115 (5):1121–9.

Gao, Y., H. T. Ravert, H. Kuwabara, Y. Xiao, C. J. Endres, J. Hilton, D. P. Holt, A. Kumar, M. Alexander, D. F. Wong, R. F. Dannals, and A. G. Horti. 2009. Synthesis and biological evaluation of novel carbon-11 labeled pyridyl ethers: candidate ligands for in vivo imaging of alpha4beta2 nicotinic acetylcholine receptors (alpha4beta2-nAChRs) in the brain with positron emission tomography. *Bioorg Med Chem* 17 (13):4367–77.

Gaspar, P., and F. Gray. 1984. Dementia in idiopathic Parkinson's disease. A neuropathological study of 32 cases. *Acta Neuropathol (Berl)* 64:43–52.

Geula, C., and M. M. Mesulam. 1989. Cortical cholinergic fibers in aging and Alzheimer's disease: a morphometric study. *Neuroscience* 33 (3):469–81.

Geula, C., and M. M. Mesulam. 1996. Systematic regional variations in the loss of cortical cholinergic fibers in Alzheimer's disease. *Cereb Cortex* 6:165–177.

Geula, C., and M. M. Mesulam. 1999. Cholinergic systems in Alzheimer's disease. In *Alzheimer disease*, edited by R. D. Terry, et al. Philadelphia, PA: Lippincott, Williams & Wilkins, pp. 69–292.

Gibb, W. R. G. 1989. Dementia and Parkinson's disease. *Br J Psychiatry* 154:596–614.

Goldman-Rakic, P. S. 1998. The cortical dopamine system: role in memory and cognition. *Adv Pharmacol* 42:707–711.

Gomperts, S. N., D. M. Rentz, E. Moran, J. A. Becker, J. J. Locascio, W. E. Klunk, C. A. Mathis, D. R. Elmaleh, T. Shoup, A. J. Fischman, B. T. Hyman, J. H. Growdon, and K. A. Johnson. 2008. Imaging amyloid deposition in Lewy body diseases. *Neurology* 71 (12): 903–10.

Gotham, A. M., R. G. Brown, and C. D. Marsden. 1988. "Frontal" cognitive function in patients with Parkinson's disease "on" and "off" levodopa. *Brain* 111:299–321.

Green, J., W. M. McDonald, J. L. Vitek, M. Evatt, A. Freeman, M. Haber, R. A. Bakay, S. Triche, B. Sirockman, and M. R. DeLong. 2002. Cognitive impairments in advanced PD without dementia. *Neurology* 59:1320–1324.

Gundisch, D., A. O. Koren, A. G. Horti, O. A. Pavlova, A. S. Kimes, A. G. Mukhin, and E. D. London. 2005. In vitro characterization of 6-[18F]fluoro-A-85380, a high-affinity ligand for alpha4beta2* nicotinic acetylcholine receptors. *Synapse* 55 (2):89–97.

Hakim, A. M., and G. Mathieson. 1979. Dementia in Parkinson's disease: A neuropathologic study. *Neurology* 29:1209–1214.

Halliday, G., M. Hely, W. Reid, and J. Morris. 2008. The progression of pathology in longitudinally followed patients with Parkinson's disease. *Acta Neuropathol* 115 (4):409–15.

Hardy, J., and D. J. Selkoe. 2002. The amyloid hypothesis of Alzheimer's disease: Progress and problems on the road to therapeutics. *Science* 297:353–356.

Heckers, S., C. Geula, and M. M. Mesulam. 1992. Cholinergic innervation of the human thalamus: Dual origin and differential nuclear distribution. *J Comp Neurol* 325:68–82.

Heckers, S., C. Geula, and M. M. Mesulam. 1992. Acetylcholinesterase-rich pyramidal neurons in Alzheimer's disease. *Neurobiol Aging* 13 (4):455–60.

Hely, M. A., W. G. Reid, M. A. Adena, G. M. Halliday, and J. G. Morris. 2008. The Sydney multicenter study of Parkinson's disease: The inevitability of dementia at 20 years. *Mov Disord* 23 (6):837–44.

Herholz, K., B. Bauer, K. Wienhard, L. Kracht, R. Mielke, M. O. Lenz, T. Strotmann, and W. D. Heiss. 2000. In-vivo measurements of regional acetylcholine esterase activity in degenerative dementia: Comparison with blood flow and glucose metabolism. *J Neural Transm* 107:1457–1468.

Hilker, R., A. V. Thomas, J. C. Klein, S. Weisenbach, E. Kalbe, L. Burghaus, A. H. Jacobs, K. Herholz, and W. D. Heiss. 2005. Dementia in Parkinson disease: Functional imaging of cholinergic and dopaminergic pathways. *Neurology* 65 (11):1716–22.

Hirsch, E. C., A. M. Graybiel, C. Duyckaerts, and F. Javoy-Agid. 1987. Neuronal loss in the pedunculopontine tegmental nucleus in Parkinson disease and in progressive supranuclear palsy. *Proc Natl Acad Sci U S A* 84 (16):5976–80.

Hughes, A. J., S. E. Daniel, L. Kilford, and A. J. Lees. 1992. Accuracy of clinical diagnosis of idiopathic Parkinson's disease: A clinicopathologic study of 100 cases. *J Neurol Neurosurg Psychiatry* 55:181–184.

Hughes, T. A., H. F. Ross, S. Musa, S. Bhattacherjee, R. N. Nathan, R. H. Mindham, and E. G. Spokes. 2000. A 10-year study of the incidence of and factors predicting dementia in Parkinson's disease. *Neurology* 54 (8):1596–602.

Hurtig, H. I., J. Q. Trojanowski, J. Galvin, D. Ewbank, M. L. Schmidt, V. M. Lee, C. M. Clark, G. Glosser, M. B. Stern, S. M. Gollomp, and S. E. Arnold. 2000. Alpha-synuclein cortical Lewy bodies correlate with dementia in Parkinson's disease. *Neurology* 54:1916–1922.

Irie, T., K. Fukushi, Y. Akimoto, H. Tamagami, and T. Nozaki. 1994. Design and evaluation of radioactive acetylcholine analogs for mapping brain acetylcholinesterase (AChE) in vivo. *Nucl Med Biol* 21 (801–808).

Irie, T., K. Fukushi, H. Namba, M. Iyo, H. Tamagami, S. Nagatsuka, and N. Ikota. 1996. Brain acetylcholinesterase activity: Validation of a PET tracer in a rat model of Alzheimer's disease. *J Nucl Med* 37: 649–655.

Irvine, G. B., O. M. El-Agnaf, G. M. Shankar, and D. M. Walsh. 2008. Protein aggregation in the brain: The molecular basis for Alzheimer's and Parkinson's diseases. *Mol Med* 14 (7–8):451–64.

Jellinger, K. 1988. The pedunculopontine nucleus in Parkinson's disease, progressive supranuclear palsy and Alzheimer's disease. *J Neurol Neurosurg Psychiatry* 51:540–543.

Jellinger, K. A. 2003. Alpha-synuclein pathology in Parkinson's and Alzheimer's disease brain: Incidence and topographic distribution—a pilot study. *Acta Neuropathol* 106 (3):191–201.

Jellinger, K. A. 2009. Significance of brain lesions in Parkinson disease dementia and Lewy body dementia. *Front Neurol Neurosci* 24: 114–25.

Jellinger, K. A., K. Seppi, G. K. Wenning, and W. Poewe. 2002. Impact of coexistent Alzheimer pathology on the natural history of Parkinson's disease. *J Neural Transm* 109 (3):329–39.

Jellinger, K. A. 2000. Morphological substrates of mental dysfunction in Lewy body disease: An update. *J Neural Transm* 59(Supp l): 185–212.

Johansson, A., I. Savitcheva, A. Forsberg, H. Engler, B. Langstrom, A. Nordberg, and H. Askmark. 2008. [(11)C]-PIB imaging in patients with Parkinson's disease: Preliminary results. *Parkinsonism Relat Disord* 14 (4):345–7.

Johnson, K. A., M. Gregas, J. A. Becker, C. Kinnecom, D. H. Salat, E. K. Moran, E. E. Smith, J. Rosand, D. M. Rentz, W. E. Klunk, C. A. Mathis, J. C. Price, S. T. Dekosky, A. J. Fischman, and S. M. Greenberg. 2007. Imaging of amyloid burden and distribution in cerebral amyloid angiopathy. *Ann Neurol* 62 (3):229–34.

Kadir, A., O. Almkvist, A. Wall, B. Langstrom, and A. Nordberg. 2006. PET imaging of cortical (11)C-nicotine binding correlates with the cognitive function of attention in Alzheimer's disease. *Psychopharmacology (Berl)* 188 (4):509–20.

Kalaitzakis, M. E., M. B. Graeber, S. M. Gentleman, and R. K. Pearce. 2008. Striatal beta-amyloid deposition in Parkinson disease with dementia. *J Neuropathol Exp Neurol* 67 (2):155–61.

Kalaitzakis, M. E., and R. K. Pearce. 2009. The morbid anatomy of dementia in Parkinson's disease. *Acta Neuropathol* 118 (5):587–98.

Kas, A., M. Bottlaender, J. D. Gallezot, M. Vidailhet, G. Villafane, M. C. Gregoire, C. Coulon, H. Valette, F. Dolle, M. J. Ribeiro, P. Hantraye, and P. Remy. 2009. Decrease of nicotinic receptors in the nigrostriatal system in Parkinson's disease. *J Cereb Blood Flow Metab* 29 (9):1601–8.

Kilbourn, M. R., S. E. Snyder, P. S. Sherman, and D. E. Kuhl. 1996. In vivo studies of acetylcholinesterase activity using a labeled substrate, N-[^{11}C]methylpiperdinyl-4-propionate ([^{11}C]PMP). *Synapse* 22:123–131.

Klunk, W. E., E. Engler, A. Nordberg, Y. Wang, G. Blomqvist, D. P. Holt, M. Bergstrom, I. Savitcheve, G. Huang, S. Estrada, B. Ausen, M. N. Debnasth, J. Barletta, J. C. Price, J. Sandell, B. J. Lopresti, A. Wall, P. Koivisto, G. Antoni, C. A. Mathis, and B. Langstrom. 2004. Imaging brain amyloid in Alzheimer's disease using the novel positron emission tomography tracer, Pittsburgh Compound-B. *Ann Neurol* 55 (3):306–19.

Kosaka, K., K. Tsuchiya, and M. Yoshimura. 1988. Lewy body disease with and without dementia: a clinicopathological study of 35 cases. *Clin Neuropathol* 7 (6):299–305.

Kuhl, D. E., R. A. Koeppe, J. A. Fessler, S. Minoshima, R. J. Ackermann, J. E. Carey, D. L. Gildersleeve, K. A. Frey, and D. M. Wieland. 1994. In vivo mapping of cholinergic neurons in the human brain using SPECT and IBVM. *J Nucl Med* 35 (3):405–10.

Kuhl, D. E., R. A. Koeppe, S. E. Snyder, S. Minoshima, K. A. Frey, and M. R. Kilbourn. 1996. Mapping acetylcholinesterase activity in human brain using PET and N-[11C]Methylpiperidinyl propionate (PMP). *J Nucl Med* 37(Suppl):21P.

Kuhl, D. E., S. Minoshima, J. A. Fessler, K. A. Frey, N. L. Foster, E. P. Ficaro, D. M. Wieland, and R. A. Koeppe. 1996. In vivo mapping of cholinergic terminals in normal aging, Alzheimer's disease, and Parkinson's disease. *Ann Neurol* 40:399–410.

Kung, M. P., Z. P. Zhuang, C. Hou, and H. F. Kung. 2004. Development and evaluation of iodinated tracers targeting amyloid plaques for SPECT imaging. *J Mol Neurosci* 24 (1):49–53.

Lange, K. W., F. R. Wells, P. Jenner, and C. D. Marsden. 1993. Altered muscarinic and nicotinic receptor densities in cortical and subcortical brain regions in Parkinson's disease. *J Neurochem* 60:197–203.

Lecourtier, L., and P. H. Kelly. 2007. A conductor hidden in the orchestra? Role of the habenular complex in monoamine transmission and cognition. *Neurosci Biobehav Rev* 31 (5):658–72.

Lee, M. S., J. O. Rinne, and C. D. Marsden. 2000. The pedunculopontine nucleus: Its role in the genesis of movement disorders. *Yonsei Med J* 41:167–184.

Lees, A. J., and E. Smith. 1983. Cognitive deficits in the early stages of Parkinson's disease. *Brain* 106:257–270.

Lewy, F. H. 1913. Zur pathologischen Anatomie der Paralysis agitans. *Dtsch Ztschr Nervenheilkunde* 50:50–55.

Libow, L. S., P. G. Frisina, V. Haroutunian, D. P. Perl, and D. P. Purohit. 2009. Parkinson's disease dementia: A diminished role for the Lewy body. *Parkinsonism Relat Disord* 15 (8):572–5.

Lieberman, A., M. Dziatolowski, M. Kupersmith, M. Serby, A. Goodgold, J. Korein, and M. Goldstein. 1979. Dementia in Parkinson's disease. *Ann Neurol* 6:355–359.

Lippa, C. F., T. W. Smith, and J. M. Swearer. 1994. Alzheimer's disease and Lewy body disease: A comparative clinicopathological study. *Ann Neurol* 35 (1):81–8.

Lockhart, A., J. R. Lamb, T. Osredkar, L. I. Sue, J. N. Joyce, L. Ye, V. Libri, D. Leppert, and T. G. Beach. 2007. PIB is a non-specific imaging marker of amyloid-beta (Abeta) peptide-related cerebral amyloidosis. *Brain* 130 (Pt 10):2607–15.

Lopez, O. L., J. T. Becker, D. I. Kaufer, R. L. Hamilton, R. A. Sweet, W. Klunk, and S. T. DeKosky. 2002. Research evaluation and prospective diagnosis of dementia with Lewy dodies. *Arch Neurol* 59:43–46.

Maetzler, W., I. Liepelt, M. Reimold, G. Reischl, C. Solbach, C. Becker, C. Schulte, T. Leyhe, S. Keller, A. Melms, T. Gasser, and D. Berg. 2009. Cortical PIB binding in Lewy body disease is associated with Alzheimer-like characteristics. *Neurobiol Dis* 34 (1):107–12.

Maetzler, W., M. Reimold, I. Liepelt, C. Solbach, T. Leyhe, K. Schweitzer, G. W. Eschweiler, M. Mittelbronn, A. Gaenslen, M. Uebele, G. Reischl, T. Gasser, H. J. Machulla, R. Bares, and D. Berg. 2008. [(11)C]PIB binding in Parkinson's disease dementia. *Neuroimage* 39 (3):1027–33.

Mahler, M. E., and J. L. Cummings. 1990. Alzheimer disease and the dementia of Parkinson disease: Comparative investigations. *Alz Dis Ass Dis* 4:133–149.

Marder, K., M-X. Tang, L. Côté, Y. Stern, and R. Mayeux. 1995. The frequency and associated risk factors for dementia in patients with Parkinson's disease. *Arch Neurol* 52:695–701.

Mash, D. C., W. F. White, and M. M. Mesulam. 1988. Distribution of muscarinic receptor subtypes within architectonic subregions of the primate cerebral cortex. *J Comp Neurol* 278 (2):265–74.

Mastaglia, F. L., R. D. Johnsen, M. L Byrnes, and B. A. Kakulas. 2003. Prevalence of amyloid-beta deposition in the cerebral cortex in Parkinson's disease. *Mov Disord* 18:81–86.

Mattila, P. M., M. Roytta, P. Lonnberg, P. Marjamaki, H. Helenius, and J. O. Rinne. 2001. Choline acetytransferase activity and striatal dopamine receptors in Parkinson's disease in relation to cognitive impairment. *Acta Neuropathol (Berl)* 102:160–166.

Mattila, P. M., M. Roytta, H. Torikka, D. W. Dickson, and J. O. Rinne. 1998. Cortical Lewy bodies and Alzheimer-type changes in patients with Parkinson's disease. *Acta Neuropathol (Berl)* 95:576–582.

Mayeux, R., Y. Stern, J. Rosen, and J. Leventhal. 1981. Depression, intellectual impairment, and Parkinson's disease. *Neurology* 31:645–650.

Mayeux, R., Y. Stern, R. Rosenstein, K. Marder, A. Hauser, L. Côté, and S. Fahn. 1988. An estimate of the prevalence of dementia in idiopathic Parkinson's disease. *Arch Neurol* 45:260–262.

Maziere, M., and J. Delforge. 1995. PET imaging [11C]nicotine: Historical aspects. In *Brain imaging of nicotine and tobacco smoking*, ed. E. Domino. Ann Arbor: NPP Books, pp. 13–28.

McKeith, I. G., D. W. Dickson, J. Lowe, M. Emre, J. T. O'Brien, H. Feldman, J. Cummings, J. E. Duda, C. Lippa, E. K. Perry, D. Aarsland, H. Arai, C. G. Ballard, B. Boeve, D. J. Burn, D. Costa, T. Del Ser, B. Dubois, D. Galasko, S. Gauthier, C. G. Goetz, E. Gomez-Tortosa, G. Halliday, L. A. Hansen, J. Hardy, T. Iwatsubo, R. N. Kalaria, D. Kaufer, R. A. Kenny, A. Korczyn, K. Kosaka, V. M. Lee, A. Lees, I. Litvan, E. Londos, O. L. Lopez, S. Minoshima, Y. Mizuno, J. A. Molina, E. B. Mukaetova-Ladinska, F. Pasquier, R. H. Perry, J. B. Schulz, J. Q. Trojanowski, and M. Yamada. 2005. Diagnosis and management of dementia with Lewy bodies: third report of the DLB Consortium. *Neurology* 65 (12):1863–72.

Merdes, A. R., L. A. Hansen, D. V. Jeste, D. Galasko, C. R. Hofstetter, G. J. Ho, L. J. Thal, and J. Corey-Bloom. 2003. Influence of Alzheimer pathology on clinical diagnostic accuracy in dementia with Lewy bodies. *Neurology* 60:1586–1590.

Mesulam, M. 2004. The cholinergic lesion of Alzheimer's disease: Pivotal factor or side show? *Learn Mem* 11 (1):43–9.

Mesulam, M. M. 1996. The systems-level organization of cholinergic innervation in the human cerebral cortex and its alterations in Alzheimer's disease. *Prog Brain Res* 109:285–97.

Mesulam, M. M., and C. Geula. 1991. Acetylcholinesterase-rich neurons of the human cerebral cortex: cytoarchitectonic and ontogenetic patterns of distribution. *J Comp Neurol* 306 (2):193–220.

Mesulam, M. M., and C. Geula. 1992. Overlap between acetylcholinesterase-rich and choline acetyltransferase-positive (cholinergic) axons in human cerebral cortex. *Brain Res* 577 (1):112–20.

Mesulam, M. M., A. Guillozet, P. Shaw, A. Levey, E. G. Duysen, and O. Lockridge. 2002. Acetylcholinesterase knockouts establish central cholinergic pathways and can use butyrylcholinesterase to hydrolyze acetylcholine. *Neuroscience* 110 (4):627–39.

Mesulam, M. M., and C. Geula. 1988. Nucleus basalis (Ch4) and cortical cholinergic innervation in the human brain: Observations based on the distribution of acetylcholinesterase and choline acetyltransferase. *J Comp Neurol* 275:216–240.

Mesulam, M. M., E. J. Mufson, B. H. Wainer, and A. I. Levy. 1983. Central cholinergic pathways in the rat: An overview based on an alternative nomenclature (CH1-CH-6). *Neurosci* 10:1185–1201.

Mesulam, M. M., D. Mash, L. Hersh, M. Bothwell, and C. Geula. 1992. Cholinergic innervation of the human striatum, globus pallidus, subthalamic nucleus, substantia nigra, and red nucleus. *J Comp Neurol* 323:252–268.

Mesulam, M. M., E. J. Mufson, A. I. Levy, and B. H. Wainer. 1983. Cholinergic innervation of cortex by the basal forebrain: Cytochemistry and cortical connections of the septal area, diagonal band nuclei, nucleus basalis (substantia innominata), and hypothalamus in the rhesus monkey. *J Comp Neurol* 214:170–197.

Meyer, P. M., K. Strecker, K. Kendziorra, G. Becker, S. Hesse, D. Woelpl, A. Hensel, M. Patt, D. Sorger, F. Wegner, D. Lobsien, H. Barthel, P. Brust, H. J. Gertz, O. Sabri, and J. Schwarz. 2009. Reduced alpha4beta2*-nicotinic acetylcholine receptor binding and its relationship to mild cognitive and depressive symptoms in Parkinson disease. *Arch Gen Psychiatry* 66 (8):866–77.

Mogg, A. J., F. A. Jones, I. A. Pullar, C. G. Sharples, and S. Wonnacott. 2004. Functional responses and subunit composition of presynaptic nicotinic receptor subtypes explored using the novel agonist 5-iodo-A-85380. *Neuropharmacology* 47 (6):848–59.

Morris, J. C., M. Storandt, D. W. McKeel, Jr., E. H. Rubin, J. L. Price, E. A. Grant, and L. Berg. 1996. Cerebral amyloid deposition and diffuse plaques in "normal" aging: Evidence for presymptomatic and very mild Alzheimer's disease. *Neurology* 46 (3):707–19.

Mulholland, G. K., D. M. Wieland, M. R. Kilbourn, K. A. Frey, P. S. Sherman, J. E. Carey, and D. E. Kuhl. 1998. [18F]fluoroethoxy-benzovesamicol, a PET radiotracer for the vesicular acetylcholine transporter and cholinergic synapses. *Synapse* 30 (3):263–74.

Musachio, J. L., V. L. Villemagne, U. A. Scheffel, R. F. Dannals, A. S. Dogan, F. Yokoi, and D. F. Wong. 1999. Synthesis of an I-123 analog of A-85380 and preliminary SPECT imaging of nicotinic receptors in baboon. *Nucl Med Biol* 26 (2):201–7.

Nakano, I., and A. Hirano. 1984. Parkinson's disease: Neuron loss in the nucleus basalis without concomitant Alzheimer's disease. *Ann Neurol* 5:415–418.

Nordberg, A. 2001. Nicotinic receptor abnormalities of Alzheimer's disease: Therapeutic implications. *Biol Psychiatry* 49 (3):200–10.

O'Brien, J. T., S. J. Colloby, S. Pakrasi, E. K. Perry, S. L. Pimlott, D. J. Wyper, I. G. McKeith, and E. D. Williams. 2008. Nicotinic alpha4beta2 receptor binding in dementia with Lewy bodies using 123I-5IA-85380 SPECT demonstrates a link between occipital changes and visual hallucinations. *Neuroimage* 40 (3):1056–63.

Oishi, N., K. Hashikawa, H. Yoshida, K. Ishizu, M. Ueda, H. Kawashima, H. Saji, and H. Fukuyama. 2007. Quantification of nicotinic acetylcholine receptors in Parkinson's disease with (123)I-5IA SPECT. *J Neurol Sci* 256 (1–2):52–60.

Perry, E. K., M. Curtis, D. J. Dick, J. M. Candy, J. R. Atack, C. A. Bloxham, G. Blessed, A. Fairbairn, B. E. Tomlinson, and R. H. Perry. 1985. Cholinergic correlates of cognitive impairment in Parkinson's disease: Comparisons with Alzheimer's disease. *J Neurol Neurosurg Psychiatry* 48:413–421.

Perry, R. H., B. E. Tomlinson, J. M. Candy, G. Blessed, J. F. Foster, C. A. Bloxham, and E. R. Perry. 1983. Cortical cholinergic deficit in mentally impaired Parkinsonian patients. *Lancet* 2 (8353):789–90.

Pichika, R., B. Easwaramoorthy, D. Collins, B. T. Christian, B. Shi, T. K. Narayanan, S. G. Potkin, and J. Mukherjee. 2006. Nicotinic alpha4beta2 receptor imaging agents: part II. Synthesis and biological evaluation of 2-[18F]fluoro-3-[2-((S)-3-pyrrolinyl)methoxy]pyridine (18F-nifene) in rodents and imaging by PET in nonhuman primate. *Nucl Med Biol* 33 (3):295–304.

Pimlott, S. L., M. Piggott, J. Owens, E. Greally, J. A. Court, E. Jaros, R. H. Perry, E. K. Perry, and D. Wyper. 2004. Nicotinic acetylcholine receptor distribution in Alzheimer's disease, dementia with Lewy bodies, Parkinson's disease, and vascular dementia: In vitro binding study using 5-[(^{125})i]-a-85380. *Neuropsychopharmacology* 29 (1):108–16.

Pirozzolo, F. J., E. C. Hansch, J. A. Mortimer, D. D. Webster, and M. A. Kuskowski. 1982. Dementia in Parkinson disease: A neuropsychological analysis. *Brain Cogn* 1:71–83.

Rogers, J. D., D. Brogan, and S. S. Mirra. 1985. The nucleus basalis of Meynert in neurological disease: A quantitative morphological study. *Ann Neurol* 17:163–170.

Rowe, C. C., S. Ng, U. Ackermann, S. J. Gong, K. Pike, G. Savage, T. F. Cowie, K. L. Dickinson, P. Maruff, D. Darby, C. Smith, M. Woodward, J. Merory, H. Tochon-Danguy, G. O'Keefe, W. E. Klunk, C. A. Mathis, J. C. Price, C. L. Masters, and V. L. Villemagne. 2007. Imaging beta-amyloid burden in aging and dementia. *Neurology* 68 (20):1718–25.

Ruberg, M., A. Ploska, F. Javoy-Agid, and Y. Agid. 1982. Muscarinic binding and choline acetyltransferase activity in Parkinsonian subjects with reference to dementia. *Brain Res* 232:129–139.

Ruberg, M., F. Rieger, A. Villageois, A. M. Bonnet, and Y. Agid. 1986. Acetylcholinesterase and butyrylcholinesterase in frontal cortex and cerebrospinal fluid of demented and non-demented patients with Parkinson's disease. *Brain Res* 362:83–91.

Samuel, W., R. Crowder, C. R. Hofstetter, and L. Hansen. 1997. Neuritic plaques in the Lewy body variant of Alzheimer disease lack paired helical filaments. *Neurosci Lett* 223 (2):73–6.

Schmaljohann, J., D. Gundisch, M. Minnerop, J. Bucerius, A. Joe, M. Reinhardt, S. Guhlke, H. J. Biersack, and U. Wullner. 2006. In vitro evaluation of nicotinic acetylcholine receptors with 2-[18F]F-A85380 in Parkinson's disease. *Nucl Med Biol* 33 (3):305–9.

Selden, N. R., D. R. Gitelman, N. Salamon-Murayama, T. B. Parrish, and M. M. Mesulam. 1998. Trajectories of cholinergic pathways within the cerebral hemispheres of the human brain. *Brain* 121:2249–2257.

Shimada, H., S. Hirano, H. Shinotoh, A. Aotsuka, K. Sato, N. Tanaka, T. Ota, M. Asahina, K. Fukushi, T. Suhara, T. Hattori, S. Kuwabara, and T. Irie. 2009. Mapping of brain acetylcholinesterase alterations in Lewy body disease by PET. *Neurology* 73 (4):273–8.

Shinotoh, H., H. Namba, M. Yamaguchi, K. Fukushi, S. Nagatsuka, M. Iyo, M. Asahina, T. Hattori, S. Tanada, and T. Irie. 1999. Positron emission tomographic measurement of acetylcholinesterase activity reveals differential loss of ascending cholinergic systems in Parkinson's disease and progressive supranuclear palsy. *Ann Neurol* 46:62–69.

Shoghi-Jadid, K., G. W. Small, E. D. Agdeppa, V. Kepe, L. M. Ercoli, P. Siddarth, S. Read, N. Satyamurthy, A. Petric, S. C. Huang, and J. R. Barrio. 2002. Localization of neurofibrillary tangles and beta-amyloid plaques in the brains of living patients with Alzheimer disease. *Am J Geriatr Psychiatry* 10 (1):24–35.

Shute, C. C., and P. R. Lewis. 1966. Electron microscopy of cholinergic terminals and acetylcholinesterase-containing neurones in the hippocampal formation of the rat. *Z Zellforsch Mikrosk Anat* 69:334–343.

Sihver, W., K. J. Fasth, A. G. Horti, A. O. Koren, M. Bergstrom, L. Lu, G. Hagberg, H. Lundqvist, R. F. Dannals, E. D. London, A. Nordberg, and B. Langstrom. 1999. Synthesis and characterization of binding of 5-[76Br]bromo-3-[[2(S)-azetidinyl]methoxy]pyridine, a novel nicotinic acetylcholine receptor ligand, in rat brain. *J Neurochem* 73 (3):1264–72.

Sihver, W., B. Langstrom, and A. Nordberg. 2000. Ligands for in vivo imaging of nicotinic receptor subtypes in Alzheimer brain. *Acta Neurol Scand Suppl* 176:27–33.

Small, G. W., V. Kepe, L. M. Ercoli, P. Siddarth, S. Y. Bookheimer, K. J. Miller, H. Lavretsky, A. C. Burggren, G. M. Cole, H. V. Vinters, P. M. Thompson, S. C. Huang, N. Satyamurthy, M. E. Phelps, and J. R. Barrio. 2006. PET of brain amyloid and tau in mild cognitive impairment. *N Engl J Med* 355 (25):2652–63.

Smid, L. M., T. D. Vovko, M. Popovic, A. Petric, V. Kepe, J. R. Barrio, G. Vidmar, and M. Bresjanac. 2006. The 2,6-disubstituted naphthalene derivative FDDNP labeling reliably predicts Congo red birefringence of protein deposits in brain sections of selected human neurodegenerative diseases. *Brain Pathol* 16 (2):124–30.

Snyder, S. E., N. Gunupudi, P. S. Sherman, E. R. Butch, M. B. Skaddan, M. R. Kilbourn, R. A. Koeppe, and D. E. Kuhl. 2001. Radiolabeled cholinesterase substrates: In vitro methods for determining structure-activity relationships and identification of a positron emission tomography radiopharmaceutical for in vivo measurement of butyrylcholinesterase activity. *J Cereb Blood Flow Metab* 21 (2):132–43.

Stein, J. F. 2009. Akinesia, motor oscillations and the pedunculopontine nucleus in rats and men. *Exp Neurol* 215 (1):1–4.

Stern, Y., R. Mayeux, J. Rosen, and J. Ilson. 1983. Perceptual motor dysfunction in Parkinson's disease: A deficit in sequential and predictive voluntary movement. *J Neurol Neurosurg Psychiatry* 46:145–151.

Sugiyama, H., J. A. Hainfellner, M. Yoshimura, and H. Budka. 1994. Neocortical changes in Parkinson's disease, revisited. *Clin Neuropathol* 13:55–59.

Tagliavini, F., G. Pilleri, C. Bouras, and J. Constantinidis. 1984. The basal nucleus of Meynert in idiopathic Parkinson's disease. *Acta Neurol Scand* 70:20–28.

Taylor, J. P., E. N. Rowan, D. Lett, J. T. O'Brien, I. G. McKeith, and D. J. Burn. 2008. Poor attentional function predicts cognitive decline in patients with non-demented Parkinson's disease independent of motor phenotype. *J Neurol Neurosurg Psychiatry* 79 (12):1318–23.

Volkow, N. D., Y. S. Ding, J. S. Fowler, and S. J. Gatley. 2001. Imaging brain cholinergic activity with positron emission tomography: its role in the evaluation of cholinergic treatments in Alzheimer's dementia. *Biol Psychiatry* 49 (3):211–20.

Weihe, E., J. H. Tao-Cheng, M. K. Schafer, J. D. Erickson, and L. E. Eiden. 1996. Visualization of the vesicular acetylcholine transporter in cholinergic nerve terminals and its targeting to a specific population of small synaptic vesicles. *Proc Natl Acad Sci U S A* 93 (8):3547–52.

Whitehouse, P. J., A. M. Martino, M. V. Wagster, D. L. Price, R. Mayeux, J. R. Atack, and K. J. Kellar. 1988. Reductions in [3H]nicotinic acetylcholine binding in Alzheimer's disease and Parkinson's disease: An autoradiographic study. *Neurology* 38 (5):720–3.

Whitehouse, P. J., J. C. Hedreen, C. L. White, and D. L. Price. 1983. Basal forebrain neurons in the dementia of Parkinson disease. *Ann Neurol* 13:243–248.

Williams-Gray, C. H., J. R. Evans, A. Goris, T. Foltynie, M. Ban, T. W. Robbins, C. Brayne, B. S. Kolachana, D. R. Weinberger, S. J. Sawcer, and R. A. Barker. 2009. The distinct cognitive syndromes of Parkinson's disease: 5 year follow-up of the CamPaIGN cohort. *Brain* 132 (Pt 11):2958–69.

Wright, C. I., G. Geula, and M. M. Mesulam. 1993. Neurological cholinesterases in the normal brain and in Alzheimer's disease: Relationship to plaques, tangles, and patterns of selective vulnerability. *Ann Neurol* 34 (3):373–84.

Xuereb, J. H., B. E. Tomlinson, D. Irving, R. H. Perry, G. Blessed, and E. K. Perry. 1990. Cortical and subcortical pathology in Parkinson's disease: Relationship to parkinsonian dementia. *Adv Neurol* 53: 35–40.

Ye, L., A. Velasco, G. Fraser, T. G. Beach, L. Sue, T. Osredkar, V. Libri, M. G. Spillantini, M. Goedert, and A. Lockhart. 2008. In vitro high affinity alpha-synuclein binding sites for the amyloid imaging agent PIB are not matched by binding to Lewy bodies in postmortem human brain. *J Neurochem* 105 (4):1428–37.

Yoshimura, M. 1988. Pathological basis for dementia in elderly patients with idiopathic Parkinson's disease. *Eur Neurol* 28 (suppl 1):29–35.

Zaccai, J., C. Brayne, I. McKeith, F. Matthews, and P. G. Ince. 2008. Patterns and stages of alpha-synucleinopathy: Relevance in a population-based cohort. *Neurology* 70 (13):1042–8.

Zubieta, J. K., R. A. Koeppe, K. A. Frey, M. R. Kilbourn, T. J. Mangner, N. L. Foster, and D. E. Kuhl. 2001. Assessment of muscarinic receptor concentrations in aging and Alzheimer disease with [^{11}C]NMPB and PET. *Synapse* 39 (4):275–87.

Zweig, R. M., W. R. Jankel, J. C. Hedreen, R. Mayeux, and D. L. Price. 1989. The pedunculopontine nucleus in Parkinson's disease. *Ann Neurol* 26 (1):41–6.

11

IMAGING INFLAMMATION IN PARKINSONIAN SYNDROMES

David J. Brooks

INTRODUCTION

Idiopathic Parkinson's disease (PD) is a neurodegenerative disorder that presents clinically with asymmetrical bradykinesia, rigidity, and resting tremor and usually responds well to dopaminergic medication (Hughes et al. 1992). The condition is neuropathologically characterized by cell loss targeting the substantia nigra pars compacta and the presence of neuronal Lewy inclusion bodies. Other brainstem nuclei—including the dorsal motor nucleus of the vagus, the locus coeruleus, the median raphe, and the nucleus basalis—are also involved, as are association cortical areas, in particular the cingulate. It has been suggested that the pathology of PD occurs in an ascending fashion from the medulla (stage 1) through to the primary cortices (stage 6) (Braak et al. 2004). Activated microglia were first reported in the substantia nigra, striatum, nucleus basalis, and hippocampus of PD patients postmortem (McGeer et al. 1988). More recently, microglial activation has also been described in the cingulate and temporal cortex of non-demented PD patients (Imamura et al. 2003).

While the nigrostriatal dopamine system is also targeted in atypical parkinsonian syndromes, they have additional clinical features and alternative pathology to PD. In multiple system atrophy (MSA), early autonomic dysfunction occurs and ataxia is a feature. Synuclein positive argyrophilic inclusions are found in glia and neurons of the substantia nigra compacta, olivopontocerebellar pathways, and the intermediolateral columns of the spinal cord associated with activated astrocytes and microglia (Papp and Lantos 1994). Progressive supranuclear palsy (PSP) is associated with early gait instability, bulbar problems, and a supranuclear gaze disorder (Steele et al. 1964). Neuronal loss is found in the oculomotor nuclei, pallidum, substantia nigra, subthalamic nucleus, and frontal cortex accompanied by microglial activation (Ishizawa and Dickson 2001). The pathologic hallmark of PSP is intraneuronal neurofibrillary tangles (NFT) composed of abnormally phosphorylated

microtubule-associated tau protein and neuropil threads. In corticobasal degeneration (CBD), limb dystonia, apraxia, and myoclonus are associated features (Gibb et al. 1989). The superior frontal gyrus and inferior parietal area atrophy while the inferior frontal gyri, temporal, and occipital lobes are spared. The atrophy is characteristically asymmetric. Microscopic findings include achromatic swollen neurons and neuronal loss with tau-positive inclusions in the affected cortices and basal ganglia (Dickson et al. 2002). These lesions are accompanied by microglial activation (Ishizawa and Dickson 2001; Rebeiz et al. 1968).

Microglia constitute 10%–20% of glial cells and are ontogenetically related to cells of mononuclear–phagocyte lineage (Kreutzberg 1996). They are the brain's resident tissue macrophages, and when resting, probably act to monitor changes in the local milieu. Any active brain pathology can lead to their activation; the transformation from a resting to an activated state takes place over minutes and often occurs before any other sign of tissue damage or cell death can be seen. Microglial activation is associated with expression of immunologically relevant molecules including HLA antigens, chemokines, and cytokines, nitric oxide, and nerve growth factors. The presence of activated microglia is, therefore, a useful indicator of ongoing neuronal injury and reflects disease activity rather than a specific etiology.

One of the molecules expressed by mitochondria during the "activation" of microglia is the translocator protein (TSPO), also known as the "peripheral benzodiazepine receptor" (Papadopoulos et al. 2006). The TSPO regulates cholesterol and steroid synthesis and is associated with the mitochondrial permeability transition pore. It contains an isoquinoline binding site and is linked to a voltage-dependent ion channel. PK11195, [1-(2-chlorophenyl)-N-methyl-N-(1-methylpropyl)-3-isoquinoline carboxamide], is a selective ligand for the TSPO. In the absence of invading blood-borne cells, the de novo expression of peripheral benzodiazepine binding sites (PBBS) occurs primarily in activated microglia (Banati et al. 1997) and, based on this relative cellular selectivity, ^{11}C-PK11195 PET has been used as a marker of in vivo microglial activation in inflammatory (Banati et al. 2000; Cagnin et al. 2001a, 2001b), ischemic (Gerhard et al. 2005; Pappata et al. 2000), and degenerative (Cagnin et al. 2001a; Turner et al. 2004) neurological disorders and can detect disease activity in asymptomatic Huntington's disease gene carriers when present (Tai et al. 2007). Other ligands of the TSPO are also now available including aryloxanilides, 2-aryl-3-indoleacetamide, pyrrolobenzoxazepine, 2-phenyl-imidazo [1,2-a]pyridine, phenoxyphenyl-acetamide, pyridazinoindole, and 8-oxodihydropurine derivatives (Papadopoulos, et al., 2006). Aryloxanilides such as PBR28 and PBR06 are higher affinity ligands than PK11195 but have a lower Bmax, apparently not binding to all subtypes of the TSPO. This results in a minority of the population being nonbinders (Brown et al. 2007; Fujimura et al. 2009).

The contribution of microglial activation to the degenerative process in parkinsonian syndromes is presently not known, but it is likely to have a damaging rather than a beneficial role (Teismann et al. 2003). There is evidence from humans (Langston et al. 1999) and monkeys (McGeer et al. 2003) exposed to the nigral toxin MPTP that, after a discrete insult, progression of parkinsonian symptoms can occur, and this is accompanied by microglial activation present years after the acute toxic exposure. Additionally, at postmortem the activated microglia present in PD are still expressing mRNA for cytokines including tumor necrosis factor (Imamura et al. 2003).

PARKINSON'S DISEASE

Ouchi and colleagues have investigated the relationship between levels of microglial activation, measured with ^{11}C-PK11195 PET, and reduction in presynaptic dopamine transporter (DAT) density, measured with ^{11}C-CFT PET, in PD (Ouchi et al. 2005). Ten drug-naive cases with early asymmetric disease, subsequently shown to be levodopa responsive, were studied and levels of tracer binding quantitated. Tracer-specific volumes of distribution—also known as binding potentials (BPs)—were computed by applying compartment analyses to PD brain time activity curves (TACs), and a normal population cerebellar cortex tissue reference was used as a measure of nonspecific binding. Levels of ^{11}C-PK11195 binding in the midbrain contralateral to the clinically more affected side were significantly raised in PD and correlated inversely with ^{11}C-CFT binding in the putamen and positively with motor severity rated with the Unified Parkinson's Disease Rating Scale. There was no correlation between midbrain ^{11}C-PK11195 binding and disease duration. The authors concluded that in vivo demonstration of parallel changes in microglial activation and dopaminergic terminal loss in the affected nigrostriatal pathway in early PD supports the view that microglial activation contributes significantly to the progressive degeneration process.

The Ouchi study did not explore the presence of cortical microglial activation in PD or follow this process longitudinally. Gerhard et al. (2006) studied 18 PD patients (13 men and 5 women, aged 50 to 69 years) with a clinical diagnosis of idiopathic Parkinson's disease according to the UK Parkinson's Disease Society Brain Bank criteria. None of the patients showed any evidence of cognitive decline nor gave a history of hallucinations. The patients ranged from mild to severe locomotor disability ("off" UPDRS motor scores 6–70; disease duration 1–20 years). Patients had both ^{11}C-PK11195 and ^{18}F-dopa PET and 8 of them had follow-up ^{11}C-PK11195 PET after 18–28 months.

Parametric images of ^{11}C-PK11195 BPs were calculated using a simplified reference tissue model (Gunn et al. 1997; Lammertsma and Hume 1996). Rather than using a normal population cerebellar cortex reference for nonspecific tracer binding, as employed by Ouchi, cluster analysis was used to extract and identify a normal brain reference input function for each individual PD case (Anderson et al. 2007; Cagnin et al. 2001a). In brief, voxels in the raw dynamic data were segmented into 10 clusters distinguished by the shape of their time-activity curves (TACs). In a normal brain, a majority of the voxels segregate into clusters representing (a) a TAC with the shape of the ligand kinetic as seen in a normal healthy cortex, (b) areas of specific brain ligand retention, (c) a TAC mainly from extracerebral structures, and (d) a cluster representing vascular binding. The PD patient cluster representing a "normal" cortical reference time activity curve (TAC) contains mainly cortical voxels.

The 18 PD patients showed significant increases in mean ^{11}C-PK11195 binding in the striatum, pallidum, thalamus, brainstem, and multiple cortical areas (precentral gyrus, frontal lobe, anterior cingulate, posterior cingulate, and hippocampus)—see Figure 1. There was a significant inverse correlation between cingulate ^{11}C-PK11195 uptake and disease duration but no correlation of regional levels of microglial activation with severity of symptoms. Although the mean BP value in the substantia nigra was raised in the PD group, the difference did not reach statistical significance, only some of the individuals showing increased signal. ^{18}F-dopa uptake was quantitated as influx constants,

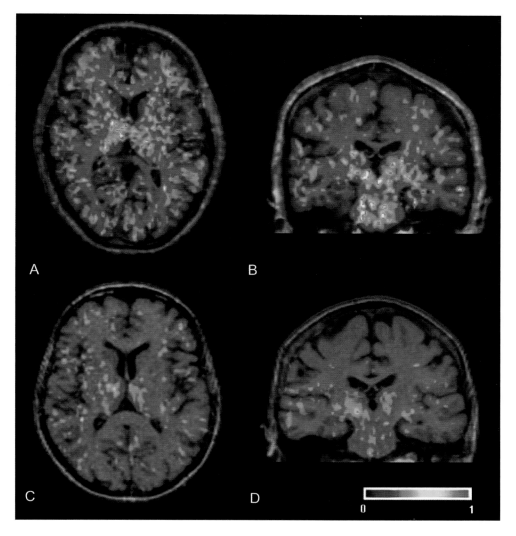

Figure 1 Transverse and coronal sections of binding potential maps co-registered to the individual MRI. In the PD patient (A, B) binding is increased in the basal ganglia, pons, and frontal regions while the healthy control subject (C, D) shows mild ^{11}C-PK11195 binding increases in the thalamus. (Figure courtesy of A Gerhard)

Ki, and the PD patients showed asymmetrically decreased mean caudate and putamen dopamine storage capacity at baseline, the putamen being most affected. There was no inverse correlation between brainstem ^{11}C-PK11195 binding and putamen ^{18}F-dopa Ki values. Eight PD patients had repeat ^{11}C-PK11195 PET after 18–28 months, and four of these also had ^{18}F-dopa PET. There was no significant change of ^{11}C-PK11195 BPs from baseline to follow-up, though UPDRS ratings measured withdrawn from medication increased and putamen ^{18}F-dopa Ki values decreased.

Gerhard's in vivo findings confirm pathological reports that microglial activation in Parkinson's disease is anatomically widespread and can be as severe in early as in late stages of the disease. Although microglial activation was initially described in the substantia nigra in PD (McGeer

et al. 1988), these workers and others also reported the presence of activated microglia in the putamen, hippocampus, transentorhinal cortex, cingulate cortex, and temporal cortex (Imamura et al. 2003). These pathological reports, however, could sample only end-stage disease.

The PD patients showed increased thalamic ^{11}C-PK11195 binding. This is most likely to reflect the presence of cortical pathology leading to disconnection of that nucleus rather than the thalamus being a primary site of pathology. Increases in thalamic signal can be seen after middle cerebral artery strokes (Gerhard et al. 2005; Pappata et al. 2000).

The mean increase in ^{11}C-PK11195 binding potential for the substantia nigra of Gerhard's PD patients failed to reach statistical significance, although individual values were increased unilaterally in 15 out of 18 patients; this individual variability may reflect the pathology of PD or reflect partial volume effects due to the 5mm resolution of the PET camera that can lead to falsely low estimates of BP measurements in this small and narrow structure.

The finding of widespread microglial activation in cortical (especially limbic) areas in PD is interesting considering that none of the patients showed signs of dementia or depression and that bedside screening tests for dementia and frontal dysfunction were normal. If ^{11}C-PK11195 PET demonstrates in vivo the presence of active cortical pathology before clinical symptoms become evident, this would imply that early PD patients can be Braak stage 5/6 pathologically by the time dopamine levels fall below the critical threshold associated with locomotor disability. Whether the staging of microglial activation follows the Braak stages is currently uncertain; Braak stage 1 and 2 PD cases are subclinical and, to date, only symptomatic subjects have been studied with ^{11}C-PK11195 PET.

The level of microglial activation appears to be static, at least over a period of two years, in PD. Despite this, the patients deteriorated clinically, and putamen ^{18}F-dopa uptake fell further. In Gerhard's baseline cross-sectional study, there was no correlation between levels of nigral and basal ganglia microglial activation and disease duration apart from in the cingulate cortex and thalamus. This would suggest that microglia are activated early and extensively in PD and then the population remains stable, possibly driving neuronal fallout via cytokine release. Experimental

studies have shown that the binding of the ^{11}C-PK11195 by activated microglia increases rapidly after neuronal injury but then stabilizes as transformation of microglia into phagocytes occurs following neuronal cell death (Banati et al. 1997).

While activated microglia may promote tissue destruction and clearance, these cells are also able to support neuronal survival by releasing growth factors and take part in remodeling of synapses. They are, thus, an integral part of brain plasticity (Banati 2002). It is, therefore, not surprising that there was no positive correlation between the clinical disability and levels of ^{11}C-PK11195 binding, as the UPDRS and F-dopa PET primarily measure clinical and dopaminergic deficits linked to the function of the nigrostriatal system.

MULTIPLE SYSTEM ATROPHY

[11]C-PK11195 PET has been used to study five cases of MSA, four clinically probable and one clinically possible based on consensus criteria (Gerhard et al. 2003). All five had parkinsonism, erectile dysfunction, and urinary incontinence. Two of the five had limb ataxia while another two had orthostatic hypotension, and all five had a poor levodopa response. ^{11}C-PK11195 BPs were calculated using a simplified reference tissue model (Gunn et al. 1997), and cluster analysis was used to extract and identify a normal

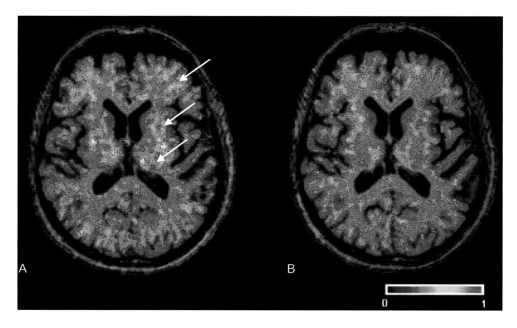

Figure 2 Transverse images of ^{11}C-PK11195 binding (arrows) in an MSA case before (A) and after (B) six months of treatment with minocycline. It can be seen that reduced microglial activation is present after chronic minocycline exposure. (Figure courtesy of A Gerhard)

brain reference input function for each individual PD case (Anderson et al. 2007).

The MSA patients had increased mean binding of ^{11}C-PK11195 in the dorsolateral prefrontal cortex, caudate, putamen, pallidum, thalamus, substantia nigra, and pons. These increases were generally greater and more extensive than those reported in Parkinson's disease, but the pattern and amplitudes were not specific enough to separate the two conditions. Increased cerebellar PET signal was seen in three patients, two of whom also had cerebellar signs. The authors concluded that the pattern of microglial activation in MSA revealed by ^{11}C-PK11195 PET agreed well with the known pathological distribution of microglial activation and provided information about the location of active disease.

In a recent small sub-study of a randomized double-blind controlled clinical trial of the efficacy of minocycline for slowing the progression of MSA, eight of 63 MSA cases had ^{11}C-PK11195 PET at baseline and again after six months of therapy (Dodel et al. 2010). Three received 200 mg of minocycline per day and five received a placebo. Two of the three cases on active treatment showed mild reductions in ^{11}C-PK11195 uptake, suggesting that minocycline could act as a microglial suppressant—see Figure 2. Clinically there was no significant effect of minocycline on disease progression.

PROGRESSIVE SUPRANUCLEAR PALSY

[11]C-PK11195 PET has been used to demonstrate in vivo the degree and distribution of the microglial response to the degenerative process in four patients (two men, two women) with a diagnosis of clinically probable PSP according to the NINDS-SPSP criteria (Gerhard et al. 2006; Litvan et al. 1996). Their mean age was 66 years and mean clinical disease duration was 3.5 years. All four had poorly levodopa responsive parkinsonism, early falls, upgaze palsies, and were impaired on tests of frontal lobe function.

Compared to healthy age-matched controls, the PSP patient group showed increased mean ^{11}C-PK11195 binding in the striatum and pallidum, thalamus, midbrain, frontal lobe, and cerebellum. Two of the patients were rescanned after 6–10 months and over that time the level of microglial activation remained stable. ^{11}C-PK11195 PET revealed a pattern of increased microglial activation in PSP patients involving cortical and subcortical regions that corresponds well with the known distribution of neuropathological changes. Again, however, the pattern of raised ^{11}C-PK11195 uptake was not specific enough to discriminate this disorder from PD or MSA.

CORTICOBASAL DEGENERATION

Four patients with CBD have been studied with ^{11}C-PK11195 PET (Gerhard et al. 2004). Their mean age was 70 years and mean clinical disease duration $3^1/_2$ years. All four had poorly levodopa associated parkinsonism and limb apraxia, three exhibited the alien limb phenomenon, two had myoclonus, and two had fixed dystonia. Compared to normal age-matched controls, the CBD patient group showed significantly increased mean ^{11}C-PK11195 binding in the caudate nucleus, putamen, substantia nigra, pons, pre- and postcentral gyrus and the frontal lobe.

CONCLUSION

In vivo markers of microglial activation, such as ^{11}C-PK11195 PET, provide a measure of disease activity and extent in parkinsonian syndromes. The pattern of microglial activation revealed by PET in these syndromes is concordant with their known pathologies and suggests widespread brain involvement even in early clinical stages. The patterns, however, are not specific enough to discriminate the different degenerative parkinsonian disorders. In the future, PET could be used to provide proof of mechanism and study efficacy of putative anti-inflammatory agents directed at microglia in parkinsonian syndromes if suitably safe medicines become available.

REFERENCES

Anderson, A. N., N. Pavese, P. Edison, Y. F. Tai, A. Hammers, A. Gerhard et al. 2007. A systematic comparison of kinetic modelling methods generating parametric maps for [(11)C]-(R)-PK11195. *Neuroimage* 36 (1): 28–37.

Banati, R. B. 2002. Brain plasticity and microglia: Is transsynaptic glial activation in the thalamus after limb denervation linked to cortical plasticity and central sensitisation? *J Physiol Paris* 96 (3–4), 289–299.

Banati, R. B., G. Goerres, D. Perkin, A. Lammertsma, V. Cunningham, R. Gunn et al. 1997. Imaging microglial activation in vivo. *J Cereb Blood Flow Metab* 17 (Supp 1): S435–S430.

Banati, R. B., J. Newcombe, R. N. Gunn, A. Cagnin, F. Turkheimer, F. Heppner et al. 2000 (Nov). The peripheral benzodiazepine binding site in the brain in multiple sclerosis: quantitative in vivo imaging of microglia as a measure of disease activity. *Brain* 123 (Pt 11): 2321–2337.

Braak, H., E. Ghebremedhin, U. Rub, H. Bratzke, and K. Del Tredici. 2004. Stages in the development of Parkinson's disease-related pathology. *Cell Tissue Res* 318 (1): 121–134.

Brown, A. K., M. Fujita, Y. Fujimura, J. S. Liow, M. Stabin, Y. H. Ryu et al. 2007. Radiation dosimetry and biodistribution in monkey and man of 11C-PBR28: A PET radioligand to image inflammation. *J Nucl Med* 48 (12): 2072–2079.

Cagnin, A., D. J. Brooks, A. M. Kennedy, R. N. Gunn, R. Myers, F. E. Turkheimer et al. 2001a (Aug 11). In-vivo measurement of activated microglia in dementia. *Lancet* 358 (9280): 461–467.

Cagnin, A., R. Myers, R. N. Gunn, A. D. Lawrence, T. Stevens, G. W. Kreutzberg et al. 2001b (Oct). In vivo visualization of activated glia by 11C(R)-PK11195-PET following herpes encephalitis reveals projected neuronal damage beyond the primary focal lesion. *Brain* 124 (Pt 10): 2014–2027.

Dickson, D. W., C. Bergeron, S. S. Chin, C. Duyckaerts, D. Horoupian, K. Ikeda et al. 2002. Office of Rare Diseases neuropathologic criteria for corticobasal degeneration. *J Neuropathol Exp Neurol* 61 (11): 935–946.

Dodel, R., A. Spottke, A. Gerhard, A. Reuss, S. Reinecker, N. Schimke et al. 2010. Minocycline 1-year therapy in multiple-system-atrophy: Effect on clinical symptoms and [(11)C] (R)-PK11195 PET (MEMSA-trial). *Mov Disord* 25 (1): 97–107.

Fujimura, Y., S. S. Zoghbi, F. G. Simeon, A. Taku, V. W. Pike, R. B. Innis et al. 2009. Quantification of translocator protein (18 kDa) in the human brain with PET and a novel radioligand, (18)F-PBR06. *J Nucl Med* 50 (7): 1047–1053.

Gerhard, A., R. B. Banati, G. B. Goerres, A. Cagnin, R. Myers, R. N. Gunn et al. 2003. [(11)C](R)-PK11195 PET imaging of microglial activation in multiple system atrophy. *Neurology* 61 (5): 686–689.

Gerhard, A., N. Pavese, G. Hotton, F. Turkheimer, M. Es, A. Hammers et al. 2006. In vivo imaging of microglial activation with [(11)C] (R)-PK11195 PET in idiopathic Parkinson's disease. *Neurobiol Dis* 21 (2): 404–412.

Gerhard, A., J. Schwarz, R. Myers, R. Wise, and R. B. Banati. 2005. Evolution of microglial activation in patients after ischemic stroke: A [(11)C](R)-PK11195 PET study. *Neuroimage* 24 (2): 591–595.

Gerhard, A., I; Trender-Gerhard, F. Turkheimer, N. P. Quinn, K. P. Bhatia, and D. J. Brooks. 2006. In vivo imaging of microglial activation with [(11)C](R)-PK11195 PET in progressive supranuclear palsy. *Mov Disord* 21 (1): 89–93.

Gerhard, A., J. Watts, I. Trender-Gerhard, F. Turkheimer, R. B. Banati, K. Bhatia et al. 2004. In vivo imaging of microglial activation with [11C](R)-PK11195 PET in corticobasal degeneration. *Mov Disord* 19 (10): 1221–1226.

Gibb, W. R. G., P. Luthert, and C. D. Marsden. 1989. Corticobasal degeneration. *Brain* 112: 1171–1192.

Gunn, R. N., A. A. Lammertsma, S. P. Hume, and V. J. Cunningham. 1997 (Nov). Parametric imaging of ligand-receptor binding in PET using a simplified reference region model. *Neuroimage* 6 (4): 279–287.

Hughes, A. J., S. E. Daniel, L. Kilford, and A. J. Lees. 1992. The accuracy of the clinical diagnosis of Parkinson's disease: A clinicopathological study of 100 cases. *J Neurol Neurosurg Psychiatr* 55: 181–184.

Imamura, K., N. Hishikawa, M. Sawada, T. Nagatsu, M. Yoshida, and Y. Hashizume. 2003. Distribution of major histocompatibility complex class II-positive microglia and cytokine profile of Parkinson's disease brains. *Acta Neuropathol (Berl)* 106 (6): 518–526.

Ishizawa, K., and D. W. Dickson. 2001. Microglial activation parallels system degeneration in progressive supranuclear palsy and corticobasal degeneration. *J Neuropathol Exp Neurol* 60 (6): 647–657.

Kreutzberg, G. W. 1996. Microglia: A sensor for pathological events in the CNS. *Trends Neurosci* 19 (8): 312–318.

Lammertsma, A. A., and S. P. Hume. 1996. Simplified reference tissue model for PET receptor studies. *Neuroimage* 4 (3) (Pt 1): 153–158.

Langston, J. W., L. S. Forno, J. Tetrud, A. G. Reeves, J. A. Kaplan, and D. Karluk, D. 1999. Evidence of active nerve cell degeneration in the substantia nigra of humans years after 1-Methyl-4-Phenyl-1,2,3,6- tetrahydropyridine exposure. *Annals of Neurology* 46 (4): 598–605.

Litvan, I., Y. Agid, D. Calne, G. Campbell, B. Dubois, R. C. Duvoisin et al. 1996. Clinical research criteria for the diagnosis of progressive supranuclear palsy (Steele-Richardson-Olszewski syndrome): Report of the NINDS-SPSP international workshop. *Neurology* 47 (1): 1–9.

McGeer, P. L., S. Itagaki, B. E. Boyes, and E. G. McGeer. 1988. Reactive microglia are positive for HLA-DR in the substantia nigra of Parkinson's and Alzheimer's disease brains. *Neurology* 38: 1285–1291.

McGeer, P. L., C. Schwab, A. Parent, and D. Doudet. 2003. Presence of reactive microglia in monkey substantia nigra years after 1-methyl-4-phenyl-1,2,3,6-tetrahydropyridine administration. *Ann Neurol* 54 (5): 599–604.

Ouchi, Y., E. Yoshikawa, Y. Sekine, M. Futatsubashi, T. Kanno, T. Ogusu et al. 2005. Microglial activation and dopamine terminal loss in early Parkinson's disease. *Ann Neurol* 57 (2): 168–175.

Papadopoulos, V., M. Baraldi, T. R. Guilarte, T. B. Knudsen, J. J. Lacapere, P. Lindemann et al. 2006. Translocator protein (18kDa): New nomenclature for the peripheral-type benzodiazepine receptor based on its structure and molecular function. *Trends Pharmacol Sci* 27 (8): 402–409.

Papp, M. I., and P. L. Lantos. 1994. The distribution of oligodendroglial inclusions in multiple system atrophy and its relevance to clinical symptomatology. *Brain* 117: 235–243.

Pappata, S., M. Levasseur, R. N. Gunn, R. Myers, C. Crouzel, A. Syrota et al. 2000. Thalamic microglial activation in ischemic stroke detected in vivo by PET and [11C]PK1195. *Neurology* 55 (7): 1052–1054.

Rebeiz, J. J., E. H. Kolodny, and E. P. Richardson. 1968. Corticodentatonigral degeneration with neuronal achromasia. *Arch Neurol* 18: 20–33.

Steele, J. C., J. C. Richardson, and J. Olszewski. 1964. Progressive supranuclear palsy. A heterogeneous degeneration involving the brain stem, basal ganglia, and cerebellum, with vertical gaze and pseudobulbar palsy. *Arch Neurol* 10: 333–359.

Tai, Y. F., N. Pavese, A. Gerhard, S. J. Tabrizi, R. A. Barker, D. J. Brooks et al. 2007. Microglial activation in presymptomatic Huntington's disease gene carriers. *Brain* 130: 1759–1766.

Teismann, P., K. Tieu, O. Cohen, D. K. Choi, D. C. Wu, D. Marks et al. 2003. Pathogenic role of glial cells in Parkinson's disease. *Mov Disord* 18 (2): 121–129.

Turner, M. R., A. Cagnin, F. E. Turkheimer, C. C. Miller, C. E. Shaw, D. J. Brooks et al. 2004. Evidence of widespread cerebral microglial activation in amyotrophic lateral sclerosis: An [11C](R)-PK11195 positron emission tomography study. *Neurobiol Dis* 15 (3): 601–609.

12

FUNCTIONAL IMAGING BIOMARKERS FOR THE ASSESSMENT OF PARKINSON'S DISEASE PROGRESSION

Chris C. Tang and David Eidelberg

IMAGING BIOMARKERS IN PD

Parkinson's disease (PD) is a progressive neurological disorder that is clinically characterized by motor manifestations, including muscle rigidity, tremor, and bradykinesia. These symptoms typically begin after a loss of more than 50% of the dopaminergic neurons in the substantia nigra pars compacta (SNc) (Bernheimer et al. 1973). Current treatment approaches allow for sufficient symptomatic relief in PD patients, especially during the early stages of the disease. However, despite treatment, continuing progression of the disease often leads to functional disability in later stages, causing decreased abilities of daily living and a growing socioeconomic burden to both the patient and his or her family.

Recent clinical studies have focused on the development of therapies designed to retard disease progression of PD. The Unified Parkinson's Disease Rating Scale (UPDRS) (Fahn et al. 1987) and the Hoehn and Yahr Scale (H&Y) (Hoehn and Yahr 1967) are the primary tools used for clinical assessment of symptom progression in PD. During the early stages of disease, UPDRS motor ratings increase on average at a rate of about 10 points each year without dopaminergic medication (Shults et al. 2002; Fahn et al. 2004). The time interval between the onset of symptoms and the development of substantial motor disability with loss of independent ambulation (H&Y stage 4) has been prolonged with currently available dopaminergic medications from about nine years in the pre-levodopa era (Hoehn and Yahr 1967) to about 26 years at the current time (Lucking et al. 2000).

Radiotracer-based imaging techniques have also been widely used to assess presynaptic dopaminergic function as a means of measuring the progression of PD (Au et al. 2005). The rate of loss of striatal dopaminergic function was thought to be dependent on disease stages with a faster decline during the early stages (Fearnley and Lees 1991;

Morrish et al. 1998), as supported by the findings of a longitudinal imaging study (Hilker et al. 2005). However, prior double-blind, randomized clinical trials (Parkinson-Study-Group 2002; Whone et al. 2003; Fahn et al. 2004) designed to assess the effects of levodopa treatment on disease progression have provided discordant presynaptic dopaminergic imaging and clinical results. These differences have been attributed to possible long-lasting influences of the symptomatic treatments on the imaging measures. Regardless of the cause, it underscores the need for alternative imaging biomarkers for accurate and objective assessment of disease progression to aid in the development of new symptomatic therapies and neuroprotective agents in PD.

In this chapter, we will briefly review recent advances in the use of metabolic imaging and network analysis in the study of the progression of PD.

ABNORMAL METABOLIC NETWORKS IN PD

Functional positron emission tomography (PET) imaging studies have provided unique insights into the mechanisms underlying the motor and non-motor manifestations of PD. The application of spatial covariance methods to analyze [18F]fluorodeoxyglucose (FDG) PET data has become an important means of assessing abnormal functional interrelationships in neurodegenerative diseases such as PD, which has led to the identification of several novel imaging biomarkers for this disorder (Eidelberg 2009; Tang and Eidelberg 2010). In recent years, three distinct spatial covariance patterns have been identified in association with PD: (1) the PD motor-related pattern (PDRP) (Eidelberg et al. 1994; Ma et al. 2007); (2) the PD cognition-related pattern (PDCP) (Huang et al. 2007a); and (3) the PD tremor-related pattern (PDTP) (Mure et al. 2011). These resting state metabolic brain networks have been separately identified and validated in independent PD patient populations.

Each represents a set of characteristic changes in regional brain function associated with the major clinical manifestations of the disorder. As we shall see, each of these metabolic patterns also exhibits a characteristic time course with advancing disease consistent with the natural history of the disorder.

PD-RELATED MOTOR PATTERN (PDRP)

Principal component analysis (PCA) of rest-state FDG PET data (Alexander and Moeller 1994; Spetsieris and Eidelberg 2011) led to the identification of a specific PD-related spatial covariance pattern associated with the motor manifestations of the disease (Eidelberg et al. 2009). This pattern (termed PDRP) is characterized by increased pallidothalamic metabolic activity associated with relative reductions in the premotor cortex, supplementary motor area, and parietal association areas. Since its original description (Eidelberg et al. 1994), the abnormal PDRP metabolic topography (Figure 1A) has been identified in seven independent patient populations (Moeller et al. 1999; Feigin et al. 2002; Lozza et al. 2004; Eckert et al. 2006; Eidelberg 2009). Network analysis has also been used to quantify the expression of a known spatial covariance pattern on a prospective single case basis. Indeed, individual case computation of PDRP expression (i.e., subject scores for the pattern) revealed that this network measure consistently exhibits test-retest reproducibility in repeat FDG PET scans separated by two months (Ma et al. 2007). PDRP expression has been consistently found to be elevated in PD patients relative to healthy controls (Lozza et al. 2004; Asanuma et al. 2006; Ma et al. 2007; 2010; Tang et al. 2010a). Subject scores for this network have also been found to correlate with Unified Parkinson's Disease Rating Scale (UPDRS) motor ratings as well as with disease duration (Feigin et al. 2002; Lozza et al. 2004; Asanuma et al. 2006). The pathophysiological basis of this functional network is supported by the relationship between individual subject PDRP expression and recordings of spontaneous single-unit activity of the subthalamic nucleus (STN) measured intraoperatively during deep brain stimulation (DBS) electrode placement (Lin et al. 2008).

The PDRP metabolic network is primarily associated with the akinetic-rigid manifestations of PD, as opposed to tremor (Mure et al. 2011). Treatment-mediated changes in PDRP expression have been found to correlate with improvement in UPDRS motor ratings during dopaminergic therapy with levodopa (Feigin et al. 2001; Asanuma et al. 2006) or following stereotaxic surgical interventions such as subthalamic nucleus DBS, lesioning, and gene therapy (Asanuma et al. 2006; Trost et al. 2006; Feigin et al. 2007).

While therapeutic approaches have been found to target different PDRP nodes, overall network modulation can be comparable, resulting in similar degrees of clinical benefit (Asanuma et al. 2006).

PD-RELATED COGNITIVE PATTERN (PDCP)

Cognitive deficits and behavioral problems also commonly affect PD patients (Schrag et al. 2000; Aarsland et al. 2005). Although the pathological basis of cognitive impairment in PD remains controversial (Hurtig et al. 2000; Jellinger et al. 2002; Braak et al. 2003; Emre 2003; Braak et al. 2005), metabolic imaging data have shed light on functional brain pathways underlying impaired cognitive functioning in PD (Mattis and Eidelberg 2010). In a recent study using rest-state FDG PET and network analysis, Huang et al. (2007a) identified a distinctive metabolic network in non-demented PD patients that is associated with performance on neuropsychological tests of executive functioning and memory. This PD cognition-related pattern (termed PDCP) is characterized by covarying reductions in the metabolic activity of the rostral supplementary motor area (pre-SMA) and medial prefrontal cortex, precuneus and inferior parietal lobule (Figure 1B). PDCP expression was abnormally elevated in both the original pattern derivation cohort and in prospective groups of non-demented PD patients. Indeed, prospectively computed PDCP scores have also been found to correlate with individual subject neuropsychological performance (Eidelberg 2009). Interestingly, PDCP expression has been found to increase incrementally with more severe cognitive dysfunction even following the onset of dementia (Huang et al. 2008; Spetsieris and Eidelberg 2011). Like the PDRP, PDCP scores exhibit excellent test-retest reproducibility in PD patients undergoing repeat FDG PET imaging over two months (Huang et al. 2007a). These results suggest that the PDCP can potentially be used as a reliable imaging biomarker of cognitive dysfunction in PD.

It remains unclear whether antiparkinsonian treatment for the motor manifestations of PD can influence cognitive functioning through modulation of individual subject PDCP expression. A previous study showed that, unlike PDRP modulation, PDCP expression was not altered by levodopa treatment in non-demented PD patients (Huang et al. 2007b). At the individual subject level, however, the cognitive response to levodopa was found to correlate with baseline performance levels and with measures of neural activity in PDCP regions (Argyelan et al. 2008). This suggests that PDCP activity may be subject to pharmacological modulation based upon the degree of network activity present in the

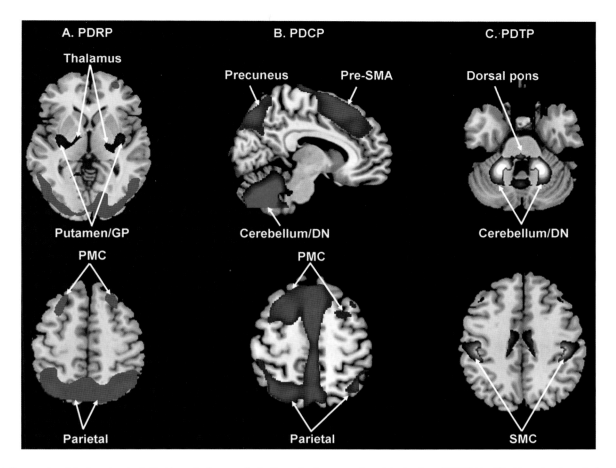

Figure 1 Abnormal metabolic networks in Parkinson's disease. **A.** Parkinson's disease motor-related pattern (PDRP) identified by network analysis of [^{18}F] fluorodeoxyglucose (FDG) PET scans from 33 PD patients and 33 age-matched normal volunteer subjects (Ma et al. 2007). This spatial covariance pattern is characterized by metabolic increases (*red*) in the putamen/globus pallidus (GP), thalamus, pons, cerebellum, and sensorimotor cortex, associated with relative decreases (*blue*) in the lateral premotor cortex (PMC) and in parieto-occipital association regions. **B.** PD cognition-related metabolic pattern (PDCP) identified in a separate network analysis of FDG PET scans from 15 non-demented PD patients (Huang et al. 2007b). This spatial covariance pattern is characterized by metabolic decreases (*blue*) in the rostral supplementary motor area (pre-SMA), precuneus, and the posterior parietal and prefrontal regions, associated with relative increases (*red*) in the dentate nucleus (DN) and cerebellar cortex. [*A, B:* Reprinted from *Trends Neurosci*, Metabolic brain networks in neurodegenerative disorders: A functional imaging approach, 548–557, Copyright 2009, with permission from Elsevier]. **C.** PD tremor-related metabolic pattern (PDTP) identified using a within-subject network analysis (Habeck et al. 2005) of FDG PET scans from nine tremor-dominant PD patients scanned at baseline and during ventral intermediate (Vim) thalamic deep brain stimulation (DBS) (Mure et al. 2011). This pattern is characterized by covarying increases in the metabolic activity of the sensorimotor cortex (SMC), cerebellum, pons, and the putamen. [*C:* Reprinted from *NeuroImage*, Parkinson's disease tremor-related metabolic network: Characterization, progression, and treatment effects, Copyright 2010, with permission from Elsevier].

unmedicated baseline condition. This possibility is currently being investigated as well as the potential utility of PDCP measurements in the assessment of novel treatments directed at the cognitive symptoms of the disorder.

PD-RELATED TREMOR PATTERN (PDTP)

Resting tremor is another cardinal motor symptom of PD that affects more than 75% of patients (Rajput et al. 1991; Hughes et al. 1993). Clinically, unlike akinesia and rigidity, PD tremor is not consistently responsive to dopaminergic treatment (Fishman 2008; Zaidel et al. 2009). This is in

accordance with the notion that the mechanism of tremor in PD is different from that of other motor signs and symptoms of the disorder (Rivlin-Etzion et al. 2006). Imaging studies have shown that elevations in PDRP expression are comparable for patients with and without parkinsonian tremor (Antonini et al. 1998; Isaias et al. 2010). Moreover, the recent observation that PDRP expression is not altered by the suppression of PD tremor by ventral intermediate (Vim) thalamic DBS (Mure et al. 2011) provides further evidence that PDRP activity is not sensitive to this disease manifestation.

In a recent study, a supervised principal component analysis (PCA) approach (Habeck et al. 2005) was used to identify a tremor-related metabolic network in tremor-dominant PD patients undergoing FDG PET on and off Vim thalamic stimulation (Mure et al. 2011). This PD tremor-related pattern (termed PDTP) was characterized by covarying metabolic increases in the cerebellum/dorsal pons, caudate/putamen, and primary motor cortex (Figure 1C). Prospectively computed PDTP scores were found to have excellent test-retest reproducibility in individual patients, consistently correlating with clinical ratings of tremor severity, but not akinesia-rigidity (Mure et al. 2011). PDTP expression was elevated only in tremor-predominant PD patients relative to the akinesia-rigid patients and healthy controls (Mure et al. 2011).

In aggregate, these findings suggest that PDTP expression is a stable and specific metabolic imaging biomarker of tremor in PD. (Please see Chapter 6 for a more detailed discussion of imaging study of PD tremor).

CHANGES IN NETWORK ACTIVITY WITH DISEASE PROGRESSION

ABNORMAL NETWORK ACTIVITY IN THE PRECLINICAL PERIOD

Experimental studies in parkinsonian animal models have suggested the presence of compensatory mechanisms prior to the development of clinically evident disease manifestations (Smith and Zigmond 2003; Bezard et al. 2003). Nonetheless, the underlying functional changes associated with the onset of clinical symptoms in PD patients remain unclear (e.g., Buhmann et al. 2003; Appel-Cresswell et al. 2010). To investigate the metabolic changes occurring during the transition from the preclinical to the symptomatic phase of PD, Tang and colleagues recently analyzed the results of a multitracer PET study in which 15 hemiparkinsonian patients (age 58.0 ± 10.2 years; H&Y Stage 1.2 ± 0.3) were followed longitudinally as symptoms bilateralized (Tang et al. 2010a). At each of the three time points (baseline, two years and four years), the subjects underwent [18F]-fluoropropyl βCIT (FP-CIT) PET to examine longitudinal changes in caudate and putamen dopamine transporter (DAT) binding as well as [18F]-fluorodeoxyglucose (FDG) PET to assess longitudinal changes in the expression of the PDRP and PDCP networks in the initially symptomatic and "preclinical" hemispheres. Over time, UPDRS motor ratings increased at similar rates for both body sides (Figure 2A). All hemiparkinsonian patients developed symptoms on the initially unaffected limbs after two years of follow-up. At all three time points, DAT binding values in the ipsilateral ("presymptomatic") putamen were higher than the contralateral ("symptomatic") values. Putamen binding declined in both hemispheres, with a faster rate on the initially presymptomatic side (Figure 2B). Interestingly, the decreases in putamen DAT binding were found to correlate negatively with concurrent increases in metabolic activity in this region. The authors suggest that the local metabolic increases represent a functional response to putamen dopamine loss exceeding a threshold of approximately 60% of the normal mean. Thus, the onset of symptoms on the initially unaffected body side was associated with critical loss of nigrostriatal dopaminergic input to the opposite putamen and with local increases in metabolic activity in this brain region.

PDRP and PDCP expression were also quantified separately on the ipsilateral and contralateral hemispheres and the time course of the network changes was assessed for each of the two disease-related patterns. PDRP expression was found to be significantly elevated at baseline in the initially presymptomatic (ipsilateral) hemisphere (Figure 2C). This change occurred approximately two years before motor signs developed on the opposite limbs. Over time, ipsilateral PDRP activity continued to rise as UPDRS motor ratings increased on the opposite body side. These findings indicate that PDRP abnormalities can be detected several years before the onset of motor signs, suggesting that this network may be suitable as a progression biomarker during the preclinical phase of the illness. By contrast, PDCP expression in both hemispheres was normal between baseline and two years and reached abnormal levels only at the 4-year time point (Figure 2D). Cingulate metabolic activity was found to be elevated prior to the rise in PDCP expression, suggesting a compensatory role for this region in the period anteceding the development of cognitive dysfunction in PD (Huang et al. 2008). In aggregate, the findings suggest that metabolic network abnormalities can be quantified and used to assess prodromal motor and non-motor features of PD prior to symptom onset. Future investigations will help determine whether network expression is also abnormal in asymptomatic carriers of PD susceptibility genes, or in individuals with specific preclinical manifestations such as REM behavioral disturbance (RBD) which is associated with an increased risk of subsequent parkinsonism.

INCREASING NETWORK ACTIVITY IN THE SYMPTOMATIC STAGE

In addition to hemispheric network changes, Huang et al. (Huang et al. 2007b) examined the time courses of whole-brain PDRP and PDCP expression in this longitudinal cohort. PDRP expression demonstrated a linear increase over time

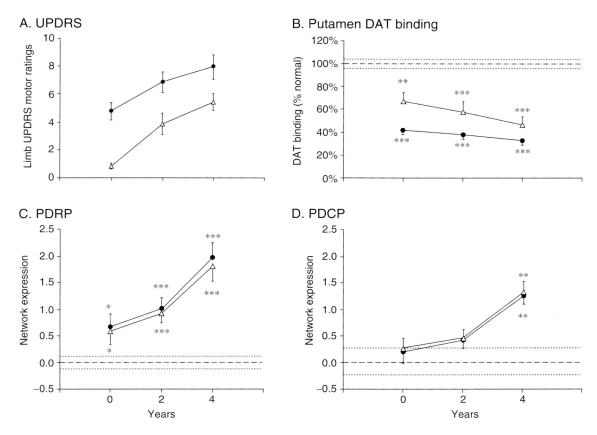

Figure 2 Changes in motor ratings, dopaminergic function, and network activity in the progression of hemiparkinsonism. **A**. Unified Parkinson's Disease Rating Scale (UPDRS) motor ratings for the limbs of the initially affected (*circles*) and non-affected (*triangles*) body sides increases in parallel over time (p < 0.001) in 15 hemiparkinsonian patients who underwent FDG PET at baseline, 2, and 4 years (Tang et al. 2010). **B**. DAT binding values for the putamen were relatively lower (p < 0.05) in the hemispheres (*circles*) contralateral to the more affected limbs at all three time points. The decline in putamen DAT binding was slower (p < 0.05) on the contralateral side. DAT binding in each hemisphere is represented as percent of the normal mean (100%, broken line) at each time point. The dotted lines represent one standard error (SE) above and below the normal mean. **C**. At baseline, PDRP expression was abnormally elevated (p < 0.05) on both contralateral (*circles*) and ipsilateral (*triangles*) hemispheres even though motor signs were evident on only one body side. Over time, network activity continued to increase in parallel (p < 0.001) for both hemispheres. **D**. PDCP expression also increased (p < 0.005) in parallel in both hemispheres, although abnormally high levels (p < 0.01) were reached only at the final time point. For both networks, subject scores in each hemisphere were z-transformed so that the normal mean was zero and the standard deviation (SD) equaled one. The error bars represent one standard error (SE) of the mean at each time point. *p < 0.05, **p < 0.01, ***p < 0.001, Student's t-tests compared to normal controls. [Tang et al. 2010 J Neurosci 30:1049–1056 with permission from Society for Neuroscience].

(Figure 3A; *red line*) and correlated with concurrent increases in UPDRS motor ratings in these patients. This correlation is not surprising in that PDRP scores have been found to correlate with clinical motor ratings in multiple cross-sectional cohorts of PD patients (e.g., Eidelberg et al. 1995; Feigin et al. 2002; Lozza et al. 2004; Asanuma et al. 2006). Striatal DAT binding (the average of left and right hemispheric values) exhibited a significant linear decrease over time, consistent with the findings reported in prior longitudinal PET studies (see Au et al. 2005 for review). There was a significant negative correlation between the decreases in putamen DAT binding and the increased UPDRS motor ratings over time. It is noteworthy that the longitudinal increases in PDRP expression, declines in striatal DAT binding, and increases in motor UPDRS ratings were intercorrelated, albeit to a modest

degree (R^2~30%), suggesting that these indices of disease progression cannot be viewed as interchangeable (Figure 3B) (Eckert et al. 2007). In other words, these measures of PD progression provide distinct, complementary information concerning the neurodegenerative process.

Whole-brain PDCP expression was also found to increase with time (Figure 3A; *blue line*). This measure, however, progressed at a slower rate than observed for the PDRP. Compared to PDRP expression, which was abnormally elevated at baseline, PDCP values exhibited a relatively late increase, reaching abnormal levels after a delay of approximately four years. Unlike the PDRP, PDCP expression did not correlate with the reductions in caudate or putamen DAT binding or with concurrent increases in UPDRS motor ratings. Rather, PDCP expression was found to be

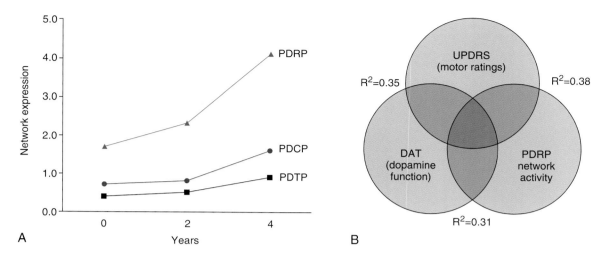

Figure 3 Changes in metabolic network activity with advancing disease. **A.** Time course of whole-brain network activity for the PDRP, PDCP, and PDTP disease patterns (see Figure 1). All three networks exhibited significant increases in activity over time (PDRP: p < 0.0001, PDCP: p < 0.0001, PDTP: p = 0.01), albeit at different rates (p < 0.01). The rate of increase in PDRP expression in these subjects was fastest, PDTP progression was slowest while PDCP expression advanced at an intermediate rate. Subject scores for each network were z-transformed so that the normal mean was zero and the standard deviation equaled one. [A: Adapted from *NeuroImage*, Parkinson's disease tremor-related metabolic network: Characterization, progression, and treatment effects, Copyright 2010 and *Brain*, Changes in network activity with the progression of Parkinson's disease, 1834–1846, Copyright 2007, with permission from Elsevier.] **B**. Schematic showing significant intercorrelations (p < 0.01) between longitudinal changes in UPDRS motor ratings, PDRP expression, and putamen DAT binding in early stage PD patients. The darker areas indicate the overlap between pairs of measures, represented by the magnitude (R^2) of their within-subject correlations. The darkest area in the center indicates the commonality (interaction effect) of the three measures (Eckert et al. 2007). [B: Reprinted from *Lancet Neurol*, Assessment of the progression of Parkinson's disease: A metabolic network approach, 926–932, Copyright 2007, with permission from Elsevier.]

elevated in anticipation of the development of cognitive dysfunction. Thus, PDCP scores were increased in patients without mild cognitive impairment (MCI). Nonetheless, network activity continued to increase as cognitive symptoms emerged in individuals with single and multiple domain MCI, reaching the highest values in PD patients with dementia (Figure 4A). Indeed, a recent analysis of cross-sectional data from a large patient cohort revealed that PDRP and PDCP expression increased linearly over time, with a relatively faster progression rate for the former disease network (Spetsieris and Eidelberg 2011) (Figure 4B). The different rate of PDRP and PDCP network progression parallels the time courses for the development of the motor and cognitive symptoms in PD. These findings support the use of PDRP and PDCP as imaging biomarkers to monitor and assess the motor and cognitive changes in PD patients.

PDTP expression has also been found to increase over time (Figure 3A, *black line*), albeit at a rate that is slower than for either PDRP or PDCP values. Interestingly, the slow progression of PDTP activity corresponds to the observed slower rate of increase in tremor ratings (as compared to akinesia and rigidity) measured in the same patients. In sum, changes in PD-related metabolic pattern expression over time can be used to assess the natural history of the major clinical manifestations of PD. Moreover, quantification of

these changes can provide estimates of the rate of progression for each disease feature in patients participating in placebo-controlled studies of potential disease-modifying agents.

MODULATION OF NETWORK ACTIVITY BY GENE THERAPY

Gene therapy with subthalamic (STN) adeno-associated virus (AAV)-borne glutamic acid decarboxylase (GAD) has been proposed as a novel treatment for advanced PD. Experiments in animal models of PD have shown reductions in overactive STN neural activity following AAV-GAD gene therapy (Luo et al. 2002; Lee et al. 2005) as well as improved motor cortical function (Emborg et al. 2007). In a subsequent phase I clinical trial of unilateral STN AAV-GAD in human subjects with advanced PD (Kaplitt et al. 2007; Feigin et al. 2007), 12 patients underwent FDG PET and clinical evaluation at baseline, and six and 12 months after surgery. In all subjects, PDRP and PDCP expression were quantified for each hemisphere and time point. This allowed for the assessment of network changes in the treated hemispheres in relation to the effects of disease progression occurring concurrently on the untreated side.

Following unilateral gene therapy, the time course of PDRP activity was different for the treated and untreated

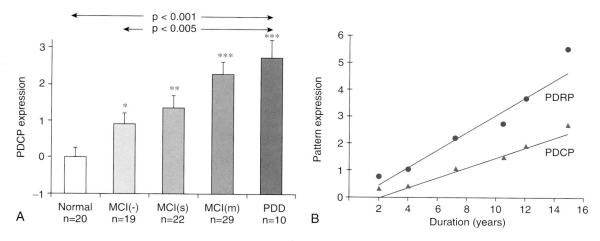

Figure 4 Increases of network activity as a function of disease duration. **A.** PDCP expression (mean±SE) in healthy control subjects, PD patients with normal cognition (MCI(−)), and with single and multiple domain mild cognitive impairment (MCI(s) and MCI(m)), and PD patients with dementia (PDD) (Eidelberg 2009). There was a significant difference in pattern expression across groups (p < 0.001), with a stepwise increase in the PD subgroups according to the degree of cognitive dysfunction that was observed at the time of imaging. The asterisks denote significant increases in network activity relative to controls (*p < 0.05, **p < 0.005, ***p < 0.0001). **B.** The PDRP (*circles*) and PDCP (*triangles*) metabolic networks increased linearly (p < 0.0001) as a function of symptom duration. The rate of progression was slower (p < 0.05), however, for the latter network. [A, B: Reprinted from *Trends Neurosci*, Metabolic brain networks in neurodegenerative disorders: A functional imaging approach, 548–557, Copyright 2009, with permission from Elsevier.]

hemispheres (Feigin et al. 2007). At baseline, PDRP expression in the treated (more clinically affected) hemisphere was abnormally elevated and declined significantly in the first six months following surgery. These values subsequently increased in parallel with the network changes observed on the unoperated side over the same time interval (Figure 5A). By contrast, PDRP expression on the unoperated side was found to increase linearly in the 12 months following surgery, consistent with disease progression. Indeed, the regression line that related PDRP progression to disease duration in the control hemispheres (Figure 5B, *open circles*) was contiguous with that determined independently in the earlier longitudinal study of early-stage PD patients (Figure 5B, *open triangles*). Interestingly, correcting PDRP scores for progression in the treated hemisphere revealed significant postsurgical declines in network activity at both six and 12 months (Figure 5C), consistent with a potential disease modifying effect. Of note, changes in hemispheric PDCP expression were also assessed as part of this clinical trial. While baseline PDCP scores were bilaterally elevated relative to healthy control subjects, there was no change in network activity in either hemisphere following gene therapy (Figure 5D). This is consistent with the absence of cognitive change after the procedure (Kaplitt et al. 2007). Further clinical studies are being conducted to evaluate the replicability of these changes in the context of a phase II sham-surgery controlled study of bilateral STN AAV-GAD in advanced PD patients (LeWitt et al. 2011).

The successful application of the PDRP and PDCP networks as biomarkers of the STN AAV-GAD treatment response serves as a model for future clinical trials of novel therapies for PD and other neurodegenerative diseases.

FUTURE DIRECTIONS

As mentioned above, in recent years substantial interest has developed in the discovery of predictive biomarkers for use in individuals at high risk for PD, such as those with rapid eye movement sleep behavior disorder (RBD). These patients have been found to exhibit cell loss in the same brain regions as in PD (Uchiyama et al. 1995; Braak et al. 2003; Boeve et al. 2004; Boeve et al. 2007). In this vein, prior imaging studies have reported deficits in presynaptic nigrostriatal dopaminergic function in RBD patients at intermediate levels between healthy controls and PD patients (Albin et al. 2000; Eisensehr et al. 2000; Stiasny-Kolster et al. 2005). It has therefore been proposed that RBD represents a prodromal form of PD. The investigation of this population with metabolic imaging and spatial covariance analysis may reveal new network biomarkers for the evaluation of preclinical disease progression and the objective assessment of potential neuroprotective therapies in at-risk individuals.

Another important area of investigation is the study of long-term washout effects on network activity. Preliminary data suggest that the standard 12-hr medication washout

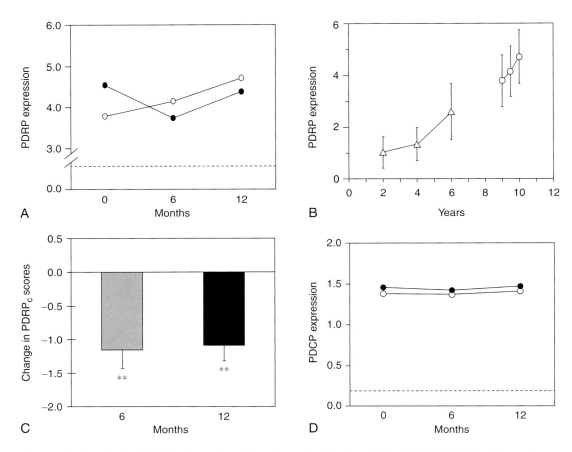

Figure 5 Changes in hemispheric network activity following unilateral gene therapy. **A.** Following unilateral STN AAV-GAD gene therapy, there was a significant difference (p < 0.002) in the postoperative time course of PDRP expression in the treated (*filled circles*) and untreated (*open circles*) cerebral hemispheres (Feigin et al. 2007). In the unoperated control hemisphere, network activity increased continuously over the 12 months after surgery. By contrast, network activity in the treated hemisphere declined during the first six months and then increased in parallel with values on the unoperated side over the subsequent six months. The dashed line represents one standard error (SE) above the normal mean value of zero. **B.** The time course of PDRP expression in the unoperated hemispheres of the patients receiving unilateral STN AAV-GAD gene therapy (*open circles*) (Feigin et al. 2007) was compared to that observed in a separate longitudinal study of early stage PD patients (*open triangles*) who underwent serial imaging over four years as part of a natural history study (Huang et al. 2007b). The rate of network progression did not differ (p = 0.60) for the two groups. Indeed, the regression line relating PDRP expression to disease duration in the gene therapy group was contiguous to that of the early stage longitudinal cohort. This substantiates the assumption that the changes in network activity observed on the unoperated hemisphere of the AAV-GAD subjects are attributable to disease progression. **C.** Progression-corrected PDRP expression (PDRP$_c$ score = PDRP score in the operated hemisphere – PDRP score in the unoperated hemisphere) representing the net effect of treatment on network expression measured for each subject and time point. Relative to baseline, PDRP$_c$ scores declined significantly at both 6 (*gray*) and 12 (*black*) months after surgery. **p < 0.005, Bonferroni tests; Bars represent standard error. **D.** In contrast to the effect of treatment on PDRP expression, there was no change in PDCP expression over time in either the operated (*filled circles*) or the unoperated (*open circles*) hemispheres (p = 0.72). The dashed line represents one standard error (SE) above the normal mean value of zero. [Feigin et al. PNAS 2007; 104:19559–19564, Copyright 2007 National Academy of Sciences, U.S.A.]

period implemented before metabolic imaging procedures is reasonable for the assessment of disease progression in chronically treated patients. This is because metabolic network activity exhibits greater sensitivity to progression than to residual medication effects at 12 hours. That said, rigorous washout studies lasting 2–4 weeks (Fahn et al. 2004) are needed to quantify the long duration effect of dopaminergic medication on network activity. This information will also provide guidance regarding the optimal choice of washout period needed to minimize the impact of

residual medication effects on estimates of the progression rate in neuroprotection trials.

Future investigations are also likely to include studies of disease progression in patients with atypical parkinsonism. Abnormal metabolic networks have been characterized for atypical forms of parkinsonism such as multisystem atrophy (MSA) and progressive supranuclear palsy (PSP) (Eckert et al. 2008). Indeed, these patterns have been used in concert with the PDRP for accurate differential diagnosis of individual cases, even at early clinical stages

(Tang et al. 2010b). Nonetheless, rates of network progression in MSA and PSP are not currently available. A recent FDG PET study of a large MSA cohort (Poston et al. 2009) suggested that disease-related network activity increases as a function of symptom duration. Longitudinal studies conducted in atypical populations will provide critical data concerning network progression in these patient groups.

CONCLUSION

There is a critical need for reliable imaging biomarkers to assess disease progression and the treatment response in PD patients. Network analysis has led to the identification and validation of three specific disease-related spatial covariance patterns associated with the clinical manifestations of the disorder. Quantification of these networks in individual subjects has helped advance current understanding of the systems-level changes that underlie the natural history of PD in both the prodromal and symptomatic phases of the illness. Ongoing studies of the long-term effects of medication on baseline network activity and longitudinal investigations in at-risk individuals will further clarify the nature of compensatory mechanisms in PD and related disorders.

ACKNOWLEDGMENTS

This work was supported by the National Institutes of Health [NINDS R01 NS 35069 and P50 NS 38370 to D.E.] and the General Clinical Research Center of The Feinstein Institute for Medical Research, North Shore-LIJ Health System [National Center for Research Resources (NCRR), a component of the National Institutes of Health, M01 RR018535]. The authors wish to thank Mr. Noam Gerber and Ms. Toni Fitzpatrick for valuable editorial assistance.

REFERENCES

Aarsland, D., J. Zaccai, and C. Brayne. 2005. A systematic review of prevalence studies of dementia in Parkinson's disease. *Mov Disord* 20:1255–63.

Albin, R. L., R. A. Koeppe, R. D. Chervin, F. B. Consens, K. Wernette, K. A. Frey et al. 2000. Decreased striatal dopaminergic innervation in REM sleep behavior disorder. *Neurology* 55:1410–2.

Alexander, G. E. and J. R. Moeller. 1994. Application of the scaled subprofile model to functional imaging in neuropsychiatric disorders: A principal component approach to modeling brain function in disease. *Hum Brain Mapp* 2:1–16.

Antonini, A., J. R. Moeller, T. Nakamura, P. Spetsieris, V. Dhawan, and D. Eidelberg. 1998. The metabolic anatomy of tremor in Parkinson's disease. *Neurology* 51:803–10.

Appel-Cresswell, S., R. de la Fuente-Fernandez, S. Galley, and M. J. McKeown. 2010. Imaging of compensatory mechanisms in Parkinson's disease. *Curr Opin Neurol* 23:407–12.

Argyelan, M., M. Carbon, M. F. Ghilardi, A. Feigin, P. Mattis, C. Tang et al. 2008. Dopaminergic suppression of brain deactivation responses during sequence learning. *J Neurosci* 25:10687–95.

Asanuma, K., C. Tang, Y. Ma, V. Dhawan, P. Mattis, C. Edwards et al. 2006. Network modulation in the treatment of Parkinson's disease. *Brain* 129:2667–78.

Au, W. L., J. R. Adams, A. R. Troiano, and A. J. Stoessl. 2005. Parkinson's disease: In vivo assessment of disease progression using positron emission tomography. *Brain Res Mol Brain Res* 134:24–33.

Bernheimer, H., W. Birkmayer, O. Hornykiewicz, K. Jellinger, and F. Seitelberger. 1973. Brain dopamine and the syndromes of Parkinson and Huntington. Clinical, morphological and neurochemical correlations. *J Neurol Sci* 20:415–55.

Bezard, E., C. E. Gross, and J. M. Brotchie. 2003. Presymptomatic compensation in Parkinson's disease is not dopamine-mediated. *Trends Neurosci* 26:215–21.

Boeve, B. F., M. H. Silber, and T. J. Ferman. 2004. REM sleep behavior disorder in Parkinson's disease and dementia with Lewy bodies. *J Geriatr Psychiatry Neurol* 17:146–57.

Boeve, B. F., M. H. Silber, C. B. Saper, T. J. Ferman, D. W. Dickson, J. E. Parisi et al. 2007. Pathophysiology of REM sleep behaviour disorder and relevance to neurodegenerative disease. *Brain* 130:2770–88.

Braak, H., K. Del Tredici, R. Rub, R. A. de Vos, E. N. Jansen Steur, E. Braak. 2003. Staging of brain pathology related to sporadic Parkinson's disease. *Neurobiol Aging* 24:197–211.

Braak, H., U. Rub, E. N. Jansen Steur, K. Del Tredici, R. A. de Vos. 2005. Cognitive status correlates with neuropathologic stage in Parkinson disease. *Neurology* 64:1404–10.

Buhmann, C., V. Glauche, H. J. Sturenburg, M. Oechsner, C. Weiller, and C. Buchel. 2003. Pharmacologically modulated fMRI—cortical responsiveness to levodopa in drug-naive hemiparkinsonian patients. *Brain* 126:451–61.

Eckert, T., T. Peschel, H. J. Heinze, and M. Rotte. 2006. Increased pre-SMA activation in early PD patients during simple self-initiated hand movements. *J Neurol* 253:199–207.

Eckert, T., C. Tang, and D. Eidelberg. 2007. Assessment of the progression of Parkinson's disease: A metabolic network approach. *Lancet Neurol* 6:926–32.

Eckert, T., C. Tang, Y. Ma, N. Brown, T. Lin, S. Frucht et al. 2008. Abnormal metabolic networks in atypical parkinsonism. *Mov Disord* 23:727–33.

Eidelberg, D. 2009. Metabolic brain networks in neurodegenerative disorders: A functional imaging approach. *Trends Neurosci* 32:548–57.

Eidelberg, D., J. R. Moeller, V. Dhawan, P. Spetsieris, S. Takikawa, T. Ishikawa et al. 1994. The metabolic topography of parkinsonism. *J Cereb Blood Flow Metab* 14:783–801.

Eidelberg, D., J. R. Moeller, T. Ishikawa, V. Dhawan, P. Spetsieris, T. Chaly et al. 1995. Assessment of disease severity in parkinsonism with fluorine-18-fluorodeoxyglucose and PET. *J Nucl Med* 36:378–83.

Eisensehr, I., R. Linke, S. Noachtar, J. Schwarz, F. J. Gildehaus, and K. Tatsch. 2000. Reduced striatal dopamine transporters in idiopathic rapid eye movement sleep behaviour disorder. Comparison with Parkinson's disease and controls. *Brain* 123 (Pt 6): 1155–60.

Emborg, M. E., M. Carbon, J. E. Holden, M. J. During, Y. Ma, C. Tang et al. 2007. Subthalamic glutamic acid decarboxylase gene therapy: Changes in motor function and cortical metabolism. *J Cereb Blood Flow Metab* 27:501–9.

Emre, M. 2003. What causes mental dysfunction in Parkinson's disease? *Mov Disord* 18 (Suppl 6): S63–71.

Fahn, S., R. Elton, and Unified Parkinson's Disease Rating Scale Development Committee. 1987. Unified Parkinson's Disease Rating Scale . In *Recent developments in Parkinson's disease*, eds. S. Fahn, C. D. Marsden, and D. Calne, pp. 153–63. New York: MacMillan.

Fahn, S., D. Oakes, I. Shoulson, K. Kieburtz, A. Rudolph, A. Lang et al. 2004. Levodopa and the progression of Parkinson's disease. *N Engl J Med* 351:2498–508.

Fearnley, J. M., and A. J. Lees. 1991. Ageing and Parkinson's disease: Substantia nigra regional selectivity. *Brain* 114:2283–301.

Feigin, A., A. Antonini, M. Fukuda, R. De Notaris, R. Benti, G. Pezzoli et al. 2002. Tc-99m ethylene cysteinate dimer SPECT in the differential diagnosis of parkinsonism. *Mov Disord* 17:1265–70.

Feigin, A., M. Fukuda, V. Dhawan, S. Przedborski, V. Jackson-Lewis, M. J. Mentis et al. 2001. Metabolic correlates of levodopa response in Parkinson's disease. *Neurology* 57:2083–8.

Feigin, A., M. G. Kaplitt, C. Tang, T. Lin, P. Mattis, V. Dhawan et al. 2007. Modulation of metabolic brain networks after subthalamic gene therapy for Parkinson's disease. *Proc Natl Acad Sci USA* 104: 19559–64.

Fishman, P. S. 2008. Paradoxical aspects of parkinsonian tremor. *Mov Disord* 23:168–73.

Habeck, C., J. W. Krakauer, C. Ghez, H. A. Sackheim, Y. Stern, D. Eidelberg et al. 2005. A new approach to spatial covariance modeling of functional brain imaging data: Ordinal trend analysis. *Neural Comp* 17:1602–45.

Hilker, R., K. Schweitzer, S. Coburger, M. Ghaemi, S. Weisenbach, A. H. Jacobs et al. 2005. Nonlinear progression of Parkinson disease as determined by serial positron emission tomographic imaging of striatal fluorodopa F 18 activity. *Arch Neurol* 62:378–82.

Hoehn, M. M., and M. D. Yahr. 1967. Parkinsonism: Onset, progression and mortality. *Neurology* 17:427–42.

Huang, C., P. Mattis, K. Perrine, N. Brown, V. Dhawan, and D. Eidelberg. 2008. Metabolic abnormalities associated with mild cognitive impairment in Parkinson disease. *Neurology* 70:1470–7.

Huang, C., P. Mattis, C. Tang, K. Perrine, M. Carbon, and D. Eidelberg. 2007a. Metabolic brain networks associated with cognitive function in Parkinson's disease. *Neuroimage* 34:714–23.

Huang, C., C. Tang, A. Feigin, M. Lesser, Y. Ma, M. Pourfar et al. 2007b. Changes in network activity with the progression of Parkinson's disease. *Brain* 130:1834–46.

Hughes, A. J., S. E. Daniel, S. Blankson, and A. Lees. 1993. A clinicopathologic study of 100 cases of Parkinson's disease. *Arch Neurol* 50:140–48.

Hurtig, H. I., J. Q. Trojanowski, J. Galvin, D. Ewbank, M. L. Schmidt, V. M. Lee et al. 2000. Alpha-synuclein cortical Lewy bodies correlate with dementia in Parkinson's disease. *Neurology* 54:1916–21.

Isaias, I. U., G. Marotta, S. Hirano, M. Canesi, R. Benti, A. Righini et al. 2010. Imaging essential tremor. *Mov Disord* 25:679–86.

Jellinger, K. A., K. Seppi, G. K. Wenning, and W. Poewe. 2002. Impact of coexistent Alzheimer pathology on the natural history of Parkinson's disease. *J Neural Transm* 109:329–39.

Kaplitt, M. G., A. Feigin, C. Tang, H. L. Fitzsimons, P. Mattis, P. A. Lawlor et al. 2007. Safety and tolerability of gene therapy with an adeno-associated virus (AAV) borne GAD gene for Parkinson's disease: An open label, phase I trial. *Lancet* 369:2097–105.

Lee, B., H. Lee, Y. R. Nam, J. H. Oh, Y. H. Cho, and J. W. Chang. 2005. Enhanced expression of glutamate decarboxylase 65 improves symptoms of rat parkinsonian models. *Gene Ther* 12:1215–22.

LeWitt, P. A., A. R. Rezai, M. A. Leehey, S. G. Ojemann, A. W. Flaherty, E. N. Eskandar et al. 2011. AAV2-GAD gene therapy for advanced Parkinson's disease: a double-blind, sham-surgery controlled, randomised trial. *Lancet Neurol* 10:309–319.

Lin, T. P., M. Carbon, C. Tang, A. Y. Mogilner, D. Sterio, A. Beric et al. 2008. Metabolic correlates of subthalamic nucleus activity in Parkinson's disease. *Brain* 131:1373–80.

Lozza, C., J. C. Baron, D. Eidelberg, M. J. Mentis, M. Carbon, and R. M. Marie. 2004. Executive processes in Parkinson's disease: FDG-PET and network analysis. *Hum Brain Mapp* 22:236–45.

Lucking, C. B., A. Durr, V. Bonifati, J. Vaughan, G. De Michele, T. Gasser et al. 2000. Association between early-onset Parkinson's disease and mutations in the parkin gene. *N Engl J Med* 342: 1560–7.

Luo, J., M. G. Kaplitt, H. L. Fitzsimons, D. S. Zuzga, Y. Liu, M. L. Oshinsky et al. 2002. Subthalamic GAD gene therapy in a Parkinson's disease rat model. *Science* 298:425–9.

Ma, Y., C. Huang, J. P. Dyke, H. Pan, A. Feigin, and D. Eidelberg. 2010. Parkinson's disease spatial covariance pattern: non-invasive quantification with perfusion MRI. *J Cereb Blood Flow Metab* 30: 505–9.

Ma, Y., C. Tang, P. G. Spetsieris, V. Dhawan, and D. Eidelberg D. 2007. Abnormal metabolic network activity in Parkinson's disease: Test-retest reproducibility. *J Cereb Blood Flow Metab* 27:597–605.

Mattis, P. and D. Eidelberg. 2010. Imaging cognition and Parkinson's disease: An overview. *US Neurol* 5:26–29.

Moeller, J. R., T. Nakamura, M. J. Mentis, V. Dhawan, P. Spetsieres, A. Antonini et al. 1999. Reproducibility of regional metabolic covariance patterns: Comparison of four populations. *J Nucl Med* 40:1264–9.

Morrish, P. K., J. S. Rakshi, D. L. Bailey, G. V. Sawle, and D. J. Brooks. 1998. Measuring the rate of progression and estimating the preclinical period of Parkinson's disease with [18F]dopa PET. *J Neurol Neurosurg Psychiatry* 64:314–9.

Mure, H., S. Hirano, C. C. Tang, I. U. Isaias, A. Antonini, Y. Ma et al. 2011. Parkinson's disease tremor-related metabolic network: Characterization, progression, and treatment effects. *Neuroimage* 54:1244–53.

Parkinson Study Group. 2002. Dopamine transporter brain imaging to assess the effects of pramipexole vs levodopa on Parkinson disease progression. *Jama* 287:1653–61.

Poston, K. L., C. Tang, T. Eckert, Y. Ma, S. Frucht, and D. Eidelberg. 2009. Longitudinal changes in regional metabolism and network activity in multiple system atrophy. *Neurology* 72(Suppl 3): A67.

Rajput, A. H., B. Rozdilsky, and L. Ang. 1991. Occurrence of resting tremor in Parkinson's disease. *Neurology* 41:1298–9.

Rivlin-Etzion, M., O. Marmor, G. Heimer, A. Raz, A. Nini, and H. Bergman. 2006. Basal ganglia oscillations and pathophysiology of movement disorders. *Curr Opin Neurobiol* 16:629–37.

Schrag, A., M. Jahanshahi, and N. Quinn. 2000. What contributes to quality of life in patients with Parkinson's disease? *J Neurol Neurosurg Psychiatry* 69:308–12.

Shults, C. W., D. Oakes, K. Kieburtz, M. F. Beal, R. Haas, S. Plumb et al. 2002. Effects of coenzyme Q10 in early Parkinson disease: Evidence of slowing of the functional decline. *Arch Neurol* 59: 1541–50.

Smith, A. D., and M. J. Zigmond. 2003. Can the brain be protected through exercise? Lessons from an animal model of parkinsonism. *Exp Neurol* 184:31–9.

Spetsieris, P. G., and D. Eidelberg. 2011. Scaled subprofile modeling of resting state imaging data in Parkinson's disease: Methodological issues. *NeuroImage* 54:2899–914.

Stiasny-Kolster, K., Y. Doerr, J. C. Moller, H. Hoffken, T. M. Behr, W. H. Oertel et al. 2005. Combination of "idiopathic" REM sleep behaviour disorder and olfactory dysfunction as possible indicator for alpha-synucleinopathy demonstrated by dopamine transporter FP-CIT-SPECT. *Brain* 128:126–37.

Tang, C. C., and D. Eidelberg. 2010. Abnormal metabolic brain networks in Parkinson's disease: From blackboard to bedside. *Prog Brain Res* 184:161–76.

Tang, C. C., K. L. Poston, V. Dhawan, and D. Eidelberg. 2010a. Abnormalities in metabolic network activity precede the onset of motor symptoms in Parkinson's disease. *J Neurosci* 30:1049–56.

Tang, C. C., K. L. Poston, T. Eckert, A. Feigin, S. Frucht, M. Gudesblatt et al. 2010b. Differential diagnosis of parkinsonism: A metabolic imaging study using pattern analysis. *Lancet Neurol* 9:149–58.

Trost, M., S. Su, P. Su, R. F. Yen, H. M. Tseng, A. Barnes et al. 2006. Network modulation by the subthalamic nucleus in the treatment of Parkinson's disease. *Neuroimage* 31:301–7.

Uchiyama, M., K. Isse, K. Tanaka, N. Yokota, M. Hamamoto, S. Aida et al. 1995. Incidental Lewy body disease in a patient with REM sleep behavior disorder. *Neurology* 45:709–12.

Whone, A. L., R. L. Watts, A. J. Stoessl, M. Davis, S. Reske, C. Nahmias et al. 2003. Slower progression of Parkinson's disease with ropinirole versus levodopa: The REAL-PET study. *Ann Neurol* 54:93–101.

Zaidel, A., D. Arkadir, Z. Israel, H. Bergman. 2009. Akineto-rigid vs. tremor syndromes in Parkinsonism. *Curr Opin Neurol* 22: 387–93.

13

EFFECTS OF TREATMENT

PHARMACOLOGIC

Alain Dagher

INTRODUCTION

Pharmacological therapy to augment dopamine neuro-transmission, either with levodopa or a dopamine agonist, relieves the motor deficits of Parkinson's disease (PD) consistently and rapidly, and for the entire duration of the illness. However, PD is also associated with cognitive and emotional disturbances, whose response to dopamine therapy is inconsistent or, in some cases, deleterious. While the neurochemical mechanism of action of levodopa or dopamine agonists is straightforward, their effect on brain networks during the performance of motor and cognitive tasks can be elucidated using functional neuroimaging.

The chief biological abnormality in PD is dopamine deficiency in the striatum, and it appears to be the cause of most of the motor, cognitive, and emotional symptoms and signs of the disease. Because the striatum is part of the neural networks involving the entire cortex, striatal dopamine deficiency has widespread functional effects. A systems neuroscience approach to understanding PD has attempted to explain the features of the disease by combining data from anatomical (Alexander et al. 1986) and neurochemical (Albin et al. 1989) studies and making predictions about the effects of dopamine deficiency on different parts of the basal ganglia and cerebral cortex. These predictions can be tested in PD patients using functional neuroimaging. By measuring cerebral blood flow (CBF), first with positron emission tomography (PET) and later with functional magnetic resonance imaging (fMRI), scientists have tried to map the neurobiological substrates of motor and cognitive symptoms in PD, and how these brain networks are affected by dopamine deficiency and therapeutic replenishment. In recent years it has become apparent that therapy may lead to excessive dopaminergic signaling in certain brain areas, most notably the mesolimbic system. Due to the variable extent of neurodegeneration in different dopamine pathways, replacing dopamine to adequate levels in the motor system may overdose other systems.

THE FUNCTIONAL NEUROANATOMY OF THE DOPAMINE SYSTEM

The basal ganglia are organized in a series of parallel cortico-striatal loops (Alexander et al. 1986). The function of each loop is determined by the cortical area it includes. Sensorimotor, cognitive, and limbic regions of the striatum can be distinguished based on their connections with cerebral cortex (Parent 1990; Haber et al. 2000) (Figure 1). Roughly speaking, these are the posterior putamen (sensorimotor), caudate plus anterior putamen (cognitive), and ventral striatum or nucleus accumbens (limbic/affective). The dorsal striatum (caudate and putamen) receives input from motor, association, and prefrontal cortex, while the ventral striatum receives input from limbic areas such as the hippocampus, amygdala, and orbitofrontal cortex.

Dopamine neuron cell bodies located in the midbrain project to the basal ganglia and cerebral cortex. Different populations send projections to the dorsal striatum (caudate and putamen), the limbic system (including the ventral striatum), and the cortex (Moore and Bloom 1978). Dopamine neurons synapse on the dendrites of medium spiny neurons in the striatum, as do glutamatergic cortical afferents. Cortical glutamate and midbrain dopamine neurons synapse in close proximity, and the two neurotransmitters can influence each other's effects (Sesack and Pickel 1992). Dopamine may act to increase the efficiency of active cortico-striatal synapses while suppressing inactive ones (Wickens and Kotter 1995). Glutamate can also directly modulate the release of dopamine (Whitton 1997).

The foregoing only partly explains how dopamine loss may lead to cortico-striatal dysfunction. Persistently low

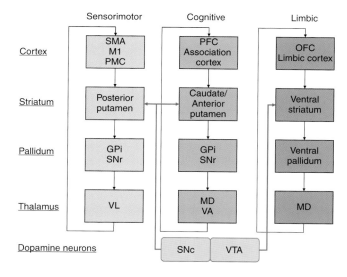

Figure 1 Cortical basal ganglia loops (based on Alexander et al. 1986; Parent 1990). The function of each of the segregated parallel loops depends on the function of the cortical regions that belong to them. Dopamine projections to the motor and cognitive loops are preferentially affected in Parkinson's disease. Abbreviations: SMA: supplementary motor area; M1: primary motor cortex; PMC: premotor cortex; PFC: prefrontal cortex; OFC: orbitofrontal cortex; GPi: Globus pallidus internal segment; SNr: Substantia nigra pars reticulata; VL: ventrolateral; MD: mediodorsal; VA: ventral anterior; SNc: Substantia nigra pars compacta; VTA: ventral tegmental area.

that dopamine neuronal firing in monkeys undergoing classical conditioning had a similar temporal pattern as a learning signal from a machine learning algorithm (Schultz et al. 1997; Schultz 1998). This signal is called a reward prediction error signal, as it signals the difference between expected and received rewards, and can be used to promote learning. These observations from neurophysiological recordings in primates have now been confirmed repeatedly in humans undergoing fMRI: a signal in dopamine projection areas (notably the striatum) can be shown to equal a reward prediction error as computed from subjects' behavior (McClure et al. 2003a; O'Doherty et al. 2003; Hare et al. 2008) (Figure 2). Thus, while dopamine deficiency in PD leads to a predominantly motor disorder, it appears that a crucial role of dopamine signaling is in reinforcement learning and motivation. Important new theoretical models have shown that dopamine has a role in reward that goes beyond learning: it also acts as a motivational signal, increasing an individual's drive and willingness to expend effort in the pursuit of rewards (McClure et al. 2003b; Niv et al. 2007). These models make predictions about cognitive and emotional function in Parkinson's disease that are just now starting to be tested using functional brain imaging.

dopamine levels are associated with increased tonic firing of inhibitory output neurons in the globus pallidus internal segment (GPi), which is thought to lead to widespread cortical dysfunction (Albin et al. 1989). This is the "functional deafferentation" hypothesis, according to which tonic GPi activity causes cortical inhibition, which leads to bradykinesia.

More recently, the role of dopamine in reward, reinforcement, learning, and motivation has received considerable attention. The seminal work of Wolfram Schultz demonstrated

FUNCTIONAL IMAGING METHODS

Brain mapping rests on the premise that synaptic neuronal activity leads to a proportionate increase in CBF (Raichle 1987). Because the signal changes that result from activation are typically quite small, data from multiple subjects must be combined into a standard coordinate space (Talairach and Tournoux 1988). This allows statistical tests to be applied at each voxel, for example by applying a general linear model

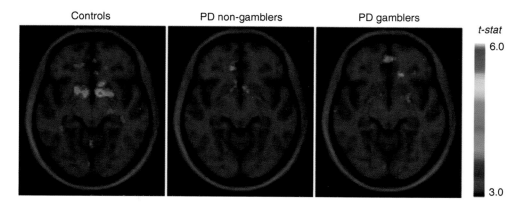

Figure 2 Reward prediction error signals detected by fMRI. Subjects performed a gambling task during fMRI. Reward prediction error signals were generated from each subject's choices and used as a covariate in the analysis of BOLD signals. In age-matched controls (n = 12), there is a clear reward prediction error signal emanating from the nucleus accumbens bilaterally. In PD patients with and without medication-induced pathological gambling (n = 12 per group), the signal is absent, supporting its dopaminergic origin in normal subjects. (Courtesy of C. Erickson)

to the functional data to yield a z or t statistical map. One can then search this statistical parametric map, which is a 3D Gaussian random field, for areas where z or t values exceed a certain threshold (Worsley et al. 2002). Importantly, it is possible to go beyond the imaging of activations and to uncover spatial patterns of correlations among brain regions, otherwise known as functional connectivity. FMRI in particular can be used to measure temporal correlations between brain areas to uncover functional brain networks.

The development of fMRI has allowed brain mapping to be performed without the injection of radioactive tracers. FMRI is based on the blood oxygen level dependent (BOLD) signal (Ogawa et al. 1990). At present, the available evidence suggests that the local BOLD signal is a function of the synaptic inputs into a brain area, and of local neuronal processing, including the activity of excitatory and inhibitory interneurons (Logothetis 2002; Logothetis and Pfeuffer 2004; Lee et al. 2010); however, while reductions in neuronal activity coincide with reduced BOLD in the visual cortex (Shmuel et al. 2006), neuronal inhibition per se may not always cause changes in BOLD (Waldvogel et al. 2000).

FMRI has several advantages over [^{15}O]H$_2$O PET for brain mapping, including greater temporal resolution (on the order of 100 ms using event-related experimental designs), slightly greater spatial resolution, and most likely greater sensitivity. All PET studies employ so-called block designs, in which the experimental conditions are separated into discrete blocks usually lasting about 60 seconds. While fMRI can use block designs, it also affords the possibility of event-related designs, in which the response associated with transient neuronal activity can be detected.

A relevant issue for PD is the attribution of fMRI signal change to dopamine activity. The neurobiological events that lead to changes in BOLD signal are complex and not yet completely understood. While BOLD is known to depend on cerebral blood flow and oxygen metabolism, the relationship of these to neurotransmitter release can only be inferred. As stated above, there is good evidence that the BOLD signal in a brain area represents the activity of neuronal inputs into this area. This suggests that increases in BOLD in the striatum could reflect firing of the plentiful glutamatergic afferents from the cortex and limbic system, rather than dopaminergic afferents, which are far sparser (Haber et al. 2000). However, two factors support an influence of dopamine on BOLD. First, extrasynaptic dopamine can augment BOLD signal by causing local vasodilatation (Choi et al. 2006). Second, dopamine acts to "gate" glutamatergic synapses, inhibiting the inactive ones and facilitating the more active ones (Horvitz 2002), and also directly

modulates excitatory postsynaptic potentials (Nicola et al. 2000), which contribute to local field potentials and hence perhaps to BOLD. Thus, the BOLD signal in the striatum depends on the activity of both glutamatergic and dopaminergic inputs, but the exact relationship is not known with certainty at this time. Although the pioneering work of Logothetis has given us an understanding of the neurobiological nature of BOLD (Logothetis 2002), work to date has not addressed this specific issue. Nonetheless, the bulk of the evidence indicates that an increase in phasic dopamine neuron firing leads to an increase in BOLD in the projection areas of the dopamine neurons. The most likely explanation for striatal BOLD signal changes in reward-related paradigms is that dopamine increases glutamate-induced dendritic currents in the striatal medium spiny neurons (Nicola et al. 2000; Knutson et al. 2004; Zink et al. 2004).

CORTICO-STRIATAL NETWORK FUNCTION IN PD

MOTOR FUNCTION

The earliest PET CBF studies in PD used simple motor tasks to determine the effect of dopamine loss on the pattern of neuronal activity during movement. A consistent finding was that PD patients demonstrated relatively deficient activation in accessory motor areas compared to control subjects (Jenkins et al. 1992; Playford et al. 1992; Rascol et al. 1992; Jahanshahi et al. 1995). For example, when the motor task consisted of moving a joystick repeatedly in one of four freely chosen directions, there was relatively less activation in PD than in controls in the supplementary motor area (SMA), anterior cingulate cortex (ACC), and dorsolateral prefrontal cortex (PFC), as well as in the contralateral putamen (Playford et al. 1992). In Stage 1 hemiparkinsonian PD patients, there was normal activation of SMA and dorsolateral PFC when patients used their clinically unaffected hand, but deficient activation in these areas when using the affected hand (Thobois et al. 2000). At first glance these results appear consistent with the model of basal ganglia function in PD, according to which an excessively high firing rate of the subthalamic nucleus (STN) and GPi results in cortical inhibition, leading to bradykinesia (Albin et al. 1989). Subsequent experiments showed that both bradykinesia and cortical underactivation were reversed by apomorphine (Jenkins et al. 1992), pallidotomy (Grafton et al. 1995; Samuel et al. 1997b), and deep brain stimulation of the GPi or STN (Limousin et al. 1997; Ceballos-Baumann et al. 1999; Fukuda et al. 2001; Strafella et al. 2003).

A notable finding from some of these studies was recruitment, in PD, of brain areas not normally activated in healthy subjects. For example, Samuel et al. (1997a), using a simple finger movement task, found relative underactivation of mesial frontal and prefrontal areas in PD patients compared to controls, but increased activation of the lateral premotor and posterior parietal cortex. The authors' explanation was that PD patients used a different brain network to perform finger movements: the lateral premotor–posterior parietal system, which is implicated in the performance of visually guided movements (Wise et al. 1997). Indeed, visually guided movements are relatively preserved in PD, and the lateral premotor cortex has direct cortico-spinal projections (Dum and Strick 2002). Haslinger et al. (2001) used the greater temporal and spatial resolution of event-related fMRI to test this hypothesis. They measured the BOLD signal in response to self-selected joystick movements in PD patients off medications and after infusion of levodopa, and in control subjects. Once again, PD patients showed reduced movement-related activation in motor areas of the mesial frontal cortex (rostral SMA) compared to controls. Moreover, when comparing PD patients on and off levodopa, they found greater activation in the on state in the caudal and rostral SMA, but greater activation in the off state in the lateral premotor cortex (PMC). In sum, PD patients show deficient activity in the mesial frontal cortex during movement, and excess activity in the lateral PMC; and this pattern is partly reversed by levodopa administration. Similarly, Hanakawa et al. (1999) described recruitment of the lateral PMC in PD patients compared to controls in a study that used SPECT scanning to measure CBF in subjects while they walked on a treadmill.

One must consider that "abnormal" cortical activation in PD may not represent recruitment, but may itself be an expression of basal ganglia dysfunction. For example, hemi-parkinsonian patients activated ipsilateral primary motor cortex (M1) when performing joystick movements with their affected hand (Thobois et al. 2000). It is not clear that ipsilateral M1 activation is beneficial (i.e., compensatory) in these patients. Peters et al. (2003) also studied hemiparkinsonian patients using fMRI while they performed simple finger oppositions off PD medications and following the administration of apomorphine. Finger movements with either hand while off medications activated contralateral M1, as well as lateral PMC, posterior parietal cortex, and cerebellum. Apomorphine significantly reduced bradykinesia and also resulted in more focused activation confined to the contralateral M1. These results are quite different than those obtained by the early PET blood flow studies cited earlier (Jenkins et al. 1992). Not only did apomorphine not

result in activation of SMA or dorsolateral PFC, it actually reduced cortical activation rather than augmenting it. This can possibly be explained by a difference in motor paradigm (Peters' subjects did not have to select or monitor their movements), but it does seem inconsistent with the functional deafferentation hypothesis. Moreover, it raises the possibility that activity in areas not normally involved in a task may not represent recruitment, which implies that it is beneficial but may be another indicator of neurological dysfunction.

As stated above, the hypothesis that excessive GPi firing in PD is responsible for both bradykinesia and blunted cortical increases in CBF during movement is not completely consistent with all the data and is now being challenged by fMRI studies. One cortical area that consistently fails to show underactivation during motor tasks in PD is M1. The early PET studies showed normal M1 CBF increases in PD patients performing freely selected movements (Jenkins et al. 1992; Playford et al. 1992), while more recent fMRI studies actually describe greater M1 activation during movement in PD patients than controls (Sabatini et al. 2000; Haslinger et al. 2001). For example, Sabatini et al. (2000), using fMRI in subjects performing a complex but well-rehearsed sequential motor task, found greater activation in PD than controls in M1, caudal SMA, cingulate cortex, and lateral PMC, all areas involved in relatively direct control of movement. The controls showed greater activation in the rostral SMA and dorsolateral PFC, areas more involved in planning, monitoring, and sequencing of movements. It is difficult to see how this difference in cortical activation patterns fits with the theory that bradykinesia is due simply to cortical hypoactivity. Both M1 and the lateral PMC, areas that show overactivation in PD, receive extensive projections from the cortico-striatal loops involving the GPI (Middleton and Strick 2000), which should be the most affected in PD. More recent methods have confirmed that dopaminergic treatment appears to reduce the extent of activation during movement, while also improving motor function (see below).

Nonetheless, other studies are consistent with the functional deafferentation hypothesis. Buhmann et al. (2003) studied early hemiparkinsonian patients with fMRI while they performed simple self-chosen paced finger movements. In distinction to the other reports already mentioned, they showed a reduced extent of BOLD activation in PD patients compared to controls in contralateral M1 when moving the affected hand, but not when moving the unaffected one. Moreover, levodopa administration increased activation in contralateral M1 and SMA when moving the affected hand, but had no effect on the cortical activation pattern during movements of the unaffected hand.

Another consistent finding in functional neuroimaging studies in PD is the identification of abnormalities involving the dorsolateral PFC. The dorsolateral PFC frequently shows underactivation during motor tasks in PD, but it is not clear how this relates to bradykinesia. The dorsolateral PFC is not involved in primary motor function, being more relevant for higher-level cognition such as planning and monitoring of working memory (Petrides 1994; Owen 1997), and even extensive lesions of the dorsolateral PFC do not impair movement in humans (Freund 1987) or animals (Goldman-Rakic 1987). It is possible that the activation of the dorsolateral PFC in motor tasks results from the need to monitor one's movements (e.g., in order to generate a random sequence). Consistent with this interpretation, Haslinger et al. (2001) found primary motor and premotor involvement during a joystick task using event-related fMRI, but not dorsolateral PFC activation, in contradistinction to the early PET studies. Most likely, this temporally precise technique detected only transient increases in neuronal activity directly related to movement, but not activity related to sustained monitoring of movements. Thus, the lack of dorsolateral PFC activation in PD may have nothing to do with bradykinesia per se, but could be explained by an attentional deficit if the neuronal activity observed in this region is involved in monitoring movements (see below).

The other cortical area consistently implicated is the SMA, although the findings are inconsistent. Several PET and fMRI studies have shown underactivation of the SMA in PD during movement (Jenkins et al. 1992; Playford et al. 1992; Jahanshahi et al. 1995; Samuel et al. 1997a; Thobois et al. 2000; Haslinger et al. 2001), but others have shown the opposite (Catalan et al. 1999; Sabatini et al. 2000), while one found normal recruitment during movement but underactivation during imagination of movement (Samuel et al. 2001). The SMA can be divided into caudal and rostral portions by a line that passes through the anterior commissure, with the rostral portion having a role in relatively higher levels of movement control and organization. The caudal SMA is thought to be involved in more basic aspects of movement (Boecker et al. 1998) and has direct cortico-spinal projections. Therefore, underactivation of the caudal rather than rostral SMA in PD could fit with the cortical deafferentation model of bradykinesia. However, Sabatini et al. (2000) found the precise opposite. When comparing PD patients to controls, they found underactivation in the rostral SMA in PD, but overactivation in caudal SMA, which again argues against SMA inhibition (deafferentation) being the direct cause of bradykinesia in PD.

These discrepancies may be reconciled by the results of another fMRI study (Rowe et al. 2002). During simple paced finger movements, PD patients had greater SMA activation than controls, consistent with Sabatini et al. However, when subjects had to attend to the movements, there was greater SMA activation in the control group. Moreover, effective connectivity between the prefrontal cortex and SMA was increased in controls but not in PD during attention to movements, suggesting the presence of a relative functional disconnection between prefrontal areas and SMA in PD. Therefore, SMA underactivation in PD is likely the result of deficient attention to movements. Indeed, in many of the tasks used in functional imaging studies of movement in PD, there is a requirement to monitor or attend to the sequence of movements. Rowe et al. also showed a defect in SMA activation during attention independent of movement in the PD group. A more recent study supports a role for the SMA in attending to one's output sequence by showing similar underactivation of the SMA during the generation of random numbers in PD (Dirnberger et al. 2005). In summary, the deficient cortical activation in the SMA and dorsolateral PFC in PD patients is not likely the neural substrate of bradykinesia. Rather, it probably represents a more general deficit in attention to movements.

Recent work shows that levodopa can normalize the deficient functional connectivity patterns seen in attentional-motor networks in PD. By measuring whole brain functional connectivity networks in PD patients performing difficult simultaneous motor tasks, Palmer et al. (2009) found numerous abnormal functional connections in PD patients compared to matched controls. In particular, normal subjects appear to increase functional connectivity between attentional regions and motor networks during dual task performance. As expected, PD patients off medications did not demonstrate this normal pattern, which likely underpins their difficulty in performing simultaneous motor tasks. Levodopa consistently normalized these attentional-motor network interactions.

In summary, the pattern of motor-induced cortical activation is different in PD patients than controls, likely reflecting a number of physiological events: disruption of cortico-striatal processing due to striatal dopamine deficiency, compensation by relatively intact neuronal circuits that do not involve the basal ganglia, and perhaps direct effects of cortical dopamine deficiency. The specific abnormalities in each experiment likely depend to a great extent on features of the motor paradigm used, including whether the movements are self-generated or automatic, and the attentional requirements of the task.

COGNITIVE FUNCTION

Cognitive dysfunction is ubiquitous in PD and contributes significantly to reduced quality of life (Schrag et al. 2000).

PD patients have cognitive deficits even in the absence of frank dementia (Dubois et al. 1991; Owen et al. 1992). In the early stages of the disease the affected domains, which are similar to those affected by frontal lobe lesions (Owen et al. 1992), include attention, planning, habit and skill learning, and cognitive flexibility. Functional imaging studies in normal subjects have shown that frontal lobe tasks, such as the Wisconsin Card Sorting Task (Monchi et al. 2001) and Tower of London (TOL) (Dagher et al. 1999), appear to involve a network of regions that include the caudate nucleus, ACC, PFC, and posterior parietal cortex. These regions make up the cognitive cortico-striatal loop (Alexander et al. 1986). However, the relative contributions to cognitive dysfunction and dementia of striatal and cortical dopamine loss, dysfunction of other neurotransmitter systems such acetylcholine and noradrenaline, and cortical neuronal loss remain to be determined.

The earliest PET CBF studies of frontal lobe tasks in PD suggested that the cognitive deficits could be explained by abnormal neural activity within the basal ganglia. For example, during performance of the TOL, a test of planning, PD patients showed normal recruitment of the PFC but abnormal CBF activation patterns in basal ganglia (Owen et al. 1998; Dagher et al. 2001). Thus, "frontal lobe" deficits may result from abnormal processing within cortico-striatal loops resulting from intrinsic striatal dopamine loss. Support for the basal ganglia being responsible for frontal lobe deficits also comes from two PET studies in PD showing a correlation between the degree of impairment on executive tasks and the reduction in caudate dopamine innervation (Marie et al. 1999; Bruck et al. 2001). However, there is also evidence of abnormal cortical activity in PD during cognitive tasks. For example, Cools et al. (2002) carried out CBF PET studies on PD patients on and off levodopa while they performed the TOL planning task. When they compared patients off medications to the controls, they found an area of dorsolateral PFC that showed greater CBF activation during planning compared to baseline in the PD group. This excessive activation disappeared when the patients were scanned after receiving levodopa, with a reduction in blood flow correlating with the improvement in performance. Mattay et al. (2002) replicated these findings using fMRI and another test of frontal lobe function: the n-back task. They found greater BOLD activation in numerous cortical areas (including dorsolateral PFC, ACC, and posterior parietal cortex) when PD patients were off compared to on levodopa. Once again the relative increase in BOLD activation and the deterioration in performance while off levodopa were correlated. Both groups of authors reason that dopamine replacement may have

caused a reduction in neuronal activity (beneficial in this case) by a direct effect on cortical neurons. There is evidence to support such a role for dopamine, which could be acting by reducing unwanted neuronal activity (Sawaguchi et al. 1990), essentially by making their target neurons less sensitive to weak inputs and more sensitive to strong excitatory afferents (Li and Sikstrom 2002). Note however that dopamine acting on the caudate nucleus could also lead to a focusing of cortical neuronal activity via the cortico-striatal system (Mink 1996). It could do this by a direct gating of cortico-striatal inputs at the level of the striatal dendrite (Sesack and Pickel 1992; Wickens and Kotter 1995), or by varying the balance of information flow between the direct and indirect pathways. It has been proposed that the arrangement of the two pathways, one designed for focused action selection and the other for broader inhibition (Hallett 1993), results in a form of center-surround inhibition, or focusing, of cortical activity (Mink 1996).

The pattern of PFC activation varies among different PD patients at the same stage of disease. Lewis et al. (2003) compared two groups of PD patients with and without executive dysfunction, but matched for disease duration, motor dysfunction, and mini-mental state exam, to age-matched controls. They performed fMRI while subjects completed a simple working memory task and found that the PD group with executive dysfunction had deficient activation in PFC and caudate bilaterally compared to the PD group without executive dysfunction. In both regions, the degree of underactivation correlated with poor performance. On the other hand, the unimpaired PD patients had an activation pattern no different than age-matched controls. This suggests that the cognitive cortico-striatal loop (PFC–caudate) may be affected in PD independently of the motor cortico-striatal loops (cortical motor areas–posterior putamen).

The studies described above demonstrate that dopamine deficiency in PD can be associated with either absent or excessive cortical activation. In fact, both patterns may coexist: during the Wisconsin Card Sorting Task, a classical frontal lobe test of set-switching and attention, PD patients displayed defective ventrolateral PFC activation but dorsolateral PFC hyperactivation (Monchi et al. 2004). We proposed that, in this task, the ventrolateral PFC was activated as part of a cortico-striatal loop, which explained why it demonstrated deficient activation in the PD patients, while the dorsolateral PFC was activated as part of a network that did not include the striatum, which explains why it showed hyperactivation in the PD group (Figure 3). This explanation was supported by a recent study using a modified card sorting task, which shows that PFC underactivation, in PD compared to controls, is seen only during those phases of

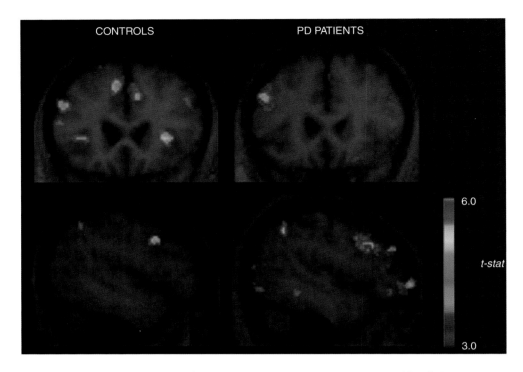

Figure 3 FMRI study showing activation during the Wisconsin Card Sorting Task (adapted from Monchi et al. 2004). fMRI study. Top panels: PD patients demonstrate a lack of activation in the ventrolateral prefrontal cortex and anterior cingulate cortex, as well as the caudate and thalamus (not shown), during set-shifting. Bottom panels: PD patients demonstrate increased activation in the dorsolateral prefrontal cortex during application of a set-shift. During this event there is no concomitant activation of the striatum in either group. This suggests that dopamine deficiency in PD causes impaired activation of cortico-striatal loops implicated in the task, but increased activation of cortical areas that are activated independently of the striatum.

the task that also recruit the caudate (Monchi et al. 2007). During the task phases that do not normally involve the caudate, the PD patients showed cortical hyperactivation compared to controls.

Note also that the hyperactivation seen in PFC in PD patients did not only involve the amplitude of BOLD signal change but also its spatial extent. Indeed, greater spatial extent of cortical activation is frequently reported in PD. Ng et al. (2010) used a novel approach to measure spatial extent of activation while PD patients and healthy controls performed a difficult motor task. PD patients off medications showed more extensive activation in SMA and M1, and this anomaly was reversed by levodopa. This is consistent with the theory that dopamine focuses cortical activity by increasing so-called signal-to-noise ratio of cortical neuronal signaling (Li and Sikstrom 2002).

Another concept that deserves mention is the overmedication hypothesis of PD, originally proposed by Gotham, Brown, and Marsden (Gotham et al. 1988). It states that an optimum dosage of dopaminergic medications to treat a patient's motor symptoms may result in side effects in the cognitive or emotional domains. This is based on the fact that, in PD, some parts of the dopamine system are preserved relative to others (Kish et al. 1988). It is thought that there

is an optimum level of dopamine for neuronal function, and that both deficiency and excess of dopamine can lead to functional deficits. Cools et al. tested this theory using fMRI and a probabilistic reversal learning task previously shown to be sensitive to levodopa in PD (Cools et al. 2007). Patients performed better at this task off medications than on. Previous work has implicated the ventral striatum and ventrolateral PFC in this task in normal subjects, and the ventral striatum has relatively preserved dopamine innervation in PD compared to the dorsal striatum (Kish et al. 1988). Thus, it is possible that a dose of levodopa adequate to treat motor symptoms may overdose the ventral PFC and ventral striatum. Indeed, an fMRI study in PD patients confirmed the authors' hypothesis: levodopa inhibited activation in the ventral striatum during the reversal learning task. The authors carefully matched performance between the two sessions, meaning that the difference in ventral striatum response cannot be due to differences in positive feedback or success rate.

The overmedication hypothesis has been rekindled recently with the emergence of a variety of impulse control disorders in PD patients. These disorders include pathological gambling, compulsive sexuality, and compulsive shopping, and also a form of addiction to dopaminergic medication referred to as the dopamine dysregulation syndrome. These syndromes are all clearly causally related to excessive intake of dopaminergic medication, especially dopamine agonists (Weintraub et al. 2006; Dagher and Robbins 2009; Weintraub et al. 2010). It is hypothesized that some individuals are vulnerable to these addictive phenomena because dopaminergic stimulation that restores motor function overdoses their mesolimbic dopamine system, leading to pathological incentive behaviors. A small number of imaging studies support this idea. A PET study showed greater dopamine release in the mesolimbic striatum in response to a single dose of levodopa in PD patients suffering from medication addiction compared to non-addicted PD patients (Evans et al. 2006). Voon et al. (2010) performed fMRI on PD patients with compulsive gambling and matched unaffected PD controls while they did a monetary reward learning task. They looked for neural signals related to learning about gains by modeling a reward prediction error signal. They found that compulsive gamblers had a reduced signal in the ventral striatum compared to non-gamblers when both were tested off medications, but that this effect was reversed by administration of a dopamine agonist. This finding was consistent with the behavioral effect, where a dopamine agonist increased gain learning only in the gamblers. One concludes that PD patients who develop addictions have a different ventral striatum dopamine innervation to start with and are somehow vulnerable to the effects of dopaminergic medication on the mesolimbic system. Two other studies demonstrated that PD patients with addictions had baseline anomalies in the ventral striatum, as assessed by measurements of dopamine D_2 receptor density (Steeves et al. 2009) and resting blood flow (Rao et al. 2010). Enhanced reward learning during dopamine agonist therapy may facilitate the progression to compulsive behavior that is a hallmark of addiction, and is also seen in non-parkinsonian vulnerable populations (Dagher and Robbins 2009).

As for motor tasks, cognitive tasks in PD may also lead to CBF changes in areas not activated in normal controls. In one study of the TOL task, PD patients had excessive activation of the hippocampus, whereas normal controls showed deactivation (reduced CBF) while performing the task (Dagher et al. 2001), findings that were replicated using fMRI with an implicit learning task that normally involves very similar brain regions as the TOL (Moody et al. 2004). The excess hippocampal activity in PD could represent recruitment of the intact declarative memory system to overcome the deficits of the impaired frontostriatal (procedural) memory system. However, evidence from animal and human also raises the possibility that hippocampal activity during the performance of "frontostriatal" tasks may actually be deleterious and need to be suppressed (Packard et al. 1989). If this is correct, the hippocampal activation seen in these PD patients could be contributing to rather than compensating for the cognitive deficits. Note that in healthy subjects, the hippocampus shows deactivation (reduced CBF) during the performance of these "frontostriatal" tasks (Dagher et al. 2001; Moody et al. 2004).

The striatum, due to its extensive connections with the entire cortex, is probably involved in numerous cognitive functions that rely on large-scale neural networks. Grossman et al. (2003) studied the processing of complex sentences in stage-I PD patients using fMRI. In normals, processing of long sentences requires working memory and grammatical processing and involves the striatum, lateral temporal cortex, ACC, and left inferior frontal cortex. PD patients showed relatively impaired activation of these areas but displayed recruitment of other cortical areas (posterior parietal and ventrolateral PFC). As in the previous studies, it is not clear whether this represents compensation or deleterious activity by a nonessential area. Nonetheless, it is likely that abnormal processing in the striatum in these early PD patients leads to significant effects on an entire neuronal network involved in linguistic processing.

Finally, Raichle has proposed that deactivations (i.e., reductions in CBF compared to baseline) in certain areas are a consistent feature in a wide range of cognitive tasks (Gusnard and Raichle 2001). These consistently deactivated brain regions are referred to as the default mode network (DMN) because they are found to have high resting activity and appear to be functionally connected with each other. The DMN includes the medial PFC and ACC, posterior cingulate cortex (PCC), precuneus, and lateral parietal and temporal cortices. Typically, DMN deactivation is proportional to task difficulty, and the DMN is anti-correlated with the so-called task positive network, consisting of brain areas involved in attention and executive function (notably the frontostriatal system that is defective in PD). There is evidence that DMN deactivation may be under the control of dopamine, as reducing dopamine levels in healthy humans disrupts DMN deactivation during an executive task (Nagano-Saito et al. 2008). In PD, several studies have demonstrated deficient deactivation of the DMN (Tinaz et al. 2008; van Eimeren et al. 2009). This deficiency is partially restored by apomorphine (Nagano-Saito et al. 2009) and levodopa (Delaveau et al. 2010), although one study demonstrated impaired ventromedial PFC deactivation induced by levodopa administration (Argyelan et al. 2008). Nonetheless, it appears that abnormal DMN deactivation in PD may contribute to cognitive deficits, is dopamine dependent, and may be partially responsive to dopaminergic medications.

In summary, PET and fMRI have demonstrated abnormal cortico-striatal function associated with cognitive deficits in PD; however, several questions remain. How many of the deficits are due to dopamine loss in the striatum as opposed to extrastriatal areas? Are some cognitive deficits worsened by dopaminergic medication? Moreover, the neurodegenerative process also affects acetylcholine, serotonin, and noradrenaline (Scatton et al. 1983) all of which play a role in cognition. There is evidence that acetylcholine loss is associated with cognitive impairment in PD (Kuhl et al. 1996; Asahina et al. 1998; Hilker et al. 2005). Finally, it is possible that cortical neurodegeneration plays a role in cognitive impairment (Nagano-Saito et al. 2005; Apostolova et al. 2010).

CONCLUSION

Early PET studies of motor and cognitive function in PD appeared to confirm a model according to which dopamine deficiency in the striatum led to widespread cortical inhibition, and hence to the well-known motor and cognitive deficits of the illness. However, fMRI, with its greater temporal resolution, has led to a reevaluation of these data. The consequences of dopamine loss in the striatum and cortex, and of pharmacological dopamine replenishment, are complex and cannot be explained by a simple functional deafferentation model. Other anomalies seen in PD, which appear to be dopamine dependent, include excessive spatial extent of cortical activation and failure to deactivate the DMN. As a general rule, dopaminergic therapy reverses many of the imaging anomalies seen in PD; however, the notion that dopamine replacement may also lead to overdosing in certain brain networks has been supported by several imaging studies.

REFERENCES

Albin, R. L., A. B. Young, J. B. Penney. 1989. The functional anatomy of basal ganglia disorders [see comments]. *Trends Neurosci* 12: 366–375.

Alexander, G. E., M. R. DeLong, and P. L. Strick. 1986. Parallel organization of functionally segregated circuits linking basal ganglia and cortex. *Annu Rev Neurosci* 9:357–381.

Apostolova, L. G., M. Beyer, A. E. Green, K. S. Hwang, J. H. Morra, Y. Y. Chou, C. Avedissian, D. Aarsland, C. C. Janvin, J. P. Larsen, J. L. Cummings, and P. M. Thompson. 2010. Hippocampal, caudate, and ventricular changes in Parkinson's disease with and without dementia. *Mov Disord* 25:687–688.

Argyelan, M., M. Carbon, M. F. Ghilardi, A. Feigin, P. Mattis, C. Tang, V. Dhawan, D. Eidelberg. 2008. Dopaminergic suppression of brain deactivation responses during sequence learning. *J Neurosci* 28: 10687–10695.

Asahina, M., T. Suhara, H. Shinotoh, O. Inoue, K. Suzuki, and T. Hattori. 1998. Brain muscarinic receptors in progressive supranuclear palsy and Parkinson's disease: A positron emission tomographic study. *J Neurol Neurosurg Psychiatry* 65:155–163.

Boecker, H., A. Dagher, A. O. Ceballos-Baumann, R. E. Passingham, M. Samuel, K. J. Friston, J. Poline, C. Dettmers, B. Conrad, and D. J. Brooks. 1998. Role of the human rostral supplementary motor area and the basal ganglia in motor sequence control: Investigations with H2 15O PET. *J Neurophysiol* 79:1070–1080.

Bruck, A., R. Portin, A. Lindell, A. Laihinen, J. Bergman, M. Haaparanta, O. Solin, and J. O. Rinne. 2001. Positron emission tomography shows that impaired frontal lobe functioning in Parkinson's disease is related to dopaminergic hypofunction in the caudate nucleus. *Neurosci Lett* 311:81–84.

Buhmann, C., V. Glauche, H. J. Sturenburg, M. Oechsner, C. Weiller, and C. Buchel. 2003. Pharmacologically modulated fMRI—cortical responsiveness to levodopa in drug-naive hemiparkinsonian patients. *Brain* 126:451–461.

Catalan, M. J., K. Ishii, M. Honda, A. Samii, and M. Hallett. 1999. A PET study of sequential finger movements of varying length in patients with Parkinson's disease. *Brain* 122:483–495.

Ceballos-Baumann, A. O., H. Boecker, P. Bartenstein, I. von Falkenhayn, H. Riescher, B. Conrad, J. R. Moringlane, and F. Alesch. 1999. A positron emission tomographic study of subthalamic nucleus stimulation in Parkinson disease: Enhanced movement-related activity of motor-association cortex and decreased motor cortex resting activity. *Arch Neurol* 56:997–1003.

Choi, J. K., Y. I. Chen, E. Hamel, and B. G. Jenkins. 2006. Brain hemodynamic changes mediated by dopamine receptors: Role of the cerebral microvasculature in dopamine-mediated neurovascular coupling. *Neuroimage* 30:700–712.

Cools, R., E. Stefanova, R. A. Barker, T. W. Robbins, and A. M. Owen. 2002. Dopaminergic modulation of high-level cognition in Parkinson's disease: The role of the prefrontal cortex revealed by PET. *Brain* 125:584–594.

Cools, R., S. J. Lewis, L. Clark, R. A. Barker, and T. W. Robbins. 2007. L-DOPA disrupts activity in the nucleus accumbens during reversal learning in Parkinson's disease. *Neuropsychopharmacology* 32: 180–189.

Dagher, A., and T. W. Robbins. 2009. Personality, addiction, dopamine: Insights from Parkinson's disease. *Neuron* 61:502–510.

Dagher, A., A. M. Owen, H. Boecker, and D. J. Brooks. 1999. Mapping the network for planning: A correlational PET activation study with the Tower of London task. *Brain* 122 (Pt 10):1973–1987.

Dagher, A., A. M. Owen, H. Boecker, and D. J. Brooks. 2001. The role of the striatum and hippocampus in planning: A PET activation study in Parkinson's disease. *Brain* 124:1020–1032.

Delaveau, P., P. Salgado-Pineda, P. Fossati, T. Witjas, J. P. Azulay, and O. Blin. 2010. Dopaminergic modulation of the default mode network in Parkinson's disease. *Eur Neuropsychopharmacol* 20(11):784–792.

Dirnberger, G., C. D. Frith, and M. Jahanshahi. 2005. Executive dysfunction in Parkinson's disease is associated with altered pallidal-frontal processing. *Neuroimage* 25:588–599.

Dubois, B., F. Boller, B. Pillon, and Y. Agid. 1991. Cognitive deficits in Parkinson's disease. In *Handbook of neuropsychology*, eds. F. Boller and J. Grafman, 195–240. New York: Elsevier Science.

Dum, R. P., and P. L. Strick. 2002. Motor areas in the frontal lobe of the primate. *Physiol Behav* 77:677–682.

Evans, A. H., N. Pavese, A. D. Lawrence, Y. F. Tai, S. Appel, M. Doder, D. J. Brooks, A. J. Lees, and P. Piccini. 2006. Compulsive drug use linked to sensitized ventral striatal dopamine transmission. *Ann Neurol* 59:852–858.

Freund, H. J 1987. Abnormalities of motor behavior after cortical lesions in humans. In *Handbook of physiology, section 1, the nervous system*, eds. V. B. Mountcastle and F. Plum, 768–810. Bethesda, MD: American Physiological Society.

between LID and cerebral blood flow–glucose metabolism dissociation.

DOPAMINERGIC SYSTEMS

PRESYNAPTIC FUNCTION

Presynaptic dopaminergic dysfunction examined by [18F]-fluorodopa in the off medication state has shown a negative correlation between putaminal uptake and dyskinesia severity (Linazasoro et al. 2004). A two-year longitudinal [18F]-fluorodopa PET study comparing patients treated with LD (−20.3%) and ropinirol (−13.4%) demonstrated a significant difference in posterolateral putamen Ki value, with concomitant difference in the incidence of dyskinesia (Whone et al. 2003). Presynaptic function measured by the dopamine transporter ligand [123I] FP-CIT and SPECT showed equally reduced striatal uptake in PD patients with and without LID off medication (Linazasoro et al. 2009). This observation was verified by the fact that PD severity was correlated with dyskinesia severity. Moreover, presynaptic dopaminergic denervation is assumed to be a prerequisite for inducing dyskinesia (Boyce et al. 1990; Peppe et al. 1993; Schneider 1989). Indeed, PD patients are far more susceptible to LID as a function of dopaminergic replacement therapy as opposed to healthy subjects (with intact presynaptic nigrostriatal projections) or atypical parkinsonian patients (with both pre- and postsynaptic dopaminergic deficits) (Constantinescu et al. 2007). While PD patients with advanced disease are predisposed to LID, and presynaptic dopaminergic deficits are required for this treatment side effect to develop, putaminal DA loss is not the only mechanism. LID has also been linked to DA turnover, defined as the proportion of presynaptic dopaminergic vesicles that undergo exocytosis per unit time. This parameter was estimated using a kinetic modeling approach applied to 18F-fluorodopa (FDOPA) PET time activity curves acquired over a long (four-hour) scanning period (Sossi et al. 2002). In these studies, increased DA turnover was evident early in the disease course, which was interpreted as a direct compensatory mechanism (Sossi et al. 2002; 2004). Additionally, DA turnover was found to be greater in early-onset PD patients relative to their older-onset counterparts (Sossi et al. 2006). The D_2 neuroreceptor ligand [11C]-raclopride exhibits less overall binding when other molecules with affinity for this receptor (including endogenous synaptic DA) are present in sufficient concentration. Indeed, changes in striatal synaptic DA levels after LD administration, measured by [11C]-raclopride PET, correlated with disease duration. Measurements of synaptic DA levels at one hour post-dose were found to be greater in PD patients with dyskinesia compared with those without motor complications. By contrast, synaptic DA levels at four hours did not differ between two groups (de la Fuente-Fernandez et al. 2004). This suggests that rapid synaptic DA overflow (i.e., pulsatile stimulation of DA receptors) following LD administration is associated with LID. Indeed, in a subsequent study, a significant correlation was reported between dyskinesia severity and the size of the levodopa-mediated change in [11C]-raclopride binding that was observed during PET imaging (Pavese et al. 2006). These observations accord well with experimental animal studies in which dyskinesias were associated with enhanced striatal production of DA following the administration of levodopa. Moreover, synaptic DA levels correlated with concurrent ratings of dyskinesia severity (Carta et al. 2006; Lee et al. 2008). Taken together, these results indicate that the prime trigger of LID is a rise in striatal DA levels following LD administration.

A recent multitracer imaging study utilizing [11C](±) dihydrotetrabenazine (DTBZ, for the vesicular monoamine transporter (VMAT2), used as an index of DA nerve terminal damage) and 11C-methylphenidate (MP, for the dopamine transporter (DAT), used as an index of DA reuptake) revealed that PD patients with LID exhibited a significant downregulation of DAT binding relative to DA nerve terminal damage compared to their counterparts without LID (Troiano et al. 2009). Nonetheless, a DAT knockout mouse exhibiting excessive and unregulated extracellular DA levels after fetal ventral mesencephalic transplantation failed to develop evidence of dyskinesia (Vinuela et al. 2008).

Abnormal DA storage is one of the major notions proposed to explain the development of LID in PD patients (Wooten 1988; Fabbrini et al. 1987; Mouradian et al. 1989). Indeed, this general hypothesis is compatible with the various PET imaging studies mentioned above. The shortening of the response duration following LD administration can be attributed to loss of presynaptic compensatory mechanisms. Likewise, the development of dyskinesias can be linked to temporary augmentation of synaptic DA levels. During the course of PD, the duration of individual doses of drug becomes limited as does the magnitude of the therapeutic response itself. Latency of the peak response is inversely correlated with off-score severity (Nutt and Holford 1996). In accord with these observations, high post-dose drug concentrations have been described in striatal extracellular fluid in a rodent dyskinesia model (Carta et al. 2006; Meissner et al. 2006).

In the advanced stages of PD, L-[11C]dopa PET showed that LD induced significant upregulation of striatal L-[11C]dopa influx rate (k_3 value, DA synthesis rate), while apomorphine (D_1/D_2 agonist) was stable. By contrast, patients with early or uncomplicated PD showed decreased influx rate by medication (Ekesbo et al. 1999; Torstenson et al. 1997). This indicates that as the nigrostriatal degeneration progresses and patients are chronically treated with DA replacement therapy, presynaptic inhibitory feedback regulation becomes disrupted. Whether this disturbed presynaptic feedback is related to development of dyskinesia is not clear and requires further research.

POSTSYNAPTIC FUNCTION

While the majority of imaging studies support a role of presynaptic function in the development of LID, it has been suggested that there is also a postsynaptic mechanism involved in the pathophysiology of this symptom. Overactivity of the direct striatal output pathway and attenuation of the indirect pathway is another well-accepted theory of LID development (Krack et al. 1999; Brotchie 2005). These two pathways have opposing functions in the control of movement. The direct pathway is responsible for execution of motor activity (Go pathway), and the indirect pathway serves an inhibitory role (No Go); this physiological balance refines the overall motor activity. Indeed, an experimental animal study suggested that chronic LD exposure would increase D_1 receptor numbers (Rioux et al. 1997). However, in vivo human studies have revealed that long-term LD treatment does not appear to be related to a change in striatal specific binding to D_1 or D_2 receptors assessed by [11C]-SCH23390 and [11C] raclopride, respectively (Dentresangle et al. 1999; Turjanski et al. 1997). These data suggest that the changes in striatal DA receptor availability are not primarily associated with the pathophysiology of LID in humans.

NON-DOPAMINERGIC SYSTEMS

Several non-dopaminergic mechanisms have been postulated for the development of LID (Brotchie 2005; Fabbrini et al. 2007). The opioid system acts as a modulator of DA in the basal ganglia (Fox et al. 2006), and opioid peptides act as co-transmitters within GABAergic neurons (Hallett and Brotchie 2007). In vivo assessment of opioid receptor binding measured by [11C] diprenorphine, a nonselective marker of μ, κ, and δ opioid sites, revealed reduced binding in the striatum, thalamus, and anterior cingulate in PD patients with LID compared to those without LID (Piccini et al. 1997). In addition, reduced binding in the putamen was associated with dyskinesia severity. Surrounding evidence

suggests that opioid transmission is increased in the basal ganglia of advanced-stage PD patients (Nisbet et al. 1995). Therefore, less [11C] diprenorphine binding in LID patients indicates an elevation of opioid receptor occupancy by endogenous ligands. This in vivo evidence suggests future use of opioid modulating agents for management options of LID in PD.

Adenosine A_{2A} receptors are G protein-coupled receptors that are predominantly found in the GABAergic striatopallidal neurons projecting from the striatum, mainly to the GPe (indirect pathway). Postmortem findings have shown that adenosine A_{2A} receptor mRNA level is increased only in the putamen of PD patients with LID compared to those without LID (Calon et al. 2004). It has been suggested that an adenosine A_{2A} receptor antagonist may be a potential candidate as an antiparkinsonian agent without the side effect of dyskinesia (Hauser and Schwarzschild 2005). Recently, the radionuclide 7-methyl-[11C]-(E)-8-(3,4,5-trimethoxystyryl)-1,3,7-trimethylxanthine ([11C]TMSX) has been developed to visualize in vivo adenosine A_{2A} receptor binding in the human brain (Mishina et al. 2007). This PET ligand could be particularly useful in future clinical trials assessing dynamic pharmacological change in PD patients.

L-aromatic amino acid decarboxylase (AADC) exists in nerve terminals of not only dopaminergic neurons, but also non-dopaminergic neurons. Growing evidence from animal studies suggests that serotonergic neurons may play an important role in the onset of LID (Carlsson et al. 2009; Carta et al. 2007). Serotonin neurons are capable of decarboxylating LD, storing DA in synaptic vesicles, and releasing it together with serotonin; however, the ability of serotonergic neurons to reuptake DA is unclear. The release of DA by these neurons without subsequent reuptake would result in unregulated DA efflux and defective DA clearance. A functional imaging study is currently in progress to elucidate this hypothesis.

α_2 adrenoreceptor is responsible for presynaptic inhibition of norepinephrine release and endothelium-dependent vasodilation by producing nitric oxide and is located within the striatum, subthalamic nucleus (STN), and substantia nigra (Bryan et al. 1996; Zou and Cowley 2000; Edvinsson and Krause 2002). By blocking α_2 adrenoreceptor in LID model animals, dyskinesia is ameliorated whereas apomorphine-induced dyskinesia is unchanged (Rascol et al. 2001; Fox et al. 2001). The striatum receives glutamatergic inputs from the cerebral cortex and the thalamus. Intracellular electrophysiological recordings from DA-depleted striatal slices have shown a significant increase in spontaneous glutamate release after DA denervation (Bezard et al. 2001). So far, there are no imaging data to support the notion that

α_2 adrenoreceptor and glutamatergic neurons are altered in LID.

CEREBRAL PERFUSION AND GLUCOSE METABOLISM

After levodopa administration, significant increases in overall brain perfusion, particularly in the basal ganglia, have been found with Xenon CT (Kobari et al. 1995; Montastruc et al. 1987). Another Xenon CT study revealed an LD-induced increase in striatal perfusion in PD but not in atypical parkinsonian subjects (Kobari et al. 1995). Furthermore, with LD administration, PD patients with good response to LD showed decrements in striatal perfusion, whereas PD patients with adverse reactions demonstrated increments in the striatum and also in the globus pallidus and thalamus (Henriksen and Boas 1985). A motor activation study reported overactivity of the supplementary motor and primary motor areas in patients with LID compared to those without LID as well as healthy control subjects (Rascol et al. 1998).

Hershey and colleagues (Hershey et al. 1998) utilized [^{15}O]H$_2$O and PET to assess perfusional changes before and after administration of LD in PD patients with and without LID. Subjects without LID showed significant perfusional increase in the left putamen and midbrain, whereas those exhibiting LID demonstrated perfusional increase in the left thalamus and putamen, and in the right globus pallidus, left hippocampus, with associated decrease in the right thalamus.

Metabolic activity in PD patients experiencing LID has been reported to be similar to that of patients with chorea (Hirato et al. 1995). Specifically, in PD patients with LID, regional cerebral glucose metabolism measured by ^{18}F-fluorodeoxyglucose (FDG) and PET was reduced in the lenticular nucleus and increased in the frontal cortex. However, in the off medication state, the same PD patients exhibited a relative metabolic increase in the lenticular nucleus. An ex vivo animal study performed with 2-deoxyglucose autoradiography designed to compare a LID model primate and non-LID primate showed that glucose utilization was significantly decreased below the normal range in the GPe and thalamus, but was increased in the STN (Guigoni et al. 2005; Mitchell et al. 1992; Mitchell et al. 1985). This indicates that afferent neurons to subthalamic nucleus overinhibit the subthalamic nucleus and thereby suppress GPi (Papa et al. 1999; Obeso et al. 2000). Since local glucose utilization reflects synaptic activity from afferent neurons, together these findings support the basal ganglia model of LID. Thus, the physiology of LID seems to be disinhibition

of neurons in the GPe, which overinhibits STN, and subsequent hypoactivity in output neurons of the basal ganglia, such as GPi and SNr (Boraud et al. 2001; Bezard et al. 2001). That said, neurophysiologic studies have demonstrated that irregular firing might be involved in the onset of dyskinesia, which complicates the interpretation of metabolic data.

Flow–metabolism dissociation in levodopa-induced dyskinesia

Investigations in normal rodents indicate that the injection of exogenous DA results in a dissociation between changes in cerebral perfusion and glucose utilization (Tuor et al. 1986). Leenders et al. (1985) reported a significant increase in perfusion (+20%) with a relative decrease of oxygen utilization (−2%) in the basal ganglia of PD patients following administration of oral LD. Generally, cerebral blood flow and metabolism are tightly coupled, except in the case of specific drug interactions (Ma and Eidelberg 2007). Along these lines, Hirano et al. (2008) compared the metabolic and neurovascular effects of antiparkinsonian LD therapy. PD patients were scanned with both [^{15}O]H$_2$O and [^{18}F]fluorodeoxyglucose PET in the unmedicated state and during intravenous LD infusion. Dyskinesia was controlled minimally by titrating LD dose. The authors found a significant dissociation between cerebral perfusion and cerebral metabolic glucose rate in the modulation of the putamen/globus pallidus, dorsal midbrain/pons, STN, and ventral thalamus (Figure 1 top). Baseline (off medication) metabolic activity in these regions was elevated in PD patients relative to healthy controls, consistent with increases in local afferent synaptic activity, represented in a PD-related metabolic spatial covariance pattern (Eidelberg et al. 1997) (See Chapter 3 for additional information on this network). This dissociation was defined by reductions (normalization) in baseline elevations in glucose metabolism occurring concurrently with increases in cerebral perfusion in the same brain regions. This flow–metabolism dissociation proved to be substantially greater in patients exhibiting LID.

It has been proposed that increased vasomotor effect of treatment seen in the putamen is associated with LD treatment, and in extreme case associates with LID (Hirano et al. 2008). Indeed, the relative increase of cerebral blood flow within the PDRP network positively correlated with disease duration. In contrast to this result, this dissociation was not observed in another group of PD patients treated with STN deep brain stimulation (DBS). Nerve terminals in these regions are known to express AADC. Even in PD patients with denervated nigrostriatal dopaminergic neurons, overall AADC levels are relatively maintained, due in all likelihood

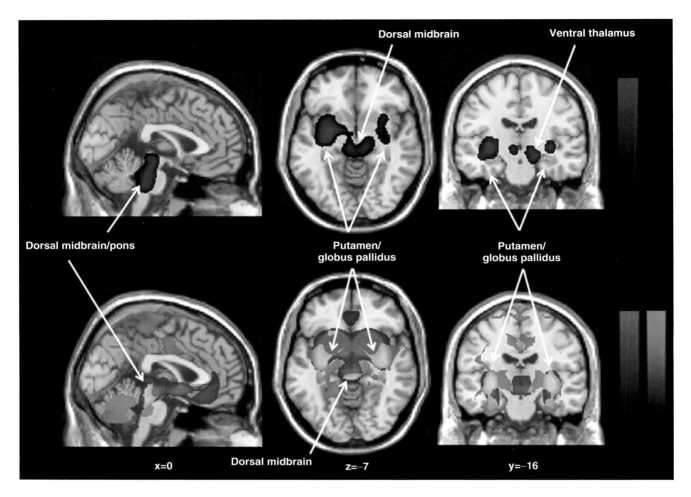

Figure 1 Top: Brain regions (blue) with increased cerebral flow ([^{15}O]H$_2$O PET) and concomitant reductions in cerebral glucose metabolism ([^{18}F]FDG PET) (dissociation) with levodopa therapy for Parkinson's disease. *Bottom*: Brain regions (red) with elevated levels of L-aromatic amino acid decarboxylase (AADC) ([^{18}F]fluorodopa) in PD patients compared to healthy subjects; brain regions (green) with relatively increased glucose metabolism ([^{18}F]FDG) in unmedicated PD patients compared to healthy subjects. Areas of overlap between the two statistical maps (yellow) indicate regions in which elevated synaptic activity and local AADC expression are both present. [Hirano et al. 2008 *J Neurosci* 28:4201-4209 with permission from the Society for Neuroscience.]

to enzyme expression in non-dopaminergic nerve terminals such as serotonergic neurons (Figure 2A). In this vein, DA agonist treatment is not dependent upon regional AADC activity and is therefore not likely to promote flow-metabolism dissociation and drug-induced dyskinesia (Figure 1 bottom). These findings suggest that flow–metabolism dissociation is a distinctive feature of LD treatment and may be especially pronounced in patients with LID. The vasoactive effects of DA may aggravate the situation by increasing the delivery of drug to AADC-rich brain regions. After quantal release of DA from the presynaptic terminal, volume transmission can occur (Agnati et al. 1995; Zoli et al. 1998), which is likely to be accentuated in PD due to concomitant reductions in DA uptake (Cragg and Rice 2004) (Figure 2C). Interestingly, the direct effects of DA on the vasculature appear to be due primarily to D$_1$-like receptors (Edvinsson and Krause 2002), which in turn have been linked to angiogenesis and

neovascularization in associated brain regions (Westin et al. 2006; Lindgren et al. 2009). While such irreversible endothelial changes can explain the priming effects seen with LID, it is not known how they relate to the development of this phenomenon in human subjects with PD. Whether flow-metabolism dissociation is itself a viable target for new antidyskinesia drug development is also unclear. That said, current data suggest that the interruption of pharamacodynamic state is of great importance in perfusion imaging studies of subjects on dopaminergic medication.

CONCLUSION

The pathophysiology of LID is complex and cannot be explained by a single factor. The phenomenon likely involves multiple interrelated mechanisms that possibly feed off of

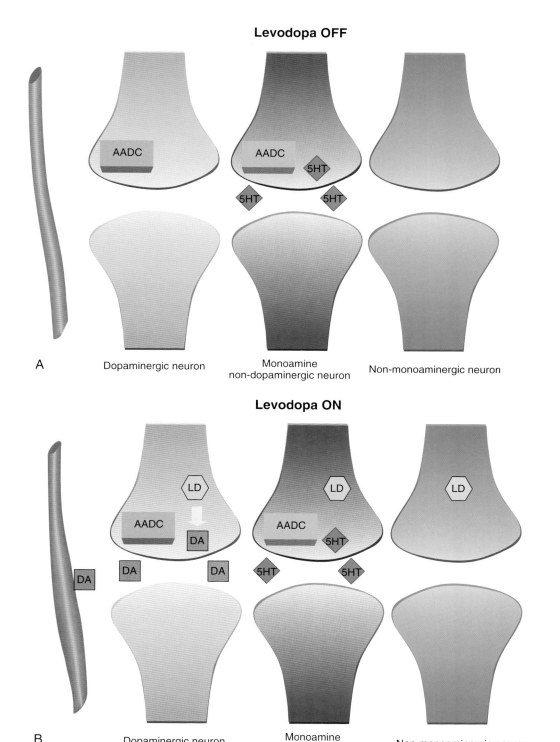

Levodopa OFF

A — Dopaminergic neuron — Monoamine non-dopaminergic neuron — Non-monoaminergic neuron

Levodopa ON

B — Dopaminergic neuron — Monoamine non-dopaminergic neuron — Non-monoaminergic neuron

Figure 2 Schematic diagram of dopaminergic, non-dopaminergic monoamine neuron (serotonin, norepinephrine), non-dopaminergic non-monoamine neuron in Parkinson's disease. L-aromatic amino acid decarboxylase exists in the presynapse of monoaminergic neuron, including dopaminergic neurons. (A) Levodopa off state: note that dopamine secretion is reduced in dopaminergic neurons. (B) Levodopa on state: levodopa is converted both in dopaminergic neurons and non-dopaminergic monoamine neurons. (C) When excessive levodopa is administered, synaptic dopamine level is abundant and spillover of dopamine (volume transmission) interacts with nearby vasculatures. Levodopa-induced hyperperfusion (or vasodilation) will locally oversupply levodopa and further aggravate the increased synaptic levodopa concentration that develops dyskinesia. LD: levodopa, DA: dopamine, AADC: L-aromatic amino acid decarboxylase, 5HT: 5 hydroxytryptamine.

(Continued)

Dyskinesia

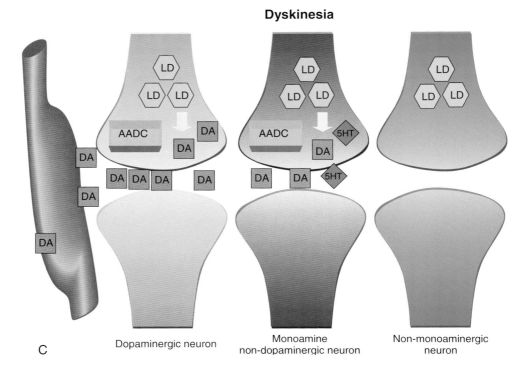

Figure 2 (Continued)

one another. Future imaging studies, particularly those that control for pharmacological state, will help clarify the cause of LID and aid in the evaluation of treatment options for this disabling side effect.

REFERENCES

Agnati, L. F., M. Zoli, I. Stromberg, and K. Fuxe. 1995. Intercellular communication in the brain: Wiring versus volume transmission. *Neuroscience* 69:711–26.

Ahlskog, J. E., and M. D. Muenter. 2001. Frequency of levodopa-related dyskinesias and motor fluctuations as estimated from the cumulative literature. *Mov Disord* 16:448–58.

Bezard, E., J. M. Brotchie, and C. E. Gross. 2001. Pathophysiology of levodopa-induced dyskinesia: Potential for new therapies. *Nat Rev Neurosci* 2:577–88.

Boraud, T., E. Bezard, B. Bioulac, and C. E. Gross. 2001. Dopamine agonist-induced dyskinesias are correlated to both firing pattern and frequency alterations of pallidal neurones in the MPTP-treated monkey. *Brain* 124:546–57.

Boyce, S., N. M. Rupniak, M. J. Steventon, and S. D. Iversen. 1990. Nigrostriatal damage is required for induction of dyskinesias by L-DOPA in squirrel monkeys. *Clin Neuropharmacol* 13:448–58.

Brotchie, J. M. 2005. Nondopaminergic mechanisms in levodopa-induced dyskinesia. *Mov Disord* 20:919–31.

Bryan, R. M. Jr., M. Y. Eichler, M. W. Swafford, T. D. Johnson, M. S. Suresh, and W. F. Childres. 1996. Stimulation of alpha 2 adrenoceptors dilates the rat middle cerebral artery. *Anesthesiology* 85: 82–90.

Calon, F., M. Dridi, O. Hornykiewicz, P. J. Bedard, A. H. Rajput, and T. Di Paolo. 2004. Increased adenosine A2A receptors in the brain of Parkinson's disease patients with dyskinesias. *Brain* 127: 1075–84.

Carlsson, T., M. Carta, A. Munoz, B. Mattsson, C. Winkler, D. Kirik et al. 2009. Impact of grafted serotonin and dopamine neurons on development of L-DOPA-induced dyskinesias in parkinsonian rats is determined by the extent of dopamine neuron degeneration. *Brain* 132:319–35.

Carta, M., T. Carlsson, D. Kirik, and A. Bjorklund. 2007. Dopamine released from 5-HT terminals is the cause of L-DOPA-induced dyskinesia in parkinsonian rats. *Brain* 130:1819–33.

Carta, M., H. S. Lindgren, M. Lundblad, R. Stancampiano, F. Fadda, and M. A. Cenci. 2006. Role of striatal L-DOPA in the production of dyskinesia in 6-hydroxydopamine lesioned rats. *J Neurochem* 96:1718–27.

Cenci, M. A. 2010. In *Dopamine Handbook*, eds L. L. Iversen, S. D. Iversen, S. E. Dunnett, and A. bjorklund, 434–44. Oxford University Press, New York.

Cenci, M. A., and M. Lundblad. 2006. Post- versus presynaptic plasticity in L-DOPA-induced dyskinesia. *J Neurochem* 99:381–92.

Constantinescu, R., I. Richard, and R. Kurlan. 2007. Levodopa responsiveness in disorders with parkinsonism: A review of the literature. *Mov Disord* 29:29.

Cragg, S. J., and M. E. Rice. 2004. DAncing past the DAT at a DA synapse. *Trends in Neurosciences* 27:270–7.

de la Fuente-Fernandez, R., V. Sossi, Z. Huang, S. Furtado, J. Q. Lu, D. B. Calne et al. 2004. Levodopa-induced changes in synaptic dopamine levels increase with progression of Parkinson's disease: Implications for dyskinesias. *Brain* 127:2747–54.

Dentresangle, C., L. Veyre, D. Le Bars, C. Pierre, F. Lavenne, P. Pollak et al. 1999. Striatal D2 dopamine receptor status in Parkinson's disease: An [18F]dopa and [11C]raclopride PET study. *Mov Disord* 14:1025–30.

Edvinsson, L., and D. Krause. 2002. Catecholamines. In *Cerebral blood flow and metabolism*, eds. L. Edvinsson and D. Krause, 191–211. Philadelphia: Lippincott Wiliams & Wilkins.

Eidelberg, D., J. R. Moeller, K. Kazumata, A. Antonini, D. Sterio, V. Dhawan et al. 1997. Metabolic correlates of pallidal neuronal activity in Parkinson's disease. *Brain* 120:1315–24.

Ekesbo, A., E. Rydin, R. Torstenson, O. Sydow, B. Laengstrom, and J. Tedroff. 1999. Dopamine autoreceptor function is lost in advanced Parkinson's disease. *Neurology* 52:120–5.

Fabbrini, G., J. M. Brotchie, F. Grandas, M. Nomoto, C. G. Goetz. 2007. Levodopa-induced dyskinesias. *Mov Disord* 22:1379–89.

Fabbrini, G., J. Juncos, M. M. Mouradian, C. Serrati, and T. N. Chase. 1987. Levodopa pharmacokinetic mechanisms and motor fluctuations in Parkinson's disease. *Ann Neurol* 21:370–6.

Fox, S. H., B. Henry, M. P. Hill, D. Peggs, A. R. Crossman, and J. M. Brotchie. 2001. Neural mechanisms underlying peak-dose dyskinesia induced by levodopa and apomorphine are distinct: Evidence from the effects of the alpha(2) adrenoceptor antagonist idazoxan. *Mov Disord* 16:642–50.

Fox, S. H., A. E. Lang, and J. M. Brotchie. 2006. Translation of nondopaminergic treatments for levodopa-induced dyskinesia from MPTP-lesioned nonhuman primates to phase IIa clinical studies: Keys to success and roads to failure. *Mov Disord* 21:1578–94.

Guigoni, C., Q. Li, I. Aubert, S. Dovero, B. H. Bioulac, B. Bloch et al. 2005. Involvement of sensorimotor, limbic, and associative basal ganglia domains in L-3,4-dihydroxyphenylalanine-induced dyskinesia. *Journal of Neuroscience* 25:2102–7.

Hallett, P. J., and J. M. Brotchie. 2007. Striatal delta opioid receptor binding in experimental models of Parkinson's disease and dyskinesia. *Mov Disord* 22:28–40.

Hauser, R. A., M. P. McDermott, and S. Messing. 2006. Factors associated with the development of motor fluctuations and dyskinesias in Parkinson disease. *Archives of Neurology* 63:1756–60.

Hauser, R. A., and M. A. Schwarzschild. 2005. Adenosine A2A receptor antagonists for Parkinson's disease: Rationale, therapeutic potential and clinical experience. *Drugs Aging* 22:471–82.

Henriksen, L., and J. Boas. 1985. Regional cerebral blood flow in hemi-parkinsonian patients. Emission computerized tomography of inhaled 133Xenon before and after levodopa. *Acta Neurol Scand* 71:257–66.

Hershey, T., K. J. Black, M. K. Stambuk, J. L. Carl, L. A. McGee-Minnich, and J. S. Perlmutter. 1998. Altered thalamic response to levodopa in Parkinson's patients with dopa-induced dyskinesias. *Proc Natl Acad Sci USA* 95:12016–21.

Hirano, S., K. Asanuma, Y. Ma, C. Tang, A. Feigin, V. Dhawan et al. 2008. Dissociation of metabolic and neurovascular responses to levodopa in the treatment of Parkinson's disease. *J Neurosci* 28:4201–9.

Hirato, M., J. Ishihara, S. Horikoshi, T. Shibazaki, and C. Ohye. 1995. Parkinsonian rigidity, dopa-induced dyskinesia and chorea—dynamic studies on the basal ganglia-thalamocortical motor circuit using PET scan and depth microrecording. *Acta Neurochir Suppl* 64:5–8.

Kobari, M., Y. Fukuuchi, T. Shinohara, K. Obara, and S. Nogawa. 1995. Levodopa-induced local cerebral blood flow changes in Parkinson's disease and related disorders. *J Neurol Sci* 128:212–8.

Kostic, V., S. Przedborski, E. Flaster, and N. Sternic. 1991. Early development of levodopa-induced dyskinesias and response fluctuations in young-onset Parkinson's disease. *Neurology* 41:202–5.

Krack, P., P. Pollak, P. Limousin, A. Benazzouz, G. Deuschl, and A. L. Benabid. 1999. From off-period dystonia to peak-dose chorea. The clinical spectrum of varying subthalamic nucleus activity. *Brain* 122 (Pt 6): 1133–46.

Lee, J., W. M. Zhu, D. Stanic, D. I. Finkelstein, M. H. Horne, J. Henderson et al. 2008. Sprouting of dopamine terminals and altered dopamine release and uptake in Parkinsonian dyskinaesia. *Brain* 131:1574–87.

Leenders, K. L., L. Wolfson, J. M. Gibbs, R. J. Wise, R. Causon, T. Jones et al. 1985. The effects of L-DOPA on regional cerebral blood flow and oxygen metabolism in patients with Parkinson's disease. *Brain* 108 (Pt 1): 171–91.

Linazasoro, G., A. Antonini, R. P. Maguire, and K. L. Leenders. 2004. Pharmacological and PET studies in patients with Parkinson's disease and a short duration-motor response: Implications in the pathophysiology of motor complications. *J Neural Transm* 111: 497–509.

Linazasoro, G., N. Van Blercom, A. Bergaretxe, F. M. Inaki, E. Laborda, and J. A. Ruiz Ortega. 2009. Levodopa-induced dyskinesias in parkinson disease are independent of the extent of striatal dopaminergic denervation: a pharmacological and SPECT study. *Clin Neuropharmacol* 32:326–9.

Lindgren, H. S., K. E. Ohlin, and M. A. Cenci. 2009. Differential involvement of D1 and D2 dopamine receptors in L-DOPA-induced angiogenic activity in a rat model of Parkinson's disease. *Neuropsychopharmacology* 34:2477–2488.

Ma, Y., and D. Eidelberg. 2007. Functional imaging of cerebral blood flow and glucose metabolism in Parkinson's disease and Huntington's disease. *Mol Imag Biol* 9:223–33.

Meissner, W., P. Ravenscroft, R. Reese, D. Harnack, R. Morgenstern, A. Kupsch et al. 2006. Increased slow oscillatory activity in substantia nigra pars reticulata triggers abnormal involuntary movements in the 6-OHDA-lesioned rat in the presence of excessive extracellular striatal dopamine. *Neurobiol Dis* 22:586–98.

Mishina, M., K. Ishiwata, Y. Kimura, M. Naganawa, K. Oda, S. Kobayashi et al. 2007. Evaluation of distribution of adenosine A2A receptors in normal human brain measured with [11C]TMSX PET. *Synapse* 61:778–84.

Mitchell, I. J., A. Boyce, M. A. Sambrook, and A. R. Crossman. 1992. A 2-deoxyglucose study of the effects of dopamine agonists on the parkinsonian primate brain. Implications for the neural mechanisms that mediate dopamine agonist-induced dyskinesia. *Brain* 115 (Pt 3): 809–24.

Mitchell, I. J., M. A. Sambrook, and A. R. Crossman. 1985. Subcortical changes in the regional uptake of [3H]-2-deoxyglucose in the brain of the monkey during experimental choreiform dyskinesia elicited by injection of a gamma-aminobutyric acid antagonist into the subthalamic nucleus. *Brain* 108 (Pt 2): 405–22.

Montastruc, J. L., P. Celsis, A. Agniel, J. F. Demonet, B. Doyon, M. Puel et al. 1987. Levodopa-induced regional cerebral blood flow changes in normal volunteers and patients with Parkinson's disease. Lack of correlation with clinical or neuropsychological improvements. *Mov Disord* 2:279–89.

Mouradian, M. M., I. J. Heuser, F. Baronti, G. Fabbrini, J. L. Juncos, and T. N. Chase. 1989. Pathogenesis of dyskinesias in Parkinson's disease. *Ann Neurol* 25:523–6.

Nisbet, A. P., O. J. Foster, A. Kingsbury, D. J. Eve, S. E. Daniel, C. D. Marsden et al. 1995. Preproenkephalin and preprotachykinin messenger RNA expression in normal human basal ganglia and in Parkinson's disease. *Neuroscience* 66:361–76.

Nutt, J. G., and N. H. Holford. 1996. The response to levodopa in Parkinson's disease: Imposing pharmacological law and order. *Ann Neurol* 39:561–73.

Obeso, J. A., M. C. Rodriguez-Oroz, M. Rodriguez, M. R. DeLong, and C. W. Olanow. 2000. Pathophysiology of levodopa-induced dyskinesias in Parkinson's disease: Problems with the current model. *Ann Neurol* 47:S22–32.

Papa, S. M., R. Desimone, M. Fiorani, and E. H. Oldfield. 1999. Internal globus pallidus discharge is nearly suppressed during levodopa-induced dyskinesias. *Ann Neurol* 46:732–8.

Pavese, N., A. H. Evans, Y. F. Tai, G. Hotton, D. J. Brooks, A. J. Lees et al. 2006. Clinical correlates of levodopa-induced dopamine release in Parkinson disease: A PET study. *Neurology* 67:1612–7.

Peppe, A., J. M. Dambrosia, and T. N. Chase. 1993. Risk factors for motor response complications in L-dopa-treated parkinsonian patients. *Adv Neurol* 60:698–702.

Piccini, P., R. A. Weeks, and D. J. Brooks. 1997. Alterations in opioid receptor binding in Parkinson's disease patients with levodopa-induced dyskinesias. *Ann Neurol* 42:720–6.

Rajput, A. H., M. E. Fenton, S. Birdi, R. Macaulay, D. George, B. Rozdilsky et al. 2002. Clinical-pathological study of levodopa complications. *Mov Disord* 17:289–96.

Rascol, O., I. Arnulf, H. Peyro-Saint Paul, C. Brefel-Courbon, M. Vidailhet, C. Thalamas et al. 2001. Idazoxan, an alpha-2 antagonist, and L-DOPA-induced dyskinesias in patients with Parkinson's disease. *Mov Disord* 16:708–13.

Rascol, O., D. J. Brooks, A. D. Korczyn, P. P. De Deyn, C. E. Clarke, A. E. Lang et al. 2006. Development of dyskinesias in a 5-year trial of ropinirole and L-dopa. *Mov Disord* 21:1844–50.

Rascol, O., U. Sabatini, C. Brefel, N. Fabre, S. Rai, J. M. Senard et al. 1998. Cortical motor overactivation in parkinsonian patients with L-dopa-induced peak-dose dyskinesia. *Brain* 121 (Pt 3): 527–33.

Rioux, L., P. A. Frohna, J. N. Joyce, and J. S. Schneider. 1997. The effects of chronic levodopa treatment on pre- and postsynaptic markers of dopaminergic function in striatum of parkinsonian monkeys. *Mov Disord* 12:148–58.

Schneider, J. S. 1989. Levodopa-induced dyskinesias in parkinsonian monkeys: Relationship to extent of nigrostriatal damage. *Pharmacol Biochem Behav* 34:193–6.

Schrag, A., and N. Quinn. 2000. Dyskinesias and motor fluctuations in Parkinson's disease. A community-based study. *Brain* 123 (Pt 11): 2297–305.

Smith, L. A., M. J. Jackson, M. J. Hansard, E. Maratos, and P. Jenner. 2003. Effect of pulsatile administration of levodopa on dyskinesia induction in drug-naive MPTP-treated common marmosets: Effect of dose, frequency of administration, and brain exposure. *Mov Disord* 18:487–95.

Sossi, V., R. de La Fuente-Fernandez, J. E. Holden, D. J. Doudet, J. McKenzie, A. J. Stoessl et al. 2002. Increase in dopamine turnover occurs early in Parkinson's disease: Evidence from a new modeling approach to PET 18 F-fluorodopa data. *J Cereb Blood Flow Metab* 22:232–9.

Sossi, V., R. de la Fuente-Fernandez, J. E. Holden, M. Schulzer, T. J. Ruth, and J. Stoessl. 2004. Changes of dopamine turnover in the progression of Parkinson's disease as measured by positron emission tomography: Their relation to disease-compensatory mechanisms. *J Cereb Blood Flow Metab* 24:869–76.

Sossi, V., R. de la Fuente-Fernandez, M. Schulzer, J. Adams, and J. Stoessl. 2006. Age-related differences in levodopa dynamics in Parkinson's: Implications for motor complications. *Brain* 129:1050–8.

Torstenson, R., P. Hartvig, B. Langstrom, G. Westerberg, and J. Tedroff. 1997. Differential effects of levodopa on dopaminergic function in early and advanced Parkinson's disease. *Ann Neurol* 41:334–40.

Troiano, A. R., R. de la Fuente-Fernandez, V. Sossi, M. Schulzer, E. Mak, T. J. Ruth et al. 2009. PET demonstrates reduced dopamine transporter expression in PD with dyskinesias. *Neurology* 72:1211–6.

Tuor, U. I., L. Edvinsson, and J. McCulloch. 1986. Catecholamines and the relationship between cerebral blood flow and glucose use. *Am J Physiol* 251:H824–33.

Turjanski, N., A. J. Lees, and D. J. Brooks. 1997. In vivo studies on striatal dopamine D1 and D2 site binding in L-dopa-treated Parkinson's disease patients with and without dyskinesias. *Neurology* 49:717–23.

Vinuela, A., P. J. Hallett, C. Reske-Nielsen, M. Patterson, T. D. Sotnikova, M. G. Caron et al. 2008. Implanted reuptake-deficient or wild-type dopaminergic neurons improve ON L-dopa dyskinesias without OFF-dyskinesias in a rat model of Parkinson's disease. *Brain* 131:3361–79.

Westin, J. E., H. S. Lindgren, J. Gardi, J. R. Nyengaard, P. Brundin, P. Mohapel et al. 2006. Endothelial proliferation and increased blood-brain barrier permeability in the basal ganglia in a rat model of 3,4-dihydroxyphenyl-L-alanine-induced dyskinesia. *J Neurosci* 26:9448–61.

Whone, A. L., R. L. Watts, A. J. Stoessl, M. Davis, S. Reske, C. Nahmias et al. 2003. Slower progression of Parkinson's disease with ropinirole versus levodopa: The REAL-PET study. *Ann Neurol* 54:93–101.

Wooten, G. F. 1988. Progress in understanding the pathophysiology of treatment-related fluctuations in Parkinson's disease. *Ann Neurol* 24:363–5.

Zoli, M., C. Torri, R. Ferrari, A. Jansson, I. Zini, K. Fuxe et al. 1998. The emergence of the volume transmission concept. *Brain Res Brain Res Rev* 26:136–47.

Zou, A. P., A. W. Cowley Jr. 2000. alpha(2)-adrenergic receptor-mediated increase in NO production buffers renal medullary vasoconstriction. *Am J Physiol Regul Integr Comp Physiol* 279: R769–77.

15

EFFECTS OF SURGICAL TREATMENT

Anna L. Bartels and Klaus L. Leenders

INTRODUCTION

This chapter summarizes the contributions of imaging to the understanding of the effects of surgical treatment in Parkinson's disease (PD). Deep brain stimulation (DBS) has been found to be an effective therapy for tremor, Parkinson's disease (PD), and dystonia. Our understanding of the pathophysiology of these movement disorders and of the mechanism of action of this form of surgical treatment has benefited from imaging studies. Structural imaging with MRI has improved precision in placement of electrodes, while functional imaging with positron emission tomography (PET), single photon emission tomography (SPECT), and recently also functional magnetic resonance imaging (fMRI) provided a method to study in vivo the involvement of different brain areas in the pathophysiology of these disorders. Furthermore, radiotracer imaging studies have been used to study the effect of several PD treatments on disease progression. This chapter will focus upon DBS and, to a lesser degree, stereotaxic lesioning procedures for the motor symptoms of PD. The role of imaging in assessing novel-cell based interventions for PD and gene therapy approaches is discussed elsewhere in this volume (see Chapters 16 and 17, respectively).

DBS IN PD: CLINICAL EFFECTS AND STRUCTURAL IMAGING

The possibility of DBS as an interventional procedure was already surmised in the 1930s. However, the precise rationale of this approach was posited only in the 1980s (Benabid et al. 2009a). Previously, neurosurgeons relied on lesioning brain structures to alleviate parkinsonian symptoms, especially tremor. In the early 1990s, DBS of the subthalamic nucleus (STN) was shown to result in effective improvement of motor function and was subsequently applied as a surgical treatment in more advanced PD patients (The Deep Brain Stimulation for Parkinson's Disease Study Group, 2001). DBS nowadays is more common, being routinely performed in approximately 5% of PD patients. However, neuropsychological unwanted effects have been shown to accompany the motor benefits of STN DBS in some advanced patients (Benabid et al. 2009b). Apart from its clinical advantages, DBS procedures have provided a rare opportunity to directly investigate the functioning of large-scale brain networks in PD through the use of imaging tools.

MODEL OF BASAL GANGLIA CIRCUITRY IN PD

Before considering changes in brain activation by DBS, it is useful to give a short overview of the organization of basal ganglia (BG) circuitry. A model of cortico-BG-cortical circuits consisting of parallel, largely segregated but interconnected closed-loop projections has first been described by Alexander and colleagues (Alexander, DeLong, and Strick 1986). Despite its simplicity, this model can be used to understand the changes in brain activation induced by DBS in PD patients (see Figure 1, adapted from Ballanger et al. (Ballanger et al. 2009b). In this model, the STN plays a critical role in the modulation of cortico-striato-pallido-thalamo-cortical (CSPTC) motor pathways. The motor symptoms of PD are related to overactivity of globus pallidus pars interna (GPi) afferents from STN and consequent increases in inhibitory pallidal outflow to the ventral thalamus and pons (Eidelberg et al. 1994, 1997). Indeed, this phenomenon in experimental models led to the development of STN surgery in PD patients (Aziz et al. 1992).

In this classical model, the basal ganglia form part of a complex network of parallel loops that integrate cerebral cortical regions (associative, oculomotor, limbic, and motor regions), basal ganglia nuclei, and the thalamus. The motor circuit within this complex consists of cortical motor areas that project to the striatum, especially the putamen. From the putamen, neurons in the "direct pathway" project to the GPi and the substantia nigra reticulata (SNr), the output nuclei of the basal ganglia. This pathway provides a direct inhibitory (GABAergic) effect on GPi/SNr neurons, hereby reducing the inhibitory effect of these nuclei on the thalamus and thus "facilitating" movement. The "indirect pathway" connects the putamen with the output nuclei via the globus pallidus pars externa (GPe) and the STN. Stimulation of striatal projection neurons in the indirect pathway leads to inhibition of the GPe, disinhibition of the STN, and excitation of the GPi/SNr, enhancing the inhibitory effect on the thalamus and "suppressing" movements (see Figure 1). In PD, bradykinesia and rigidity are related to a lack of activation of the dorsolateral prefrontal cortex (DLPFC), the supplementary motor area (SMA), and the anterior cingulated cortex (ACC) through inhibition of the thalamocortical excitatory pathway (Jenkins et al. 1992). In addition to the motor circuit, there are at least three other circuits connecting the basal ganglia to the thalamus and cortex: associative loops, projecting from the caudate to the DLPFC; limbic loops from the ventral striatum to the ACC; and the orbital frontal cortex and oculomotor circuit, involved in control of saccadic eye movements. The dorsolateral prefrontal circuit is involved in aspects of memory and orientation in space, and the lateral orbitofrontal circuit is thought to be involved in the ability to change behavioral sets, signaling changes in reinforcement contingencies, and behavioral control. Of note, motor, associative, and limbic territories are represented in each nucleus of the BG and DBS can affect motor as well as cognitive and emotional disease manifestations. Cognitive and emotional symptoms in PD may also relate to lesions in the mesocortical dopaminergic system, projecting from the ventral tegmental area (VTA) to the frontal regions (Javoy-Agid and Agid 1980). Moreover, apart from the dopamine system, PD symptoms may be the consequence of progressive degeneration in other ascending subcortical neurotransmitter systems (Braak and Braak 2000).

It is still unclear how the denervation in PD alters the normal functioning of the BG-cortical loops. It has been suggested that after nigrostriatal dopamine depletion, cross-connection between "segregated" BG subcircuits becomes more active, resulting in abnormal synchronized activity within the BG (Hammond, Bergman, and Brown 2007).

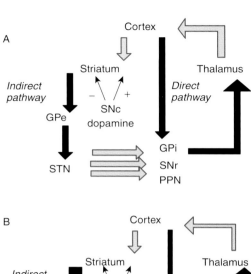

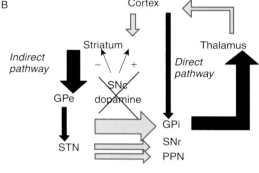

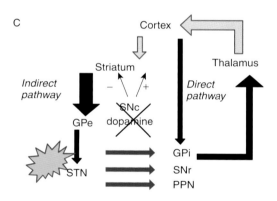

Figure 1 (adapted from Ballanger et al. (2009b) PET functional imaging of deep brain stimulation in movement disorders and psychiatry. Cortical-basal ganglia loops in **A)** normal situation, **B)** Parkinson's disease, and **C)** Parkinson's disease with STN DBS. Gray arrows indicate glutamatergic pathways, black arrows GABAergic pathways. In PD, dopaminergic degeneration in SNc leads to hyperactivity of the indirect pathway and reduced activity of the direct pathway. STN DBS reverses the inhibitory output from the GPi to the thalamus and increases cortical activation.

DBS IN PD: FUNCTIONAL EFFECTS

STN DBS produces a change in the pattern and periodicity of neuronal activity in the basal ganglia-thalamic network. The results of several studies are consistent with the explanation that stimulation raises output from the STN, with activation of the inhibitory basal ganglia output nuclei and subsequent deactivation of the thalamic anteroventral and ventrolateral nuclei and the supplementary motor area (Geday et al. 2009) (see Figure 1). The changes also include cerebellar pathways likely via activation of adjacent cerebello-thalamic fiber bundles (Xu et al. 2008). Most functional imaging studies in the context of surgery have investigated modification of brain perfusion or energy metabolism by DBS.

[^{18}F]fluorodeoxyglucose (FDG) uptake of the brain, as a measure of energy metabolism, is thought to be primarily determined by local afferent synaptic activity. Increased FDG uptake is suggested to reflect the perpetuation of neuronal membrane depolarization in response to excitation (Gjedde, Marrett, and Vafaee 2002). In PD patients without treatment, increased metabolism is found in the main BG output nuclei, namely the pallidum and the SN, which get strong glutamatergic projections from the excessively firing STN (see Figure 1). Increased BG FDG uptake in PD patients is explained by loss of inhibitory nigrostriatal dopaminergic input, leading to functional overactivation of the putamen (Eidelberg et al. 1994; Eidelberg et al. 1997; Eggers

et al. 2009; Tang et al. 2010). Metabolic studies using FDG-PET in resting PD patients have shown that STN DBS reduces this increased glucose metabolism in the putamen and GPi, thereby modulating the basal ganglia-cortical networks (Asanuma et al. 2006; Trost et al. 2006; Lin et al. 2008; Wang et al. 2010) (see Figures 2 and 3 for examples of network effects as measured with FDG-PET).

Recent FDG-PET studies showed increased energy metabolism in the area of the STN electrode and in the GP during active STN stimulation. This suggests that DBS exerts activation of the electrode area downstream in the GPi (Hilker et al. 2008). This may imply a mechanism of DBS action that is fundamentally different from lesional surgery. An FDG-PET study after unilateral subthalamotomy in PD patients showed decreased cerebral metabolic activity in the STN and GPi (Su et al. 2001; Trost et al. 2003). However, in another FDG-PET study it was found that lesioning and stimulation of the STN were mechanistically similar at a system level (Trost et al. 2006).

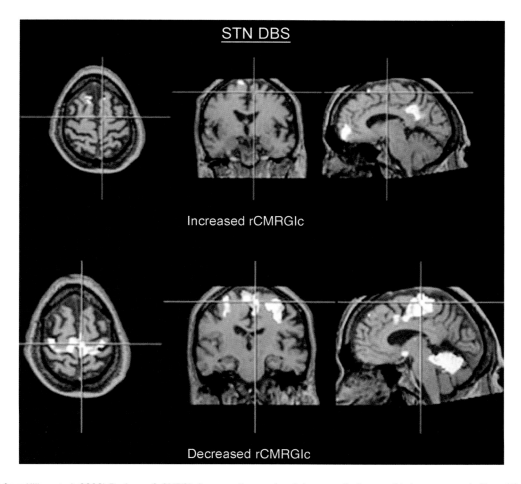

Figure 2 (adapted from Hilker et al. 2002) Regions of rCMRGlc increase (top row) and decrease (bottom row) between on- and off-conditions of bilateral STN DBS, matched to a T1-weighted MRI scan. Increases were seen in left premotor cortex, right SMA, bilaterally in the frontomesial cortex, (pre) cuneus, posterior temporal gyrus, posterior cingulate and right caudal cerebellum, and cerebellar vermis. Decreases with DBS-on were seen in bilateral primary motor cortex, left hypothalamus, and bilateral rostral cerebellum.

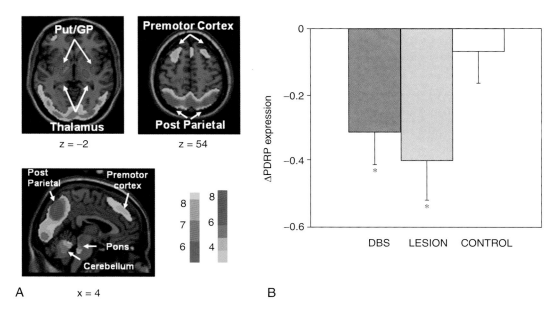

Figure 3 (Reprinted with permission from Trost et al. (2006) Network modulation by the subthalamic nucleus in the treatment of Parkinson's disease.) (A) Parkinson's disease-related pattern (PDRP) identified by network analysis of [^{18}F]fluorodeoxyglucose (FDG) PET scans from 30 PD patients and 30 age-matched normal volunteer subjects. This pattern was characterized by relative metabolic increases in the pallidum and thalamus (left) and in the pons and cerebellum (bottom). These changes covaried with metabolic decreases in the lateral premotor and parieto-occipital association areas (right). Voxels with positive region weights (metabolic increases) are color-coded from red to yellow; those with negative region weights (metabolic decreases) are color-coded from blue to purple. (B) Bar histogram of the change in PDRP expression (ΔPDRP; mean $\pm$ SE) quantified in hemispheres undergoing either STN deep brain stimulation (DBS, filled bar) or lesioning (LESION, shaded bar), and in non-operated control hemispheres (CONTROL, open bar). Significant reductions in network activity were observed with both interventions ($p < 0.05$). However, the degree of network modulation was not different for the two treatment groups ($p = 0.58$). [Asterisks refer to comparisons with control hemispheres; $p < 0.05$].

FDG-PET scans showed metabolic declines in the midbrain, GPi, and the cingulate motor region (BA 24/6) after both interventions. Metabolic increases seen in the parietal cortex (BA 7/39/40) were also common in both surgical procedures, although more pronounced following STN stimulation. Indeed, the presence of metabolic reductions in the rostral pons and midbrain, in proximity to the pedunculopontine nucleus (PPN), suggest diminished outflow from the STN target to the brainstem following both interventions (see Figure 3). The main difference in metabolic changes between the two procedures was that metabolic declines in the pallidum were greater in the STN lesioned patients.

Although the therapeutic outcome and functional mechanisms of stimulation and lesioning seem similar, the neural mechanisms underlying the two interventions may be different. Evidence from experimental animal models has suggested that neurochemical and physiologic changes with stimulation at the target site may not be explained simply by inhibition (Windels et al. 2000). On the other hand, neural recordings during DBS have indicated that local inhibition is an important feature of therapeutic DBS (Dostrovsky and Lozano 2002). According to the so-called dual concept of DBS action, the effect of DBS depends on the electrical properties of the stimulated target and on its position within the electrical field. In the immediate proximity of the electrode tip, depolarization blockade of cell somata inhibits neuronal firing (Filali et al. 2004). Conversely, farther away from the epicenter of the electrical field the stimulation current activates axons passing nearby. The subthalamic-pallidal bundle connecting the STN with the main outflow pathway of the BG is thus activated in STN DBS, resulting in high-frequency glutamatergic inputs to the GPe and GPi (McIntyre et al. 2004). Finally, it was hypothesized that DBS overrides synchronized bursts of the BG in the parkinsonian state with a high-frequent, more regular activity pattern in the gamma frequency range (neuronal jamming) (Meissner et al. 2005). Tonic driving of fibers crossing the subthalamic area may cause the increased subthalamic and pallidal energy metabolism under STN stimulation. This likely occurs in excitatory glutamatergic efferents of STN neurons to the GPi, as well as pallidothalamic fibers and GPe-STN outflow connections.

STN DBS has furthermore been shown to enhance glucose consumption in cortical association regions (Hilker et al. 2004), which is consistent with STN inhibition and consequent reduction in inhibitory output from the GPi and SNr on the thalamus. The reported effects of STN stimulation on thalamic activity have been variable, with regional increases (Hilker et al. 2004; Goerendt et al. 2006; Karimi et al. 2008), as well as decreases (Geday et al. 2009). In the simplified cortico-BG-cortical circuitry model, increased activity of the thalamus would lead to decreased cortical activation, while decreased thalamic activation would result in cortical increases. However, discrepant findings relating to subcortical increases and cortical decreases in activation are difficult to reconcile in this simplified model. The postulated overactivation of basal ganglia output in the parkinsonian condition, as represented by high firing rates in the GPi and SNr and low firing rates in the motor thalamus, may not be the pathophysiological attribute responsive to DBS treatment. A reduced burst firing pattern during DBS (Hashimoto, Goto, and Hongo 2009) may support the notion that DBS may exert its therapeutic effects via a modulation of basal ganglia firing patterns rather than by changing firing rates. Most likely, DBS-induced metabolic activation in midbrain and thalamic areas reflects neuronal jamming of ascending and descending fiber bundles in the pallidothalamic bundle and zona incerta, and their projection sites.

Furthermore, methodological differences may account for some of the differences in subcortical activations found in several studies. Recently, it has been suggested that increases in subcortical regions are an artefactual product of ratio normalization to the global mean FDG-PET uptake values (Borghammer et al. 2009). In simulation studies comparing two groups, even small, statistically insignificant differences in cortical activity resulted in subcortical increases after normalization of the uptake values to the global mean. Nonetheless, the relevance of this concern to the interpretation of metabolic data from human PD subjects is not clear. Due to intersubject variability, absolute measures of glucose uptake have not shown significant differences in subcortical structures between PD and control subjects (Ma et al. 2009). Moreover, there is a paucity of evidence indicating substantial deficits in global glucose metabolism (a potential source of normalization bias) in non-demented PD patients (Spetsieris and Eidelberg 2011). That said, animal studies using 2-DG autoradiography in 6-OHDA induced parkinsonism have demonstrated absolute metabolic increases in the GPi and GPe, STN, PPN, and thalamus (Carlson et al. 1999). Furthermore, in MPTP-lesioned macaque monkeys, chronic STN-HFS reversed abnormally decreased 2-DG uptake in the STN and reversed abnormally increased 2-DG accumulation in the GPi (Meissner et al. 2007), demonstrating pathophysiological changes in metabolic activity in the BG in parkinsonism.

Finally, the spatial resolution of most PET tomographs is currently 4 mm, which can be improved by 3D volumetric acquisition. However, this may not permit detailed examination of small structures like the STN or GPi. Studies performed on new, high-resolution PET scanners may improve the quantification of tracer metabolism in these small subcortical regions (Eggers et al. 2009).

In addition to radiotracer imaging studies, a number of studies have investigated the pattern of functional MR imaging activation during STN DBS using an externalized pulse generator. Activation as measured with fMRI is based on hemodynamic responses with oximetric changes that reflect changes in neuronal firing activity. One initial study in five PD patients showed activation in the ipsilateral GP and thalamus and in the contralateral superior cerebellum (Phillips et al. 2006). In a case report, right STN DBS with the electrode placed more laterally to the intended STN site showed less extensive changes in motor regions, but increases in the superior prefrontal cortex, ACC, anterior thalamus, caudate, and brainstem, and marked decreases in the medial prefrontal cortex, which was clinically associated with transient depression (Stefurak et al. 2003).

Besides functional imaging studies in rest, activation studies with radiotracer imaging during performance of specific tasks have also been performed in DBS-treated PD patients. In DBS-treated PD patients at rest, a decrement of cerebral blood flow (rCBF) in motor and premotor regions was seen, while a unimanual motor task gave increased rCBF in the SMA, anterior cingulate gyrus, and dorsolateral prefrontal cortex (DLPFC) in PD patients with STN stimulation, and a moderate but non-significant increase in the SMA and anterior cingulate in patients with GPi stimulation (Limousin et al. 1997).

RELATION OF REGIONAL EFFECTS TO PARKINSONIAN SYMPTOMS

Several studies investigated the relation of specific brain regions with functional changes after DBS with changes in specific symptoms. Correlations were found between STN DBS-induced improvement of rigidity and decreased rCBF in the SMA, and between improvement of bradykinesia and increased rCBF in the thalamus (Karimi et al. 2008). Remarkably, bilateral STN stimulation resulted in right-sided midbrain and premotor rCBF increases (Hilker et al. 2004; Karimi et al. 2008). On the other hand, unilateral STN DBS led to bilateral basal ganglia and thalamus changes (Arai et al. 2008). The reduction of contralateral GPi activity by STN DBS induces contralateral thalamic disinhibition, causing contralateral motor cortical activation and improving ipsilateral motor symptoms. Contralateral GPi activation by STN DBS may be explained by effects on brainstem structures, such as the pedunculopontine nucleus (PPN), which has connections to the basal ganglia in both hemispheres.

Because the STN plays an important role not only in motor, but also in limbic and associative BG circuits (Alexander, Crutcher, and DeLong 1990), neuropsychological effects may be related to stimulation-induced alterations of neuronal activity in these non-motor BG networks. STN DBS was found to activate glucose metabolism in the frontal limbic and associative territory (Hilker et al. 2004), areas that are involved in the regulation of cognition, mood, and behavior. Interestingly, dorsal neocortical areas that get activated in patients with depression (Mayberg 1994) are similar to the regions that show restored glucose metabolism after STN DBS (Hilker et al. 2004). This finding agrees with the clinical observation that PD-related depression tends to improve after STN DBS (Ardouin et al. 1999). Transient neuropsychiatric side effects after device implantation have also been reported, but could in the few patients studied to date not be related to specific alterations in glucose metabolism.

Finally, a clear influence of STN DBS is seen upon the activity of cerebellar neurons. Cerebellar hypermetabolism in PD disappears with STN stimulation (Hilker et al. 2004). Suppression of parkinsonian tremor in the DBS-on condition was found to be associated with an increase of glucose metabolism in the posterior cingulate, as well as a marked cerebellar decrease, corroborating the concept of cerebellar involvement in parkinsonian tremor. Additional PET studies showed decreased cerebellar blood flow with suppression of parkinsonian tremor by DBS of the thalamic ventral intermediate nucleus (Vim) (Deiber et al. 1993; Parker et al. 1992; Fukuda et al. 2004; Mure et al. 2011). Both STN and Vim DBS likely deactivate the cerebellum via an antidromic (from axon to soma) effect in dentate-thalamic fibers.

STN DBS thus interacts with widespread cortical and cerebellar pathways. These alterations of neuronal resting energy metabolism were reversible after turning the devices off. This indicates a temporary functional phenomenon in line with the relapse of parkinsonism in the DBS-off condition.

PPN-DBS

It has been supposed that brainstem structures such as the PPN play an important role in axial and gait disturbances in PD. Recent work suggests that PPN-DBS may be beneficial in the treatment of axial symptoms and especially freezing of gait, although (a combination with) lower frequency STN stimulation was more effective in alleviating gait disturbance (Moreau et al. 2009). The mechanisms underlying these

effects are unknown. In PD, the increased inhibitory GABAergic activity from the GPi is believed to inhibit the PPN (see Figure 1) (Pahapill and Lozano 2000). One group used [^{15}O]H$_2$O-PET to investigate regional cerebral blood flow (rCBF) in three advanced PD patients who underwent unilateral PPN-DBS (Ballanger et al. 2009a). Stimulation revealed increase in rCBF bilaterally in the thalamus and cerebellum and ipsilateral in the ventral midbrain. This is consistent with anatomical reports demonstrating descending PPN projections to the cerebellum and ascending fibers through the dorsal tegmental pathway to the thalamus (Pahapill and Lozano 2000). At the cortical level, increases were found in the contralateral dorsolateral prefrontal cortex, anterior cingulated cortex, orbitofrontal cortex, temporal gyrus, and occipital cortex. Furthermore, PPN stimulation resulted in lower frequency and increase in amplitude of self-paced lower limb movements, which was associated with increased blood flow in medial sensorimotor areas (Ballanger et al. 2009b). These findings are in line with the idea that PPN-DBS induces functional changes in neural networks involved in locomotion and possibly also in executive function and arousal (Alessandro et al. 2010).

EFFECT OF SURGERY ON DISEASE PROGRESSION

Numerous SPECT and PET studies have investigated the nigrostriatal dopaminergic system in PD patients (Leenders et al. 1986). Presynaptic dopaminergic function is mostly studied with [^{18}F]fluorodopa (FDOPA), a substrate for dopa-decarboxylase in catecholaminergic neurons, and PET. More recently, tracers for dopamine presynaptic reuptake sites (dopamine transporter or DAT sites) were also developed for SPECT imaging. FDOPA uptake in the putamen was found to be inversely correlated with motor disability and with duration of illness, while caudate uptake showed more specific correlation with the occurrence of cognitive deficits (van Beilen et al. 2008). Follow-up studies with FDOPA-PET reported an annual decrement of the FDOPA uptake of 9% in the putamen and 3% in the caudate (Morrish, Sawle, and Brooks 1996), while another study measured a 13% decrease in dopamine transporter density in the putamen (Nurmi et al. 2000). Furthermore, sequential FDOPA-PET scanning was performed to evaluate the efficacy of intrastriatal grafting of mesencephalic neurons before and after transplantation (Pogarell et al. 2006; Remy et al. 1995; Sawle et al. 1992; Ma et al. 2010).

Hilker et al. (Hilker et al. 2005) have investigated 30 PD patients using FDOPA-PET before and 12 to 36 months after succesful STN DBS. STN DBS has been proposed to potentially slow disease progression since STN DBS is supposed to reduce glutamatergic hyperactivity from the STN toward, e.g., the substantia nigra pars compacta. Glutamatergic hyperactivity is under certain circumstances excitotoxic. Reducing this hyperactivity would then perhaps result in less dopaminergic cell loss in the SNc. If true, striatal FDOPA-PET would demonstrate a slower annual decline of the nigrostriatal dopamine system.

Nonetheless, the annual decline proved to be in a similar range as in unoperated PD patients, negating a neuroprotective influence of STN on these neurons.

REFERENCES

Alessandro, S., R. Ceravolo, L. Brusa, M. Pierantozzi, A. Costa, S. Galati, F. Placidi, A. Romigi, C. Iani, F. Marzetti, and A. Peppe. 2010. Non-motor functions in parkinsonian patients implanted in the pedunculopontine nucleus: Focus on sleep and cognitive domains. *J Neurol Sci* 289 (1–2): 44–8.

Alexander, G. E., M. D. Crutcher, and M. R. DeLong. 1990. Basal ganglia-thalamocortical circuits: Parallel substrates for motor, oculomotor, "prefrontal" and "limbic" functions. *Prog Brain Res* 85: 119–46.

Alexander, G. E., M. R. DeLong, and P. L. Strick. 1986. Parallel organization of functionally segregated circuits linking basal ganglia and cortex. *Annu Rev Neurosci* 9:357–81.

Arai, N., F. Yokochi, T. Ohnishi, T. Momose, R. Okiyama, M. Taniguchi, H. Takahashi, H. Matsuda, and Y. Ugawa. 2008. Mechanisms of unilateral STN-DBS in patients with Parkinson's disease: A PET study. *J Neurol* 255 (8): 1236–43.

Ardouin, C., B. Pillon, E. Peiffer, P. Bejjani, P. Limousin, P. Damier, I. Arnulf, A. L. Benabid, Y. Agid, and P. Pollak. 1999. Bilateral subthalamic or pallidal stimulation for Parkinson's disease affects neither memory nor executive functions: A consecutive series of 62 patients. *Ann Neurol* 46 (2): 217–23.

Asanuma, K., C. Tang, Y. Ma, V. Dhawan, P. Mattis, C. Edwards, M. G. Kaplitt, A. Feigin, and D. Eidelberg. 2006. Network modulation in the treatment of Parkinson's disease. *Brain* 129 (Pt 10): 2667–78.

Aziz, T. Z., D. Peggs, E. Agarwal, M .A. Sambrook, and A. R. Crossman. 1992. Subthalamic nucleotomy alleviates parkinsonism in the 1-methyl-4-phenyl-1,2,3,6-tetrahydropyridine (MPTP)-exposed primate. *Br J Neurosurg* 6 (6): 575–82.

Ballanger, B., A. M. Lozano, E. Moro, T. van Eimeren, C. Hamani, R. Chen, R. Cilia, S. Houle, Y. Y. Poon, A. E. Lang, and A. P. Strafella. 2009a. Cerebral blood flow changes induced by pedunculopontine nucleus stimulation in patients with advanced Parkinson's disease: A [(15)O] H2O PET study. *Hum Brain Mapp* 30 (12): 3901–9.

Ballanger, B., M. Jahanshahi, E. Broussolle, and S. Thobois. 2009b. PET functional imaging of deep brain stimulation in movement disorders and psychiatry. *J Cereb Blood Flow Metab* 29 (11): 1743–54.

Benabid, A. L., S. Chabardes, J. Mitrofanis, and P. Pollak P. 2009. Deep brain stimulation of the subthalamic nucleus for the treatment of Parkinson's disease. *Lancet Neurol* 8 (1): 67–81.

Borghammer, P., P. Cumming, J. Aanerud, S. Forster, and A. Gjedde. 2009. Subcortical elevation of metabolism in Parkinson's disease—a critical reappraisal in the context of global mean normalization. *Neuroimage* 47 (4): 1514–21.

Braak, H., and E. Braak. 2000. Pathoanatomy of Parkinson's disease. *Journal of Neurology* 247:3–10.

Carlson, J. D., R. D. Pearlstein, J. Buchholz, R. P. Iacono, and G. Maeda. 1999. Regional metabolic changes in the pedunculopontine nucleus of unilateral 6-hydroxydopamine Parkinson's model rats. *Brain Res* 828 (1–2): 12–9.

Deiber, M. P., P. Pollak, R. Passingham, P. Landais, C. Gervason, L. Cinotti, K. Friston, R. Frackowiak, F. Mauguiere, and A. L. Benabid. 1993. Thalamic stimulation and suppression of parkinsonian tremor. Evidence of a cerebellar deactivation using positron emission tomography *Brain* 116 (Pt 1): 267–79.

Dostrovsky, J. O., and A. M. Lozano. 2002. Mechanisms of deep brain stimulation. *Mov Disord* 17 Suppl 3:S63–S68.

Eggers, C., R. Hilker, L. Burghaus, B. Schumacher, and W. D. Heiss. 2009. High resolution positron emission tomography demonstrates basal ganglia dysfunction in early Parkinson's disease. *J Neurol Sci* 276 (1–2): 27–30.

Eidelberg, D., J. R. Moeller, V. Dhawan, P. Spetsieris, S. Takikawa, T. Ishikawa, T. Chaly, W. Robeson, D. Margouleff, S. Przedborski, and S. Fahn. 1994. The metabolic topography of parkinsonism. *J Cereb Blood Flow Metab* 14:783–801.

Eidelberg, D., J. R. Moeller, K. Kazumata, A. Antonini, Sterio Djordje, V. Dhawan, P. Spetsieris, R. Alterman, P. J. Kelly, M. Dogali, E. Fazzini, and A. Beric. 1997. Metabolic correlates of pallidal neuronal activity in Parkinson's disease. *Brain* 120:1315–24.

Filali, M., W. D. Hutchison, V. N. Palter, A. M. Lozano, and J. O. Dostrovsky. 2004. Stimulation-induced inhibition of neuronal firing in human subthalamic nucleus. *Exp Brain Res* 156 (3): 274–81.

Fukuda, M., A. Barnes, E. S. Simon, A. Holmes, V. Dhawan, N. Giladi, Y. Fodstad, Y. Ma, and D. Eidelberg. 2004. Thalamic stimulation for parkinsonian tremor: Correlation between regional cerebral blood flow and physiological tremor characteristics. *NeuroImage* 21(2):608–15.

Geday, J., K. Ostergaard, E. Johnsen, and A. Gjedde. 2009. STN-stimulation in Parkinson's disease restores striatal inhibition of thalamocortical projection. *Hum Brain Mapp* 30 (1): 112–21.

Gjedde, A., S. Marrett, and M. Vafaee. 2002. Oxidative and nonoxidative metabolism of excited neurons and astrocytes. *J Cereb Blood Flow Metab* 22 (1): 1–14.

Goerendt, I. K., A. D. Lawrence, M. A. Mehta, J. S. Stern, P. Odin, and D. J. Brooks. 2006. Distributed neural actions of anti-parkinsonian therapies as revealed by PET. *J Neural Transm* 113 (1): 75–86.

Hammond, C., H. Bergman, and P. Brown. 2007. Pathological synchronization in Parkinson's disease: Networks, models and treatments. *Trends Neurosci* 30 (7): 357–64.

Hashimoto, T., T. Goto, and K. Hongo. 2009. Neuronal responses to high-frequency stimulation in human subthalamic nucleus. *Mov Disord* 24 (12): 1860–2.

Hilker, R., A. T. Portman, J. Voges, M. J. Staal, L. Burghaus, T. van Laar, A. Koulousakis, R. P. Maguire, J. Pruim, B. M. de Jong, K. Herholz, V. Sturm, W. D. Heiss, and K. L. Leenders. 2005. Disease progression continues in patients with advanced Parkinson's disease and effective subthalamic nucleus stimulation. *J Neurol Neurosurg Psychiatry* 76 (9): 1217–21.

Hilker, R., J. Voges, S. Weisenbach, E. Kalbe, L. Burghaus, M. Ghaemi, R. Lehrke, A. Koulousakis, K. Herholz, V. Sturm, and W. D. Heiss. 2004. Subthalamic nucleus stimulation restores glucose metabolism in associative and limbic cortices and in cerebellum: Evidence from a FDG-PET study in advanced Parkinson's disease. *J Cereb Blood Flow Metab* 24 (1): 7–16.

Hilker, R., J. Voges, T. Weber, L. W. Kracht, J. Roggendorf, S. Baudrexel, M. Hoevels, V. Sturm, and W. D. Heiss. 2008. STN-DBS activates the target area in Parkinson disease: An FDG-PET study. *Neurology* 71 (10): 708–13.

Hilker, R., J. Voges, A. Thiel, M. Ghaemi, K. Herholz, V. Sturm, and W. D. Heiss.2002. Deep brain stimulation of the subthalamic nucleus versus levodopa challenge in Parkinson's disease: Measuring the on- and off-conditions with FDG-PET. *J Neural Transm* 109(10): 1257–64.

Jahanshahi, M., C. M. Ardouin, R. G. Brown, J. C. Rothwell, J. Obeso, A. Albanese, M. C. Rodriguez-Oroz, E. Moro, A. L. Benabid, P. Pollak, and P. Limousin-Dowsey. 2000. The impact of deep brain stimulation on executive function in Parkinson's disease. *Brain* 123 (Pt 6): 1142–54.

Javoy-Agid, F., and Y. Agid. 1980. Is the mesocortical dopaminergic system involved in Parkinson disease? *Neurology* 30 (12): 1326–30.

Jenkins, I. H., W. Fernandez, E. D. Playford, A. J. Lees, R. S. Frackowiak, R. E. Passingham, and D. J. Brooks. 1992. Impaired activation of the supplementary motor area in Parkinson's disease is reversed when akinesia is treated with apomorphine. *Ann Neurol* 32 (6): 749–57.

Karimi, M., N. Golchin, S. D. Tabbal, T. Hershey, T. O. Videen, J. Wu, J. W. Usche, F. J. Revilla, J. M. Hartlein, A. R. Wernle, J. W. Mink, and J. S. Perlmutter. 2008. Subthalamic nucleus stimulation-induced regional blood flow responses correlate with improvement of motor signs in Parkinson disease. *Brain* 131 (Pt 10): 2710–9.

Leenders, K. L., A. J. Palmer, N. Quinn, J. C. Clark, G. Firnau, E. S. Garnett, C. Nahmias, T. Jones, and C. D. Marsden. 1986. Brain dopamine metabolism in patients with Parkinson's disease measured with positron emission tomography. *Journal of Neurology Neurosurgery and Psychiatry* 49 (8): 853–60.

Limousin, P., J. Greene, P. Pollak, J. Rothwell, A. L. Benabid, R. Frackowiak. 1997. Changes in cerebral activity pattern due to subthalamic nucleus or internal pallidum stimulation in Parkinson's disease. *Ann Neurol* 42 (3): 283–91.

Lin, T., M. Carbon, C. Tang, A. Mogilner, D. Sterio, A. Beric, V. Dhawan, and D. Eidelberg. 2008. Metabolic correlates of subthalamic nucleus activity in Parkinson's disease. *Brain* 131 (Pt 5): 1373–80.

Ma, Y., C. Tang, J. R. Moeller, and D. Eidelberg. 2009. Abnormal regional brain function in Parkinson's disease: Truth or fiction? *Neuroimage* 45 (2): 260–6.

Ma, Y., C. Tang, T. Chaly, P. Greene, R. Breeze, S. Fahn, C. Freed, V. Dhawan, and D. Eidelberg. 2010. Dopamine cell implantation in Parkinson's disease: long-term clinical and ^{18}F-FDOPA PET outcomes. *J Nucl Med* 51: 7–15.

Mayberg, H. S. 1994. Frontal lobe dysfunction in secondary depression. *J Neuropsychiatry Clin Neurosci* 6 (4): 428–42.

McIntyre, C. C., M. Savasta, L. Kerkerian-Le Goff, and J. L. Vitek. 2004. Uncovering the mechanism(s) of action of deep brain stimulation: Activation, inhibition, or both. *Clin Neurophysiol* 115 (6): 1239–48.

Meissner, W., A. Leblois, D. Hansel, B. Bioulac, C. E. Gross, A. Benazzouz, and T. Boraud. 2005. Subthalamic high frequency stimulation resets subthalamic firing and reduces abnormal oscillations. *Brain* 128 (Pt 10): 2372–82.

Meissner, W., C. Guigoni, L. Cirilli, M. Garret, B. H. Bioulac, C. E. Gross, E. Bezard, and A. Benazzouz. 2007. Impact of chronic subthalamic high-frequency stimulation on metabolic basal ganglia activity: A 2-deoxyglucose uptake and cytochrome oxidase mRNA study in a macaque model of Parkinson's disease. *Eur J Neurosci* 25 (5): 1492–500.

Moreau, C., L. Defebvre, D. Devos, F. Marchetti, A. Destee, A. Stefani, A. Peppe. 2009. STN versus PPN-DBS for alleviating freezing of gait: Toward a frequency modulation approach? *Mov Disord* 24 (14): 2164–6.

Morrish, P. K., G. V. Sawle, and D. J. Brooks. 1996. The rate of progression of Parkinson's disease. A longitudinal [18F]DOPA PET study. *Adv Neurol* 69: 427–31.

Mure, H., S. Hirano, C. C. Tang, I. U. Isaias, A. Antonini, Y. Ma, V. Dhawan, and D. Eidelberg. 2011. Parkinson's disease tremor-related metabolic network: characterization, progression, and treatment effects. *NeuroImage* 54 (2): 1244–53.

Nurmi, E., H. M. Ruottinen, V. Kaasinen, J. Bergman, M. Haaparanta, O. Solin, and J. O. Rinne. 2000. Progression in Parkinson's disease: A positron emission tomography study with a dopamine transporter ligand [18F]CFT. *Ann Neurol* 47 (6): 804–8.

Pahapill, P. A., and A. M. Lozano. 2000. The pedunculopontine nucleus and Parkinson's disease. *Brain* 123 (Pt 9): 1767–83.

Parker, F., N. Tzourio, S. Blond, H. Petit, and B. Mazoyer. 1992. Evidence for a common network of brain structures involved in parkinsonian tremor and voluntary repetitive movement. *Brain Res* 584 (1–2): 11–7.

Phillips, M. D., K. B. Baker, M.J. Lowe, J. A. Tkach, S. E. Cooper, B. H. Kopell, and A. R. Rezai. 2006. Parkinson disease: Pattern of functional MR imaging activation during deep brain stimulation of subthalamic nucleus—initial experience. *Radiology* 239 (1): 209–16.

Pogarell, O. W. Koch, F. J. Gildehaus, A. Kupsch, O. Lindvall, W. H. Oertel, and K. Tatsch. 2006. Long-term assessment of striatal dopamine transporters in Parkinsonian patients with intrastriatal embryonic mesencephalic grafts. *Eur J Nucl Med Mol Imaging* 33 (4): 407–11.

Remy, P., Y. Samson, P. Hantraye, A. Fontaine, G. Defer, J. F. Mangin, G. Fenelon, C. Geny, F. Ricolfi, and V. Frouin. 1995. Clinical correlates of [18F]fluorodopa uptake in five grafted parkinsonian patients. *Ann Neurol* 38 (4): 580–8.

Sawle, G. V., P. M. Bloomfield, A. Bjorklund, D. J. Brooks, P. Brundin, K. L. Leenders, O. Lindvall, C. D. Marsden, S. Rehncrona, and H. Widner. 1992. Transplantation of fetal dopamine neurons in Parkinson's disease: PET [18F]6-L-fluorodopa studies in two patients with putaminal implants. *Ann Neurol* 31 (2): 166–73.

Spetsieris, P. G., and D. Eidelberg. 2011. Scaled subprofile modeling of resting state imaging data in Parkinson's disease: methodological issues. *NeuroImage* 54:2899–14.

Stefurak, T., D. Mikulis, H. Mayberg, A. E. Lang, S. Hevenor, P. Pahapill, J. Saint-Cyr, and A. Lozano. 2003. Deep brain stimulation for Parkinson's disease dissociates mood and motor circuits: A functional MRI case study. *Mov Disord* 18 (12): 1508–16.

Su, P. C., H. M. Tseng, H. M. Liu, R. F. Yen, and H. H. Liou. 2003. Treatment of advanced Parkinson's disease by subthalamotomy: one-year results. *Mov Disord* 18 (5): 531–8.

Su, P. C., Y. Ma, M. Fukuda, M. J. Mentis, H. M. Tseng, R. F. Yen, H. M. Liu, J. R. Moeller, and D. Eidelberg. 2001. Metabolic changes following subthalamotomy for advanced Parkinson's disease. *Ann Neurol* 50 (4): 514–20.

Tang, C., K. Poston, V. Dhawan, and D. Eidelberg. 2010. Abnormalities in metabolic network activity precede the onset of motor symptoms in Parkinson's disease. *J Neurosci* 30 (3): 1049–56.

Trošt, M., P. C. Su, A. Barnes, S. L. Su, R-F. Yen, H. Tseng, Y. Ma, and D. Eidelberg. 2003. Subthalamotomy: Evolving metabolic changes during the first postoperative year. *J Neurosurg* 99 (5): 872–78.

Trost, M., S. Su, P. Su, R. F. Yen, H. M. Tseng, A. Barnes, Y. Ma, and D. Eidelberg. 2006. Network modulation by the subthalamic nucleus in the treatment of Parkinson's disease. *Neuroimage* 31 (1): 301–7.

van Beilen, M., A. T. Portman, H. A. Kiers, R. P. Maguire, V. Kaasinen, M. Koning, J. Pruim, and K. L. Leenders. 2008. Striatal FDOPA uptake and cognition in advanced non-demented Parkinson's disease: A clinical and FDOPA-PET study. *Parkinsonism Relat Disord* 14 (3): 224–8.

Wang, J., Y. Ma, Z. Huang, B. Sun, Y. Guan, and C. Zuo. 2010. Modulation of metabolic brain function by bilateral subthalamic nucleus stimulation in the treatment of Parkinson's disease. *J Neurol* 257 (1): 72–8.

Windels, F., N. Bruet, A. Poupard, N. Urbain, G. Chouvet, C. Feuerstein, and M. Savasta. 2000. Effects of high frequency stimulation of subthalamic nucleus on extracellular glutamate and GABA in substantia nigra and globus pallidus in the normal rat. *Eur J Neurosci* 12 (11): 4141–6.

Xu, W., G. S. Russo, T. Hashimoto, J. Zhang, and J. L. Vitek. 2008. Subthalamic nucleus stimulation modulates thalamic neuronal activity. *J Neurosci* 28 (46): 11916–24.

CELL-BASED THERAPIES
IMAGING OUTCOMES

Paola Piccini and Marios Politis

Transplantation of human fetal DA neurons grafted in the striatum of Parkinson's disease (PD) patients has been investigated for over two decades. The pattern of recovery has varied between cases, with some patients exhibiting significant symptomatic relief with reduced "off-phase" severity and decreased requirement for dopaminergic replacement therapy while others have not benefited as much or have developed adverse effects such as "off-medication" dyskinesias (off-dyskinesias). These dyskinesias have became a major roadblock for the further development of DA cell replacement strategies for PD, including stem cells (Lindvall and Hagell 2000; Lindvall and Björklund 2004).

Clinical trials assessing the efficacy and safety of intrastriatal transplantation of fetal ventral mesencephalic (VM) tissue in patients with PD rely on the rationale that the grafted tissue will restore the striatal DA transmission and improve striatal-cortical circuitries, thereby producing long-lasting clinical improvement. However, despite the current scientific developments, the mechanisms responsible for the success or failure of grafting human fetal VM tissue are only partly understood.

Positron emission tomography (PET) with the use of specific radioligands has been proven to be a useful in vivo tool for the development of a clinically competitive cell replacement therapy in PD. PET with ^{18}F-fluorodopa (^{18}F-Fdopa) has been used to monitor survival and storage of DA in grafted neurons and can be used for screening patients who are not suitable for transplantation. PET with ^{11}C-raclopride and pharmacological challenge with levodopa or amphetamine can assess the ability of the grafted DA cells to increase synaptic levels of DA. Activation studies with PET and O^{15} labeled water (H$_2$^{15}O) allow measures of regional changes in brain metabolism and blood flow (Brooks 2004). Functional magnetic resonance imaging (fMRI) and diffusion tensor imaging (DTI) techniques can also assess the effect of the transplanted DA cells on the basal ganglia–cortical networks and the relevance of the restoration of these circuitries on the clinical outcome. PET with ^{11}C-DASB can provide insight on the role of serotonergic terminals into the mechanisms underlying postoperative off-dyskinesias by providing means of the amount of serotonergic component present in the dopaminergic-rich transplanted graft.

MONITORING SURVIVAL AND GROWTH OF GRAFTED DA CELLS

The survival and growth of grafted DA cells can be assessed in vivo by measuring the striatal uptake of ^{18}F-dopa using PET. After intravenous administration, ^{18}F-dopa is taken up by the dopaminergic terminals and stored as ^{18}F-dopamine and its metabolites (Firnau et al. 1987). ^{18}F-dopa uptake reflects both transport into the DA vesicles and decarboxylation by dopa decarboxylase (DDC), and within a 90-minute PET scan the uptake can be represented kinetically by an influx constant, Ki (Patlak and Blasberg 1985; Brooks et al. 1990). The fact that ^{18}F-dopa is taken up presynaptically provides a good measure of the number of viable nigrostriatal DA terminals. In PD patients, putaminal ^{18}F-dopa uptake correlates inversely with the degree of motor impairment (Remy et al. 1995; Morrish et al. 1996), whereas the same correlation is weaker for the caudate (Morrish et al. 1996).

PET and single photon emission computed tomography (SPECT) techniques can also evaluate the number of functionally intact dopaminergic terminals within the striatum by measuring the availability of presynaptic DA transporter (DAT) (PET tracers: ^{11}C-CFT, ^{18}F- CFT, ^{11}C-RTI-121, and ^{11}C-RTI-32; SPECT tracers: ^{123}I-β-CIT, ^{123}I-FP-CIT, ^{123}I-altropane, and ^{99m}Tc-TRODAT-1) or by measuring the density of vesicular monoamine transporter (such as ^{11}C-dihydrotetrabenazine PET). PET studies with ^{11}C-RTI-121 in rats have shown a correlation between the survival of grafted striatal DA cells and striatal binding of the tracer (Sullivan et al. 1998). Currently, there are no reported ^{11}C-dihydrotetrabenazine PET data on the expression and survival of vesicular monoamine transporter in VM tissue grafts. Also, it is uncertain whether the grafted dopaminergic neurons express or retain the function of the DAT. PET studies have been unable to detect significant increases in DAT binding after implantation of fetal VM tissue, even though putaminal ^{18}F-dopa uptake was found increased (Cochen et al. 2003) and two postmortem studies have reported conflicting results regarding the DAT expression in grafted neurons (Kordower et al. 1996, 2008). Therefore, ^{18}F-dopa PET remains today the standard for monitoring survival and growth of grafted DA cells.

Survival of human fetal VM dopaminergic neurons transplanted into the striatum of patients with PD has been documented. Significant increases in ^{18}F-dopa uptake in the grafted striatum have been observed in several open-label trials (Lindvall et al. 1990, 1994; Sawle et al. 1992; Peschanski et al. 1994; Freeman et al. 1995; Remy et al. 1995; Wenning et al. 1997; Hagell et al. 1999; Hauser et al. 1999; Piccini et al. 1999; Brundin et al. 2000; Mendez et al. 2000, 2002; Cochen et al. 2003), even after several years despite disease progression and discontinuation of antiparkinsonian drug treatment (Piccini et al. 1999). These data are compatible with evidence from histopathological studies, which have confirmed survival of DA neurons and their ability to reinnervate the striatum (Kordower et al. 1995, 1996, 1998). The majority of grafted cells remain functionally unimpaired after a decade (Mendez et al. 2008; Li et al. 2008) although it was recently shown that transplanted VM dopaminergic neurons can develop α-synuclein-positive Lewy bodies (Kordower et al. 2008; Li et al. 2008). Several studies have also shown that the levels of increased striatal ^{18}F-dopa uptake after transplantation are correlated to the degree of clinical improvement (Hagell et al. 1999; Hauser et al. 1999). These reports are in line with results in rats, which suggest a correlation between behavioral effects and survival of grafted DA neurons (Brundin et al. 1994).

Serial ^{18}F-dopa PET results were initially reported for a small cohort of PD patients who had received unilateral or bilateral transplantation of fetal VM tissue using different surgical techniques and methods of cell suspension and preparation. Most of these studies showed evidence of restored dopaminergic innervation in the grafts as assessed by ^{18}F-dopa for up to 10 years (Freed et al. 1992; Widner et al. 1992; Lindvall et al. 1994, 1999; Freeman et al. 1995; Remy et al. 1995; Wenning et al. 1997; Hagell et al. 1999; Hauser et al. 1999; Brundin et al. 2000).

Remy and colleagues (1995) reported up to two-year data on five PD patients following unilateral intraputaminal (in two cases also in caudate) fetal VM tissue transplantation. One year postoperatively, ^{18}F-dopa PET showed a mean 61% increase in grafted putaminal ^{18}F-dopa uptake with no significant changes in ^{18}F-dopa uptake in the grafted caudate in the two cases. Individual putaminal ^{18}F-dopa values pre- and post-operation correlated with percentage times "on," and timed finger dexterity in "off." This study concluded that the increase of putaminal ^{18}F-dopa uptake to normal levels after transplantation seems sufficient to restore normal limb function in patients with PD.

Freeman and colleagues (1995) presented data from four PD patients who had received bilateral intraputaminal fetal VM tissue transplantation. By six months postoperatively, ^{18}F-dopa PET showed mean increases of 53% and 33% in the right and left putamen, respectively. All four patients improved clinically with a mean 37% decrease in total Unified Parkinson's Disease Rating Scale (UPDRS) score, a mean 41% increase in Schwab and England disability scores, a mean 65% decrease of time spent "off," and a mean 92% decrease of "on" time with dyskinesias.

Wenning and colleagues (1997) reported up to six-year data on six PD patients receiving unilateral intraputaminal (in two cases also in caudate) fetal VM tissue grafts. After one year postoperatively, mean ^{18}F-dopa uptake was increased by 68% in the grafted putamen with only minor changes in the grafted and non-grafted caudate. The non-grafted putamen showed a corresponding mean decrease of 25% in ^{18}F-dopa uptake. The PET data from this study were mirrored by a mean improvement in "off-phase" UPDRS motor score of 18% and 26%, a 10% and 20% reduction in levodopa dose, a 34% and 44% reduction in the "off" time, and a 45% and 58% increase in the duration of response after a single levodopa dose during the first and second years after transplantation, respectively. Overall, there was therapeutically valuable improvement in four patients, but only modest changes in the other two, which subsequently developed atypical features.

Five of these six PD patients subsequently received transplantation of fetal VM tissue in the non-grafted putamen (and in one case also in the non-grafted caudate) (Hagell et al. 1999). After an additional 12 to 18 months, ^{18}F-dopa PET showed a mean 85% increase in radiotracer uptake in the putamen receiving the second graft, whereas there was no significant further change in the previously transplanted putamen. Two of the five patients receiving the second graft were judged to have marked additional improvements as evidenced by reduced "on-off" fluctuations, bradykinesia, time in "off," and lower levodopa requirements (one withdrawn and the other reduced by 70%). Improvement in the third patient was moderate, while the two patients with atypical features, who responded poorly to the first graft, worsened following the second transplantation with one of them developing features suggestive of multiple-system atrophy. The major conclusion from this study was that putaminal grafts that are able to restore ^{18}F-dopa uptake can produce improvements of major therapeutic value.

Brundin and colleagues (2000) assessed four advanced PD patients following bilateral putamen and caudate transplantations of fetal VM tissue treated with tirilazad mesylate, a lipid peroxidation inhibitor. Six months after transplantation the mean ^{18}F-dopa uptake rose by 53% in the putamen and by 24% in the caudate. Twenty months after there was a further increase of 4% in ^{18}F-dopa uptake in the putamen and caudate (Figure 1) while UPDRS motor scores fell by 50% and levodopa requirements were reduced by 50% (one of the patients was withdrawn from dopaminergic therapy), suggesting that graft integration continued to mature despite the stabilization of dopaminergic reinnervation.

Following the encouraging results from these open clinical trials, two double-blind sham-surgery controlled trials were conducted on PD (Freed et al. 2001; Olanow et al. 2003). Freed and colleagues (2001) studied 40 subjects with advanced PD. Patients were randomized to receive either bilateral intraputaminal transplantation of human fetal VM tissue or sham surgery. The results were analyzed as a whole and also with the patients divided into groups according to age (young group: equal or less than 60 years of age *vs.* older group: more than 60 years of age). This study did not reach its primary endpoint, and the transplanted patients showed no significant improvement in clinical global impression scores scored by patients themselves at year one. Secondary outcomes included clinical and PET imaging measures such as UPDRS, Schwab and England scores assessed in "off," and putaminal ^{18}F-dopa uptake. Mean UPDRS motor scores and Schwab and England scores were significantly reduced in the transplanted patients compared with the sham-surgery group. This was mostly due to improvements observed in the transplanted patients under 60 years of age who showed a mean 34% reduction in the UPDRS motor scores and strong significant reductions in Schwab and England scores. ^{18}F-dopa uptake increased a mean 40% in the putamen of the transplanted patients, while there was no difference from baseline in the sham-surgery group. Tertiary outcomes included changes in drug doses and neuropsychological assessments. No significant differences between the treatment groups were observed one year after surgery. This study first brought to light the problem of "off" dystonia and dyskinesias, as 15% of grafted patients experienced these adverse effects one year after surgery even after reduction or termination of levodopa. In a recent report, Ma and colleagues (2010) have retrospectively analyzed the long-term clinical and PET outcome in 33 of the original trial participants who were followed for two years after transplantation, with 15 of these subjects having been followed for two additional years. The authors reported that UPDRS motor scores in these patients improved over time after transplantation, and the differences between the younger and older group seen at one year after transplantation were no longer evident at longer-term follow-up. ^{18}F-dopa uptake in the transplanted putamen correlated with these clinical changes,

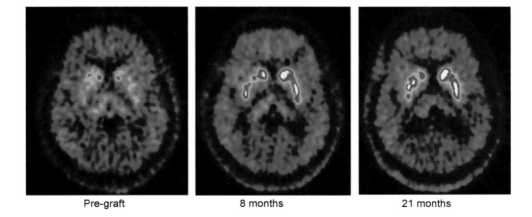

| Pre-graft | 8 months | 21 months |

Figure 1 Serial ^{18}F-dopa PET scans in a PD patient transplanted with human fetal VM tissue in caudate and putamen bilaterally. Pre-graft and 8 and 21 months after transplantation.

suggesting overall that clinical benefit and graft viability are sustained up to four years after transplantation and that clinical outcome over the long term is not dependent on subject age.

The second double-blind controlled trial studied 34 patients who were randomized into three groups to receive either bilateral intraputaminal transplantation of human fetal VM tissue derived from one fetus per side or four fetuses per side, or to receive sham surgery (Olanow et al. 2003). The primary outcome was set as the change in the UPDRS motor score in the "off" at the second year after transplantation. This study also did not achieve its primary endpoint, and the transplanted patients showed no significant improvement in the "off-phase" UPDRS motor scores compared to the sham-surgery group. No significant differences were evident between groups for Activities of Daily Living, total "off" time, "on" time without dyskinesias, and levodopa dose requirements. Interestingly, patients with less severe PD who received transplantation with four donors per side showed significant reductions in UPDRS motor scores compared to the sham-surgery group. However, no age effect was noted. The mean putaminal ^{18}F-dopa uptake was unchanged in the sham-surgery group, whereas there was a significant mean increase of 20% and 30% in patients receiving tissue from one and four donors, respectively. This study also further highlighted the problem of "off-medication" dyskinesias, as this adverse effect was present in 57% of the transplanted patients but was not seen in the sham-surgery group.

Overall, the double-blind trials failed to replicate the hopeful results shown in the open clinical trials. Despite both PET and in some cases histological evidence of graft function, neither of the double-blind trials demonstrated clinical efficacy, as they did not reach their primary endpoints while the improvements varied according to the secondary and tertiary measures. There were, however, some indications that the patients with less severe disease and those with age less than 60 years could benefit from intraputaminal transplantation of human fetal VM tissue. In both of these trials, "off-medication" dyskinesias, probably graft related, were major concerns, while the role of immunosuppression was not fully understood.

ASSESSMENT OF GRAFT FUNCTION

PET imaging has been proven a useful technique for assessing the function of the graft after transplantation of human fetal VM tissue in the striatum of patients with PD. Studies from our unit have indeed shown that graft-derived

dopaminergic cells were able to restore the release of endogenous DA in the striatum to an almost normal level and also that grafted cells can form connections in the host brain and are able to restore activation of motor cortical areas during movements (Piccini et al. 1999, 2000).

Both PET and SPECT ligands have been used to look into postsynaptic DA receptors. ^{11}C-raclopride is a low-affinity D_2 receptor ligand subjected to competitive displacement by endogenous DA (Volkow et al. 1994). Amphetamine and its derivatives are known to increase the levels of synaptic DA neurotransmission and result in reduced striatal ^{11}C-raclopride binding (Laruelle et al. 1995; de la Fuente-Fernandez et al. 2001; Goerendt et al. 2003). In normal subjects, a 0.3 mg/kg infusion of amphetamine results in a 25% reduction in striatal ^{11}C-raclopride binding, which has been estimated to represent at least a 10-fold increase in synaptic DA levels (Morris et al. 1995). In PD patients, infusion of amphetamine resulted in, on average, only 40% of the DA release seen in normal subjects (Piccini et al. 2003).

Piccini and colleagues (1999) demonstrated that grafts of human fetal VM tissue can restore the release of endogenous DA in the putamen. In one PD patient who had received human fetal VM tissue 10 years previously and had shown major clinical improvement, putamen ^{18}F-dopa PET uptake on the grafted side rose to normal values while ^{18}F-dopa uptake in the non-grafted putamen was only about 10% of, normal level. DA release, evaluated using a double ^{11}C-raclopride PET scan after placebo or methamphetamine administration, was also within normal range in the grafted putamen but very low in the non-grafted side. The results of this study suggested that it is very likely that the efficient restoration of DA release in large parts of the grafted putamen underlies this patient's major clinical improvement.

$H_2{}^{15}O$ and FDG PET studies have shown increased levels of oxygen and glucose metabolism in the contralateral striatum of hemiparkinsonian patients with early disease (Wolfson et al. 1985; Miletich et al. 1988). Patients with advanced PD and established bilateral symptoms have normal levels of striatal metabolism (Wolfson et al. 1985; Eidelberg et al. 1994). However, covariance analysis has revealed relatively raised striatal and lower frontal cortex metabolism in PD patients, and the degree of these changes correlated with clinical disease severity (Eidelberg et al. 1994, 1995). $H_2{}^{15}O$ PET studies have demonstrated that normal subjects—after paced movements of a joystick in freely selected directions—show increases in regional cerebral blood flow (rCBF) in the contralateral sensorimotor cortex and lentiform nucleus and bilaterally in the anterior cingulate, supplementary motor area, lateral premotor cortex, and dorsolateral prefrontal cortex (Playford et al. 1992; Jahanshahi et al. 1995).

Piccini and colleagues (2000) studied four PD patients with serial $H_2^{15}O$ PET scans over a period of two years following implantation with human fetal VM tissue into both caudate and putamen. Changes in rCBF were measured while the subjects performed paced joystick movements every four seconds in freely selected directions using their right hand. The movement-related activation in dorsolateral prefrontal cortex and SMA increased linearly over the course of the two years, at which time it reached a significant level of increase in comparison to the preoperative condition (Figure 2). The significant increase in activation shown with $H_2^{15}O$ PET at two years was delayed in comparison to the increase in ^{18}F-dopa uptake in the implanted striatum, already present six months after transplantation, but it was associated with significant clinical improvements in motor function. The fact that clinical improvement paralleled the restoration of levels of frontal activation rather than improvements in striatal dopaminergic reinnervation

suggests that relief of motor symptoms after transplantation of human fetal VM tissue requires functional reafferentation of striato-thalamocortical circuitries, along with an increased ability to produce and store DA.

IMAGING TO IMPROVE PATIENT SELECTION

Transplantation of human fetal VM tissue has been reported as one of the most effective reparative therapies in PD patients to date, although different studies have shown inconsistent results (Freed et al. 1992; Defer et al. 1996; Hagell et al. 1999; Hauser et al. 1999; Brundin et al. 2000; Mendez et al. 2002). The reasons behind this heterogeneity of outcomes are still not well understood. PET imaging has been used to try and identify some of the mechanisms underlying the inconsistent outcomes. Piccini and colleagues (2005) retrospectively studied nine PD patients who had received intraputaminal transplantation of human fetal VM tissue. These authors observed that the patients with the best functional outcome after transplantation did not show dopaminergic denervation, as measured by ^{18}F-dopa, in areas outside the striatum either preoperatively or at one or two years postoperatively. Conversely, transplanted patients with no or modest clinical benefit had, prior to transplantation, significant reduction of ^{18}F-dopa uptake in ventral striatal areas (Figure 3). Withdrawal of immunosuppression at 29 months after transplantation caused no reduction in ^{18}F-dopa uptake or worsening of UPDRS motor score, indicating continued survival and function of the graft. The findings from this study indicated that poor outcome after transplantation is connected with progressive dopaminergic denervation in areas outside the grafts that could have started before surgery. Also, the authors suggested that long-term immunosuppression can be withdrawn without interfering with graft survival or the motor recovery induced by transplantation.

Another recent PET study (Ma et al. 2010) retrospectively assessed long-term clinical and PET outcomes in 33 of the original participants in the trial by Freed and colleagues (2001). Similarly to the previously mentioned study, these authors found that superior clinical outcomes after transplant surgery were associated with the degree of ^{18}F-dopa uptake that was present preoperatively in the ventrorostral putamen. These findings suggest that subjects with terminal loss restricted to the dorsoposterior putamen appear to respond well to tissue engraftment that targets this area, whereas individuals with more extensive nigrostriatal attrition are less likely to exhibit a clinically meaningful response to such local engraftment.

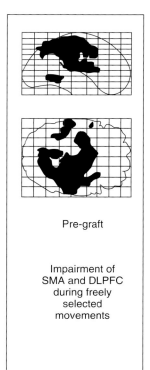

Pre-graft

Impairment of SMA and DLPFC during freely selected movements

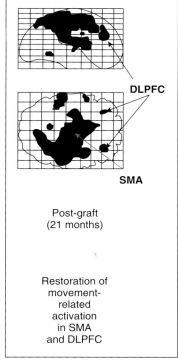

DLPFC

SMA

Post-graft (21 months)

Restoration of movement-related activation in SMA and DLPFC

Figure 2 $H_2^{15}O$ PET scans in 4 PD patients transplanted with human fetal VM tissue in caudate and putamen bilaterally. SPM analysis shows significantly decreased activation of supplementary motor area (SMA) and dorsolateral prefrontal cortex (DLPFC) during paced movements of a joystick in freely selected directions in the four patients before transplantation (left panel) and significant restoration of movement-related activation in the same areas 21 months after transplantation (right panel).

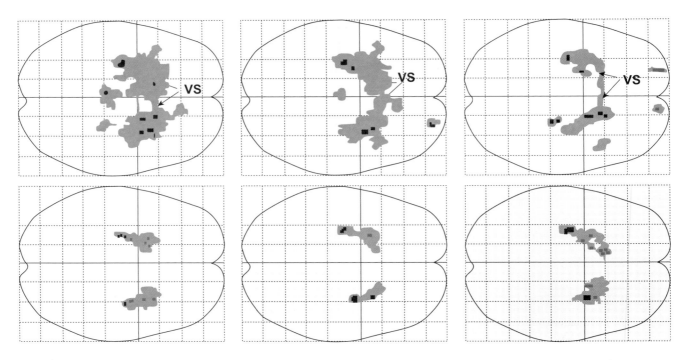

Figure 3 ^{18}F-dopa PET scans in six patients who received implantation of human fetal VM tissue bilaterally to the putamen. Upper panels: SPM analysis shows significant reduction of ^{18}F-dopa uptake in the ventral striatal areas (VS) in three patients. These patients showed modest or no benefit following transplantation. Lower panels: SPM analysis shows reduction of ^{18}F-dopa uptake confined to dorsal striatum in 3 additional patients who subsequently showed good clinical outcome following transplantation.

Taken together, these reports raise the possibility of a time window for optimal transplantation outcomes. Preoperative preservation of dopaminergic innervation in ventral striatal areas seems to be predictive of a better outcome; therefore, measures of ^{18}F-dopa uptake can provide valuable information to assist in the selection of patients for future trials of cell-based dopaminergic therapies for PD.

GRAFT-RELATED DYSKINESIAS

The further development and refinement of transplantation therapies in Parkinson's disease has been hindered by the occurrence of "off-medication" dyskinesias in a percentage of the grafted patients (Freed et al. 2001; Hagell et al. 2002; Olanow et al. 2003).

The pathogenesis of this type of dyskinesias is not well understood. One of the possibilities includes an excessive dopaminergic stimulation from the grafted cells, and this viewpoint is supported by two studies. In the first study, patients with persistent "off-medication" dyskinesias after transplantation showed unexpected and asymmetric increases in ^{18}F-dopa uptake in the ventral striatum (Freed et al. 2001; Ma et al. 2002). In the second study, the "off-medication" dyskinesias observed in two patients were associated with an increased caudate ^{18}F-dopa uptake in one and greater than expected striatal ^{11}C-raclopride displacement after levodopa in both cases. Also, in both patients, ^{11}C-raclopride binding in the "off" state was reduced below normal, suggesting that striatal D_2 receptors were occupied by excessive release of DA both basally and after levodopa (Olanow et al. 2003; Huanz et al. 2003). Conversely, two other studies using PET have shown that "off-medication" dyskinesias are not the consequence of graft-derived dopaminergic overgrowth or excessive release of dopamine (Hagell et al. 2002; Piccini et al. 2005). In support of these latter observations, Olanow and colleagues (2003) reported no obvious relationship between the emergence of off-dyskinesia and increases in ^{18}F-dopa uptake.

Another possible hypothesis indicates that the mishandling of DA by serotonin neurons in the graft could be responsible for the dyskinesias. Animal models of PD indicate that serotonergic neurons may play a role in levodopa-induced dyskinesias by releasing DA as a false transmitter (Carlsson et al. 2007, 2009; Carta et al. 2007; Munoz et al. 2008). In addition, serotonergic neurons have been found at postmortem in the grafted tissue of PD patients (Mendez et al. 2008). PET with ^{11}C-DASB, a specific tracer for the serotonin transporter (SERT), allows for study of the density of serotonin neurons within the graft, and a blockade of the serotonin transmitter-dependant release of DA with serotonin agonists will allow for the exploration of whether these terminals are responsible for that effect.

In conclusion, functional imaging, particularly with PET, has provided paramount information in clinical trials assessing the efficacy and safety of human fetal VM cells transplanted in the striatum of PD patients. More refined imaging techniques and novel radioligands will allow further development in the field of cell transplantation therapy, including stem cells.

REFERENCES

Brooks, D. J., E. P. Salmon, C. J. Mathias et al. 1990. The relationship between locomotor disability, autonomic dysfunction, and the integrity of the striatal dopaminergic system, in patients with multiple system atrophy, pure autonomic failure, and Parkinson's disease, studied with PET. *Brain* 113:1539–1552.

Brooks, D. J. 2004. Positron emission tomography imaging of transplant function. *NeuroRx* October, 1 (4): 482–91.

Brundin, P., W. M. Duan, and H. Sauer. 1994. Functional effects of mesencephalic dopamine neurons and adrenal chromaffin cells grafted to the rodent striatum. In *Functional neural transplantation*, eds. S. B. Dunnett and A. Bjorklund, 9–46. New York: Raven Press.

Brundin, P., O. Pogarell, P. Hagell et al. 2000. Bilateral caudate and putamen grafts of embryonic mesencephalic tissue treated with lazaroids in Parkinson's disease. *Brain* 123:1380–90.

Carlsson, T., M. Carta, C. Winkler, A. Björklund, and D. Kirik. 2007. Serotonin neuron transplants exacerbate L-DOPA-induced dyskinesia in a rat model of Parkinson's disease. *J Neurosci* July 25, 27 (30): 8011–22.

Carlsson, T., M. Carta, A. Muñoz, B. Mattsson, C. Winkler, D. Kirik, and A. Björklund. 2009. Impact of grafted serotonin and dopamine neurons on development of L-DOPA-induced dyskinesias in parkinsonian rats is determined by the extent of dopamine neuron degeneration. *Brain* February, 132 (Pt 2): 319–35.

Carta, M., T. Carlsson, D. Kirik, and A. Björklund. 2007. Dopamine released from 5-HT terminals is the cause of L-DOPA-induced dyskinesia in parkinsonian rats. *Brain* July, 130 (Pt 7): 1819–33.

Cochen, V., M. J. Ribeiro, J. P. Nguyen, J. M. Gurruchaga, G. Villafane, C. Loc'h et al. 2003. Transplantation in Parkinson's disease: PET changes correlate with the amount of grafted tissue. *Mov Disord* 18: 928–932.

De La Fuente-Fernandez, R., J. Q. Lu, V. Sossi et al. 2001. Biochemical variations in the synaptic level of dopamine precede motor fluctuations in Parkinson's disease: PET evidence of increased dopamine turnover. *Ann Neurol* 49:298–303.

Defer, G. L., et al. 1996. Long-term outcome of unilaterally transplanted parkinsonian patients. I. Clinical approach. *Brain* 119:41–50.

Eidelberg, D., J. R. Moeller, V. Dhawan et al. 1994. The metabolic topography of parkinsonism. *J Cereb Blood Flow Metab* 14: 783–801.

Eidelberg, D., J. R. Moeller, T. Ishikawa et al. 1995. Assessment of disease severity in Parkinsonism with fluorine-18-fluorodeoxyglucose and PET. *J Nucl Med* 36:378–383.

Firnau, G., S. Sood, R. Chirakal et al. 1987. Cerebral metabolism of 6-[18F] fluoro-L-3,4-dihydroxyphenylalanine in the primate. *J Neurochem* 48: 1077–1082.

Freed, C. R., R. E. Breeze, N. L. Rosenberg et al. 1992. Survival of implanted fetal dopamine cells and neurologic improvement 12 to 46 months after transplantation for Parkinson's disease. *N Engl J Med* 327:1549–1555.

Freed, C. R., P. E. Greene, R. E. Breeze et al. 2001. Transplantation of embryonic dopamine neurons for severe Parkinson's disease. *N Engl J Med* 344:710–719.

Freeman, T. B., C. W. Olanow, R. A. Hauser, G. M. Nauert, D. A. Smith, C. V. Borlongan et al. 1995. Bilateral fetal nigral transplantation into the postcommissural putamen in Parkinson's disease. *Ann Neurol* 38: 379–388.

Goerendt, I. K., C. Messa, A. D. Lawrence et al. 2003. Dopamine release during sequential finger movements in health and Parkinson's disease: A PET study. *Brain* 126:312–325.

Hagell, P., A. Schrag, P. Piccini, M. Jahanshahi, R. Brown, S. Rehncrona et al. 1999. Sequential bilateral transplantation in Parkinson's disease: Effects of the second graft. *Brain* 122:1121–1132.

Hagell, P., P. Piccini, A. Björklund, P. Brundin, S. Rehncrona, H. Widner, L. Crabb, N. Pavese, W. H. Oertel, N. Quinn, D. J. Brooks, and O. Lindvall. 2002. Dyskinesias following neural transplantation in Parkinson's disease. *Nat Neurosci* 5:627–8.

Hauser, R. A., T. B. Freeman, B. J. Snow, M. Nauert, L. Gauger, J. H. Kordower et al. 1999. Long-term evaluation of bilateral fetal nigral transplantation in Parkinson disease. *Arch Neurol* 56:179–187.

Huang, Z., R. De la Fuente-Fernandez, R. A. Hauser et al. 2003. Dopaminergic alteration in Parkinson's patients with "off period" dyskinesia following striatal embryonic mesencephalic transplant. *Neurology* 60 (Suppl 1): A126. (Abstract).

Jahanshahi, M., I. H. Jenkins, R. G. Brown et al. 1995. Self-initiated versus externally-triggered movements: Measurements of regional cerebral blood flow and movement-related potentials in normals and Parkinson's disease. *Brain* 118:913–933.

Kordower, J. H., T. B. Freeman, B. J. Snow, F. J. Vingerhoets, E. J. Mufson, P. R. Sanberg et al. 1995. Neuropathological evidence of graft survival and striatal reinnervation after the transplantation of fetal mesencephalic tissue in a patient with Parkinson's disease. *N Engl J Med* 332:1118–1124.

Kordower, J. H., J. M. Rosenstein, T. J. Collier, M. A. Burke, E. Y. Chen, J. M. Li et al. 1996. Functional fetal nigral grafts in a patient with Parkinson's disease: Chemoanatomic, ultrastructural, and metabolic studies. *J Comp Neurol* 370:203–230.

Kordower, J. H., T. B. Freeman, E. Y. Chen, E. J. Mufson, P. R. Sanberg, R. A. Hauser et al. 1998. Fetal nigral grafts survive and mediate clinical benefit in a patient with Parkinson's disease. *Mov Disord* 13: 383–393.

Kordower, J. H., Y. Chu, R. A. Hauser, T. B. Freeman, and C. W. Olanow. 2008. Lewy body-like pathology in long-term embryonic nigral transplants in Parkinson's disease. *Nat Med* 14:504–506.

Laruelle, M., A. Abi-Dargham, C. H. van Dyck et al. 1995. SPECT imaging of striatal dopamine release after amphetamine challenge. *J Nucl Med* 36:1182–1190.

Li, J. Y. et al. 2008. Lewy bodies in grafted neurons in subjects with Parkinson's disease suggest host-to-graft disease propagation. *Nat Med* 14:501–503.

Lindvall, O., P. Brundin, H. Widner, S. Rehncrona, B. Gustavii, R. Frackowiak et al. 1990. Grafts of fetal dopamine neurons survive and improve motor function in Parkinson's disease. *Science* 247: 574–577.

Lindvall, O., G. Sawle, H. Widner, J. C. Rothwell, A. Bjorklund, D. Brooks et al. 1994. Evidence for long-term survival and function of dopaminergic grafts in progressive Parkinson's disease. *Ann Neurol* 35:172–180.

Lindvall, O. 1999. Cerebral implantation in movement disorders: State of the art. *Mov Disord* 14:201–205.

Lindvall, O., and P. Hagell. 2000. Clinical observations after neural transplantation in Parkinson's disease. *Prog Brain Res* 127:299–320.

Lindvall, O. and A. Björklund. 2004. Cell therapy in Parkinson's disease. *NeuroRx* 1:382–393.

Ma, Y., A. Feigin, V. Dhawan, M. Fukuda, Q. Shi, P. Greene, R. Breeze, S. Fahn, C. Freed, D. Eidelberg. 2002. Dyskinesia after fetal cell transplantation for parkinsonism: A PET study. *Ann Neurol* November, 52(5): 628–34.

Ma, Y., C. Tang, T. Chaly, P. Greene, R. Breeze, S. Fahn, C. Freed, V. Dhawan, D. Eidelberg. 2010. Dopamine cell implantation in Parkinson's disease: Long-term clinical and (18)F-FDOPA PET outcomes. *J Nucl Med* January, 51(1): 7–15.

Mendez, I., A. Dagher, M. Hong et al. 2000. Enhancement of survival of stored dopaminergic cells and promotion of graft survival by exposure of human fetal nigral tissue to glial cell line-derived neurotrophic factor in patients with Parkinson's disease. Report of two cases and technical considerations. *J Neurosurg* 92:863–69.

Mendez, I., A. Dagher, M. Hong, P. Gaudet, S. Weerasinghe, V. McAlister et al. 2002. Simultaneous intrastriatal and intranigral fetal dopaminergic grafts in patients with Parkinson disease: A pilot study. Report of three cases. *J Neurosurg* 96:589–596.

Mendez, I. et al. 2008. Dopamine neurons implanted into people with Parkinson's disease survive without pathology for 14 years. *Nat Med* 14:507–509.

Miletich, R. S., T. Chan, M. Gillespie et al. 1988. Contralateral basal ganglia metabolism is abnormal in hemiparkinsonian patients. An FDG-PET study. *Neurology* 38:S260.

Morris, E. D., R. E. Fisher, N. M. Alpert et al. 1995. In vivo imaging of neuromodulation using positron emission tomography: Optimal ligand characteristics and task length for detection of activation. *Hum Brain Mapp* 3:35–55.

Morrish, P., G. V. Sawle, D. J. Brooks. 1996. An [18F] dopa-PET and clinical study of the rate of progression in Parkinson's disease. *Brain* 119:585–91.

Muñoz, A., Q. Li, F. Gardoni, E. Marcello, T. Qin, T. Carlsson, D. Kirik, M. Di Luca, A. Björklund, E. Bezard, M. Carta M. 2008. Combined 5-HT1A and 5-HT1B receptor agonists for the treatment of L-DOPA-induced dyskinesia. *Brain* December, 131 (Pt 12): 3380–94.

Olanow, C. W., C. G. Goetz, J. H. Kordower et al. 2003. A double-blind controlled trial of bilateral fetal nigral transplantation in Parkinson's disease. *Ann Neurol* 54:403–414.

Patlak, C., R. G. Blasberg. 1985. Graphical evaluation of blood-to-brain transfer constants from multiple-time uptake data. Generalisations. *J Cereb Blood Flow Metab* 5:584–590.

Peschanski, M., G. N. Defer, J. P. Guyen, J. Ricolfi, J. C. Monfort, P. Remy et al. 1994. Bilateral motor improvement and alteration of L-dopa effect in two patients with Parkinson's disease following intrastriatal transplantation of foetal ventral mesencephalon. *Brain* 117:487–499.

Piccini, P., D. J. Brooks, A. Bjorklund, R. N. Gunn, P. M. Grasby, O. Rimoldi et al. 1999. Dopamine release from nigral transplants visualized in vivo in a Parkinson's patient. *Nat Neurosci* 2: 1137–1140.

Piccini, P., O. Lindvall, A. Bjorklund et al. 2000. Delayed recovery of movement-related cortical function in Parkinson's disease after striatal dopaminergic grafts. *Ann Neurol* 48: 689–695.

Piccini, P., N. Pavese, D. J. Brooks. 2003. Endogenous dopamine release after pharmacological challenges in Parkinson's disease. *Ann Neurol* 53:647–653.

Piccini, P., N. Pavese, P. Hagell, J. Reimer, A. Björklund, W. H. Oertel, N. P. Quinn, D. J. Brooks, and O. Lindvall. 2005. Factors affecting the clinical outcome after neural transplantation in Parkinson's disease. *Brain*, December 128 (Pt 12): 2977–86.

Playford, E. D., I. H. Jenkins, R. E. Passingham et al. 1992. Impaired mesial frontal and putamen activation in Parkinson's disease: A PET study. *Ann Neurol* 32:151–161.

Remy, P., Y. Samson, P. Hantraye et al. 1995. Clinical correlates of [18F] fluorodopa uptake in five grafted parkinsonian patients. *Ann Neurol* 38:580–88.

Sawle, G. V., P. M. Bloomfield, A. Bjorklund, D. J. Brooks, P. Brundin, K. L. Leenders et al. 1992. Transplantation of fetal dopamine neurons in Parkinson's disease: PET [18F]6-L-fluorodopa studies in two patients with putaminal implants. *Ann Neurol* 31:166–173.

Sullivan, A. M., J. Pohl, S. B. Blunt. 1998. Growth/differentiation factor 5 and glial cell line-derived neurotrophic factor enhance survival and function of dopaminergic grafts in a rat model of Parkinson's disease. *Eur J Neurosci* 10:3681–88.

Volkow, N. D., G.-J. Wang, J. S. Fowler et al. 1994. Imaging endogenous dopamine competition with [11C]raclopride in the human brain. *Synapse* 16:255–262.

Wenning, G. K., P. Odin, P. Morrish, S. Rehncrona, H. Widner, P. Brundin et al. 1997. Short- and long-term survival and function of unilateral intrastriatal dopaminergic grafts in Parkinson's disease. *Ann Neurol* 42:95–107.

Widner, H., J. Tetrud, S. Rehncrona et al. 1992. Bilateral fetal mesencephalic grafting in two patients with parkinsonism induced by 1-methyl-4-phenyl-1,2,3,6-tetrahydro-pyridine (MPTP). *N Engl J Med* 327:1556–1563.

Wolfson, L. I., K. L. Leenders, L. L. Brown, and T. Jones. 1985. Alterations of regional cerebral blood flow and oxygen metabolism in Parkinson's disease. *Neurology* 35:1399–1405.

17

IMAGING APPLICATIONS TO PARKINSON'S DISEASE CLINICAL TRIALS

Martin Niethammer and Andrew Feigin

INTRODUCTION

Clinical trials of new treatments for Parkinson's disease (PD) can be categorized into those that seek to improve the signs and symptoms of PD, and those that seek to modify the progression of the disease. While clinical measures are typically used as the primary determinants of outcome, these may be confounded by potential variability in assessments (e.g., inter- and intra-investigator variability in performing clinical scales, effects of therapy); small effect sizes, especially early in the disease; or placebo effects (Goetz et al. 2008). Thus, objective markers have been sought that might be used as surrogates for standard clinical measures to optimize the conduct of the clinical trials (Ravina et al. 2009). Though there has been debate on the role of such markers beyond Phase II trials (De Gruttola et al. 2001), they may have relevance for many aspects of clinical trials, including confirmation of diagnosis during the screening process, and as adjunctive objective means for assessing efficacy. Brain imaging in particular has been utilized as an outcome measure in several clinical trials of PD. This chapter will review the use of brain imaging in prior clinical trials and will assess potential novel applications of imaging to the experimental therapeutics of PD.

WHAT IS A BIOMARKER?

The National Institutes of Health's Biomarkers Definitions Working Group defines a biomarker as

"a characteristic that is objectively measured and evaluated as an indicator of normal biological processes, pathogenic processes, or pharmacologic responses to a therapeutic intervention" (Biomarkers Definitions Working Group 2001).

However, not all available biomarkers are typically usable as surrogate endpoints in clinical trials. Use as a surrogate endpoint requires that it be

"expected to predict clinical benefit (or harm or lack of benefit or harm) based on epidemiologic, therapeutic, pathophysiologic, or other scientific evidence" (Biomarkers Definitions Working Group 2001).

In PD, neuroimaging may be useful for differential diagnosis (Eckert et al. 2004, 2005; Tang et al. 2010), measuring pathological severity (e.g., loss of dopaminergic nerve terminals) (Dhawan and Eidelberg 2006), and assessing treatment response (Hilker et al. 2003; Pavese et al. 2006; Piccini et al. 2005; Ma et al. 2007). To date, however, no biomarker, including imaging measures, has risen to the level of a true surrogate endpoint in PD trials, though imaging has been used as an adjunctive outcome measure in several clinical trials (Table 1).

IMAGING IN PD CLINICAL TRIALS

DISEASE MODIFICATION

The primary pathology in PD involves the abnormal loss of nigrostriatal dopaminergic neurons. While this process inexorably progresses over time (though at a variable rate among patients), the signs and symptoms of PD may vary considerably over time due to changes in medication and other factors. In fact, PD patients may appear clinically to have milder PD after being started on dopaminergic therapy or after dopaminergic therapy is increased. As a result, utilizing clinical measures to assess progression in clinical trials may be problematic. One of the first trials to attempt

Trial name (year published[*])	Trial design/Primary outcome measure	Imaging method	Aim
CALM-PD (2000)	Double-blind, controlled/Efficacy	β-CIT SPECT	Disease modification
REAL-PET (2003)	Double-blind, controlled/Efficacy	FDOPA PET	Disease modification
ELLDOPA (2004)	Double-blind, controlled/Efficacy	β-CIT SPECT	Disease modification
PELMOPET (2006)	Double-blind, controlled/Efficacy	FDOPA PET	Disease modification
Fetal Cell (2001)	Double-blind, controlled/Efficacy	FDOPA PET	Disease modification
Riluzole (2005)	Double-blind, controlled/Efficacy	FDOPA PET	Disease modification
GDNF (2003)	Open-label/Safety-Tolerability	FDOPA PET	Disease modification
GDNF (2006)	Open-label/Efficacy	FDOPA PET	Disease modification
PRECEPT (2007)	Double-blind, controlled/Efficacy	β-CIT SPECT	Disease modification
GAD (2007)	Open-label/Safety-Tolerability	FDG PET	Symptomatic treatment
Neurturin (2008)	Open-label/Safety-Tolerability	FDOPA PET	Disease modification
AADC (2009)	Open-label/Safety-Tolerability	FMT PET	Symptomatic treatment
Spheramine (2005)	Open-label/Safety-Tolerability	FDOPA PET	Disease modification
STEPS (not yet published)	Double-blind, controlled/Efficacy	FDOPA PET	Disease modification

β-CIT = [^{123}I]-2-β-carbomethoxy-3-β-[4-iodophenyl]tropane

FDOPA = [^{18}F]-6-fluorodopa

FDG = [^{18}F]fluorodeoxyglucose

FMT = [^{18}F]fluoro-L-m-tyrosine

PET = Positron Emission Tomography

SPECT = Single Photon Emission Tomography

[*]See bibliography for full study citations

to study modification of disease progression in PD, the DATATOP (Deprenyl and Tocopherol Antioxidative Therapy of Parkinsonism) trial, serves as a good example of this dilemma (Parkinson Study Group 1989a, b). Eight hundred early untreated PD subjects were randomly assigned to receive the MAO-B inhibitor deprenyl, vitamin E, both, or neither (placebo) in a 2×2 factorial design. Over the course of the study, subjects taking deprenyl (selegiline) were less likely to reach the study endpoint, which was defined as need for dopaminergic therapy, than those on placebo. The study concluded

". . . deprenyl . . . delays the onset of disability associated with early, otherwise untreated cases of Parkinson's disease," but "the mechanism (symptomatic, protective, or both) of the effect is unclear" (Parkinson Study Group 1989b).

When the study was conceived it had been assumed that deprenyl had little or no effect on PD symptoms (Parkinson Study Group 1989a, b), but subsequent analysis demonstrated a small but significant symptomatic benefit.

This led to debate regarding the meaning of the DATATOP results. An editorial critiquing the study wrote,

"The null hypothesis of this protocol is the investigational drugs do not retard the pathologic process . . . The null hypothesis may validly be rejected *only* if there is a significant difference between control and treated groups in the *absence of symptomatic effects* . . . This restrictive stipulation is essential because the protocol's *only* significant measure of pathologic process is symptom severity" (Landau 1990).

Though attempts have been made to develop novel clinical trial designs to address this issue, most notably the delayed-start design of the TEMPO and ADAGIO trials (Olanow et al. 2009), the problem of symptomatic effects confounding potential neuroprotective effects continues to be a source of controversy in the interpretation of these and other trials (Ahlskog and Uitti 2010; Olanow and Rascol 2010).

Given the difficulty encountered in studying disease modification solely with clinical measures, several clinical trials since DATATOP have utilized imaging methods to quantify dopaminergic nerve terminals and their rate of loss over time, in an effort to objectively measure disease progression independent of changes in clinical status. The dopaminergic imaging methods that have been used in such clinical trials include dopamine transporter (DAT) imaging with [123I]-2-β-carbomethoxy-3-β-[4-iodophenyl]tropane (β-CIT) and SPECT, and dopa-decarboxylase imaging with [18F]-6-fluorodopa (FDOPA) and PET.

MEDICAL THERAPIES

Among medication trials, the CALM-PD (Parkinson Study Group 2000, 2002; Holloway et al. 2004; Parkinson Study Group CALM Cohort Investigators 2009), PRECEPT (The Parkinson Study Group PRECEPT Investigators 2007), and ELLDOPA (Fahn et al. 2004) trials utilized β-CIT SPECT, whereas REAL-PET (Whone et al. 2003), PELMOPET (Oertel et al. 2006), and a riluzole trial utilized FDOPA PET (Table 1) (Figure 1). All of these trials sought to measure the rate of change in dopamine neuronal loss over time and to compare these rates among treatment groups (e.g., active treatment vs. placebo in ELLDOPA or dopamine agonists vs. levodopa in CALM-PD, REAL-PD, or PELMOPET).

In the PRECEPT and riluzole trials, the imaging findings conformed to the clinical findings, confirming a lack of therapeutic neuromodulating benefit of the drugs under study. Both trials examined drugs that were not expected to have symptomatic effects in PD, but were expected to exert disease-modifying effects (i.e., to slow PD progression). In PRECEPT, the study drug was a c-Jun kinase inhibitor; the study failed to demonstrate changes in PD progression utilizing either clinical or imaging (β-CIT SPECT) outcomes. A double-blind, placebo-controlled trial of riluzole, a Na+ channel blocker that had been shown to have neuroprotective activity in animal models of PD (Obinu et al. 2002), showed no clinical or imaging (FDOPA PET) differences between the treatment groups over the course of the study. The trial was thus halted after the first ad interim analysis (Pavese et al. 2005, 2009).

In the CALM-PD, REAL-PET, and ELLDOPA trials, however, the imaging results appeared to contradict the clinical results, highlighting the potential complications of utilizing adjunctive secondary outcome measures. In CALM-PD and REAL-PET, subjects randomized to dopamine agonists (pramipexole and ropinirole, respectively) demonstrated more functional disability and worse motor performance than subjects randomized to levodopa, yet the imaging studies suggested a slower rate of decline in the dopamine agonist groups. Similarly, the PELMOPET study demonstrated greater clinical improvement with levodopa than pergolide (Oertel et al. 2006) with a trend toward a slower rate of decline in FDOPA uptake with

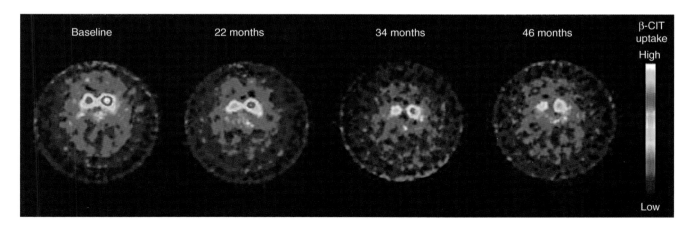

Figure 1 Dopaminergic Imaging in Parkinson's Disease. An example from the CALM-PD trial (Parkinson Study Group, 2002) demonstrates progressive loss of striatal β-CIT uptake in a patient with Parkinson's disease. Single-photon emission computed tomography (SPECT) β-CIT images from a single patient show progressive striatal dopamine transporter loss during the 46-month evaluation period. Loss of activity is greater in the putamen than in the caudate. Levels of SPECT activity are color-encoded from low (black) to high (yellow/white). [Reprinted from *JAMA*, April 3, 2002, 287, p. 1657, Copyright © (2002) American Medical Association. All rights reserved.]

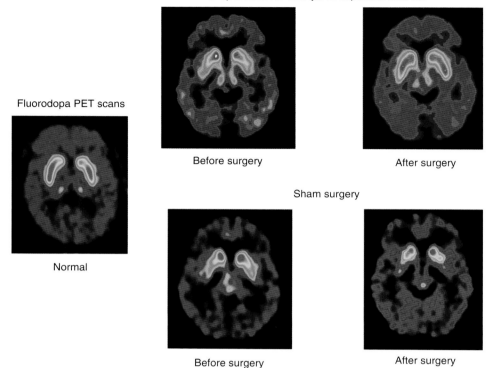

Transplantation of embryonic dopamine neurons

Fluorodopa PET scans

Before surgery

After surgery

Sham surgery

Normal

Before surgery

After surgery

Figure 2 Change in FDOPA Uptake in the Brains of Patients with Parkinson's Disease after Fetal Dopaminergic Transplantation, as Shown in FDOPA PET Scans. In the panel on the far left, an axial section through the caudate and putamen of a normal subject shows intense uptake of FDOPA (red). On the right side, the upper panels show preoperative and 12-month postoperative scans in a patient in the transplantation group. Before surgery, the uptake of FDOPA was restricted to the region of the caudate. After transplantation, there was increased uptake of FDOPA in the putamen bilaterally. In contrast, the lower panels show FDOPA scans in a patient in the sham-surgery group, with no postoperative change in FDOPA uptake. [Reprinted from *N Engl J Med*, March 8, 2001, 344, p. 715, Copyright © 2001 Massachusetts Medical Society. All rights reserved.]

pergolide (Oertel et al. 2001; Pavese et al. 2009). Given the lack of a placebo group, it remains uncertain whether these results indicate that dopamine agonists slow progression, levodopa hastens progression, or alternatively, these drugs directly alter imaging ligand binding. In ELLDOPA, subjects randomized to levodopa were clinically better than those randomized to placebo after nine months of therapy even after up to four weeks of washout, yet the imaging (β-CIT SPECT) indicated a faster rate of decline in the levodopa group.

Taken together, these results raise questions about whether dopaminergic imaging provides an independent measure of nigrostriatal integrity even when contradicting clinical results, or if the imaging measures, like the clinical measures, can be affected by dopaminergic (or other) therapies. For example, in the ELLDOPA trial, did levodopa actually hasten progression of nigrostriatal cell loss, or did it simply cause downregulation of the dopamine transporter

as measured by β-CIT binding and SPECT? The results of these trials have led to a rethinking of the use of neuroimaging in clinical trials aimed at disease modification.

SURGICAL THERAPIES

A small number of surgical PD clinical trials have sought to evaluate potential neuromodulation or neurorestoration using FDOPA PET imaging. Two of these trials involved forms of cell transplantation, and two involved the use of glial derived neurotrophic factor (GDNF).

In a double-blind, randomized sham-surgery controlled trial of fetal dopaminergic cell transplantation (Freed et al. 2001), FDOPA PET demonstrated increased uptake in the treated group (Figure 2), although the clinical results of the study were less compelling. That is, despite increases in FDOPA uptake, in subjects over age 60, clinical improvement was not demonstrated after one year. This was the

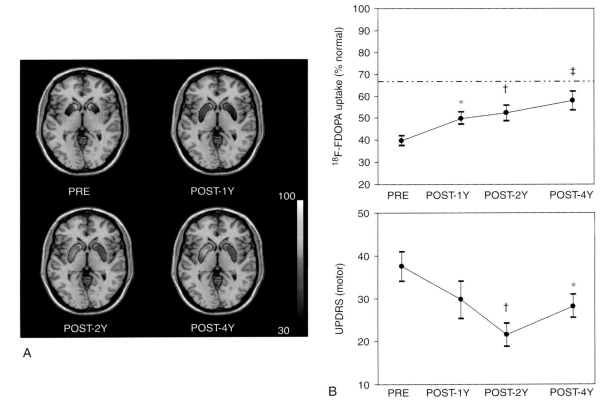

Figure 3 Sustained Increase in FDOPA Uptake after Fetal Dopaminergic Transplantation. **A.** Maps of mean FDOPA uptake in transplant recipients scanned at baseline (pre) and at 1 (post-1Y), 2 (post-2Y), and 4 (post-4Y) years after surgery. Postoperative scans showed sustained increases in putamen FDOPA uptake after transplantation. [Maps were created on a voxel basis from spatially normalized images of FDOPA uptake ratio, presented as percentage of normal value in 15 healthy subjects and displayed on a standard MRI brain template. Color stripe represents normalized values of FDOPA uptake in striatal regions thresholded at 30%.] **B.** Striatal FDOPA uptake (*top*) and off-state UPDRS motor ratings (*bottom*) (mean ± SE) at baseline (pre) and at 1 (post-1Y), 2 (post-2Y), and 4 (post-4Y) years after bilateral implantation of fetal dopaminergic cells into the putamen of PD patients. Significant treatment effect was noted over 2 years ($p < 0.0001$; RMANOVA) in the whole group and over 4 years ($p < 0.001$) in 15 participants who were evaluated at all four time points. [Reprinted by permission of the Society of Nuclear Medicine from Ma et al. 2010: Figure 1 and 2].

case even though significant dopaminergic complications, namely dyskinesias, were noted.

However, on follow-up, increases in FDOPA uptake were sustained over four years, and clinical benefit was also evident in the older patients, at least in the subgroup still followed at that time (Ma et al. 2010) (Figure 3).

In a second cell transplantation study, retinal pigment epithelial cells attached to gelatin microcarriers (Spheramine®; Titan Pharmaceuticals, Inc, Somerville, NJ) were transplanted into the striatum of PD patients, and dopaminergic reinnervation was assessed utilizing FDOPA PET (Stover et al. 2005). This Phase I open-label study demonstrated almost a 50% improvement in clinical motor scores lasting up to 24 months. A subsequent Phase IIb randomized placebo-controlled trial (the STEPS trial), however, failed to demonstrate statistically significant

clinical improvement (Watts et al. 2009), though the FDOPA PET results have not yet been presented or published.

Likewise, studies of putaminal infusion of GDNF have yielded inconsistent results. In an unblinded Phase I trial, GDNF was infused into the striatum of PD subjects (Gill et al. 2003). The treatment resulted in clinical improvements and significant increases in FDOPA uptake. A subsequent placebo-controlled trial, however, did not demonstrate clinical improvement despite confirming increases in FDOPA uptake in the treatment group relative to the placebo group (Lang et al. 2006).

This is in contrast to an open-label gene therapy trial of the gene for the GDNF analog, Neurturin, delivered via an adeno-associated virus vector (AAV-NRTN, CERE-120) (Marks et al. 2008). Here, significant improvements in motor function were found, but FDOPA failed to demonstrate an increase in dopaminergic terminals. As with the medical therapy clinical trials described above, the contradictory clinical and imaging results of these surgical trials make it difficult to come to definitive conclusions regarding these therapies. Interestingly, a subsequent double-blind sham-surgery controlled clinical trial of Neurturin demonstrated a lack of clinical benefit (http://www.ceregene.com/press_112608.asp, results not yet published), suggesting that perhaps the FDOPA PET results from the Phase I trial provided a reliable assessment of the experimental therapy in the setting of unreliable uncontrolled clinical results.

SYMPTOM RELIEF

Two early-phase gene therapy clinical trials aimed at improving the signs and symptoms of PD have utilized imaging as a secondary outcome measure. These trials were primarily designed to test the safety and tolerability of gene therapy approaches, but secondary clinical and imaging assessments were also used. One study examined the effect of unilateral administration of the gene for glutamic acid decarboxylase delivered with an adeno-associated virus vector (AAV-GAD) in advanced PD, and utilized [^{18}F]fluorodeoxyglucose (FDG) PET to measure changes in regional brain metabolism. The untreated hemisphere served as a control for the imaging comparisons. The study demonstrated a statistically significant improvement in motor function on the body side contralateral to the side of the brain that received AAV-GAD (Kaplitt et al. 2007). In concordance with this, FDG PET demonstrated reductions in thalamic metabolism consistent with predicted changes from known effective symptomatic therapies (Feigin et al. 2007) (Figure 4A). This trial also demonstrated hemispheric suppression of a PD-specific metabolic brain network, termed PDRP (Ma et al. 2007; Eidelberg 2009) (see Chapters 3 and 12 for further detail of disease-specific patterns), on the operated side (Figure 4B–C). Furthermore, for individual subjects, changes in network activity correlated with improvements in Unified Parkinson's Disease Rating Scale (UPDRS) scores (Feigin et al. 2007).

In another gene therapy trial testing the safety and tolerability of AAV-amino acid decarboxylase gene (AADC) in 10 advanced PD patients (Eberling et al. 2008; Christine et al. 2009), [^{18}F]fluoro-L-m-tyrosine (FMT) PET was utilized to directly measure changes in AADC activity. This open-label study found significant improvements in clinical motor ratings, and the imaging documented increases in AADC activity. This study is notable in that it

is the only gene therapy clinical trial that has utilized an imaging measure to directly document increased expression of the gene being delivered.

Both of these trials suggest that imaging may be a powerful adjunctive tool in small early-phase trials. In fact, the imaging data, when supportive of unblinded clinical results, may be critical for deciding whether to pursue a larger, more expensive, and time-consuming efficacy trial.

DEEP BRAIN STIMULATION

To date, imaging has not been used as part of formal clinical trials evaluating the clinical efficacy of deep brain stimulation (DBS) (e.g., Benabid et al. 1987, 2001; Deuschl et al. 2006; Follett et al. 2010). Nevertheless, though not strictly as part of a clinical trial, imaging has been utilized extensively to investigate the mechanisms of DBS surgery (Hilker et al. 2003; Fukuda et al. 2004; Karimi et al. 2008; Hilker et al. 2008; Asanuma et al. 2006; Kalbe et al. 2009). One small prospective open-label trial of subthalamic nucleus (STN) DBS, however, did utilize FDOPA PET to assess PD progression over 16 months following DBS surgery (Hilker et al. 2005). The study found a rate of progression comparable to that observed in other longitudinal studies.

FUTURE APPLICATIONS

As discussed above, PD clinical trials that have utilized imaging as an outcome measure have largely focused on the dopaminergic system. Future applications of imaging to PD clinical trials will likely include confirmation of diagnosis during screening (e.g., idiopathic PD versus atypical parkinsonism) and assessments of non-dopaminergic systems. Significant progress has been made in both of these areas, and clinical trials are likely to incorporate these methods.

Clinical criteria alone may not be satisfactory for diagnosing idiopathic PD. It is estimated that approximately 20% of patients diagnosed with PD will be found to have atypical parkinsonism (e.g., progressive supranuclear palsy [PSP], multiple system atrophy [MSA], or corticobasal degeneration [CBD]) on postmortem examination (Hughes et al. 1992). In addition, past clinical trials that utilized dopaminergic imaging found that up to 15% of subjects did not appear to have a dopaminergic deficit (Whone et al. 2003; Fahn et al. 2004). In most cases, follow-up scans up to four years later remained normal. Moreover, clinical follow-up on 150 patients with normal

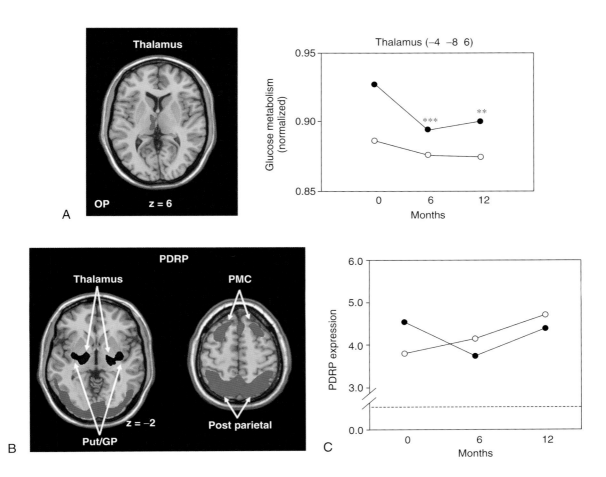

Figure 4 Changes in regional metabolism and network activity after gene therapy. **A.** *Left:* Voxel-based analysis of changes in regional metabolic activity after unilateral STN AAV-GAD gene therapy for advanced PD. After unilateral gene therapy, a significant reduction in metabolism was found in the operated thalamus, involving the ventrolateral and mediodorsal nuclei. Shown are representative axial T1-weighted MRI with merged FDG PET slices; the operated (OP) side is signified on the left. Metabolic declines are displayed by using a blue–purple scale. The displays were thresholded at p < 0.05, corrected for multiple comparisons. *Right:* Display of the metabolic data for this region at each time point exhibited significant changes over time. These regional changes were present on the operated side (filled circles) but not in homologous regions of the unoperated side (open circles). **p < 0.005; ***p < 0.001; Bonferroni tests relative to baseline values. **B.** The PD-related metabolic pattern (PDRP). This motor-related spatial covariance pattern (Ma et al. 2007) is characterized by relative pallidothalamic hypermetabolism (left) associated with relative metabolic reductions in the lateral premotor and posterior parietal areas (right). Put/GP: putamen/globus pallidus; PMC: premotor cortex. **C.** Changes in mean PDRP network activity over time for the operated (filled circles) and the unoperated (open circles) hemispheres. After gene therapy, there was a significant difference (p < 0.002) in the time course of PDRP activity across the two hemispheres. In the unoperated hemisphere, network activity increased continuously over the 12 months after surgery. By contrast, in the operated hemisphere, a decline in network activity was evident during the first 6 months. Over the subsequent 6 months, network activity on this side increased in parallel with analogous values on the unoperated side. The dashed line represents one standard error above the normal mean value of zero. [A–C: Reprinted from *PNAS*, Modulation of metabolic brain networks after subthalamic gene therapy for Parkinson's disease, 19559–19564, Copyright 2007, with permission from The National Academy of Sciences.]

N-ω-fluoropropyl-2β-carboxymethoxy-3β-(4-[^{123}I]iodo-phenyl) nortropane (^{123}I-FP-CIT) SPECT imaging (since termed "scans without evidence of dopaminergic deficit" [SWEDD]) showed that 97% did not have a neurodegen-erative parkinsonian disorder (Marshall et al. 2006).

Taken together, these observations suggest that up to one-third of subjects entering PD clinical trials (especially trials enrolling early untreated subjects) may not have idio-pathic PD. Though the validity of these trials is maintained

through the process of randomization (i.e., equal numbers of PD/non-PD subjects are randomized to treatment and control groups), power is sacrificed, and more subjects need to be enrolled in trials, escalating costs. Therefore, a reliable and objective screening diagnostic procedure would be of potentially great value in conducting clinical trials.

Several imaging measures have been studied for their utility in differentiating idiopathic PD from atypical par-kinsonism. Presynaptic dopaminergic imaging is generally not useful in this regard, since both PD and atypical parkinsonism result in the loss of dopaminergic nerve terminals and cannot be accurately distinguished by β-CIT, FDOPA, or other presynaptic dopaminergic ligands (Eerola et al. 2005). Postsynaptic dopaminergic imaging, however, might be helpful in this regard. For example, recent data suggests that [^{18}F]desmethoxyfallypride (DMFP) PET (a measure of dopamine D_2-like receptors) can distinguish PD from atypical parkinsonism (la Fougere et al. 2010), though this does not appear to be useful for distinguishing among the atypical parkinsonian disorders. A more widely available PET imaging ligand, [^{18}F]fluorodeoxyglucose (FDG), however, appears to have the potential to accurately discriminate PD from other causes of parkinsonism, such as MSA, PSP, or CBD (Eckert et al. 2005; Tang et al. 2010). FDG PET is relatively inexpensive and widely available, making it a potentially viable method for screening subjects in clinical trials. This may have greater importance in early-stage trials involving relatively few subjects, where a small number of misdiagnosed individuals could have a significant impact on such studies. In a currently ongoing Phase II double-blind sham-surgery controlled trial of AAV-GAD, FDG PET is being utilized for screening to assure that all subjects entering the trial have idiopathic PD. In addition, this trial is using FDG PET as an outcome measure so that scans are being repeated at 6 and 12 months after therapy.

Moreover, FDG PET scans can be used in conjunction with spatial covariance analysis to quantify disease-specific regional metabolic patterns that correlate with clinical disease progression, and may prove useful as secondary outcome measures in clinical trials (see Figure 4 in Eidelberg 2009 for example).

In vivo imaging of substantia nigra structural integrity might also be of use in the clinical trial setting. For example, diffusion-weighted MR imaging may have utility in distinguishing between MSA and PD (Seppi and Schocke 2005). Magnetic transfer imaging (MTI) and susceptibility-weighted MRI (SWI) likewise appear to have the ability to help distinguish PD from atypical parkinsonism (Hanyu et al. 2001; Anik et al. 2007; Gupta et al. 2010). Substantia nigra iron content can be directly imaged and potentially quantified using MRI (Martin 2009) and might serve as a measure of disease severity. Magnetic resonance spectroscopy (MRS) (Henchcliffe et al. 2008) and transcranial sonography (Walter 2009) have also shown promise in differentiating PD from atypical parkinsonism. Though these methods and others may be of value in future clinical trials, to date none of these modalities have been validated for their ability to provide a reliable and reproducible marker for diagnosis or disease progression.

Other modalities of imaging in clinical trials are likely to be utilized in the future. Specifically, more direct measure of PD pathology may be useful for assessing disease progression, thereby allowing for better evaluations of disease modification or neuroprotection. A potential example of this would be in vivo imaging of Lewy body pathology. Such imaging of Lewy bodies may be accomplished with α-synuclein ligands such as 2-(1-[6-[(2-[^{18}F]fluoroethyl)(methyl)amino]-2-naphthyl]ethylidene) malononitrile (FDDNP) (Smid et al. 2006), or [^{18}F]-BF22 (Fodero-Tavoletti et al. 2009). However, neither of these ligands are specific for α-synuclein, and both ligands also bind to β-amyloid, necessitating separate imaging and image subtraction with ligands specific for β-amyloid, such as [^{11}C] benzothiazole-aniline (Pittsburgh Compound B, PIB) (Maetzler et al. 2008; Gomperts et al. 2008; Burack et al. 2010). Development of ligands specific for Lewy bodies would greatly aid in this approach.

Lastly, imaging may also be used in future PD clinical trials to assess mechanisms of action of specific drugs. For example, neuroinflammation has been hypothesized to contribute to the neurodegenerative process underlying PD. A small study involving five PD patients assessed the effects of the cyclooxygenase-2 inhibitor celecoxib on microglial activation utilizing [^{11}C]-PK-11195 and PET (Bartels et al. 2010). The study failed to demonstrate a decrease in microglial activation with therapy, but similar imaging methods might be utilized in the future (especially in small pilot trials) for assessing specific drug mechanisms of action and efficacy.

CONCLUSION

Imaging has been utilized in PD clinical trials to investigate both symptomatic and potentially disease-modifying therapies. Most of these trials have focused on dopaminergic imaging as a secondary outcome measure, though other modalities such as FDG PET have also been utilized. Some of these studies have raised doubts about the utility of these measures because of contradicting imaging and clinical outcomes. Nonetheless, imaging may provide important insights into the efficacy (or lack thereof) of new therapies. Increasingly, imaging is being utilized in early-phase clinical trials to provide supplemental neurophysiological evidence of efficacy, potentially where imaging is of greatest value. As new imaging modalities become more widely available, they are likely to be increasingly used in

whereas characteristic abnormalities in CBD include asymmetric *hypo*metabolism in the hemispheric cortex and striatum contralateral to the more affected limbs (Hosaka et al. 2002; Nagahama et al. 1997; Eidelberg et al. 1991). While identification of the characteristic abnormalities can be used to assist in the diagnosis of individual patients (Antonini et al. 1997; Foster et al. 1988; Otsuka et al. 1991), more subtle abnormalities often require further quantitative analysis, such as SPM (Ghaemi et al. 2002; Hosaka et al. 2002). In addition, although FDG PET is commonly available, neuroradiologists with experience in movement disorders-specific abnormalities are rare, even at many academic medical centers.

When available, quantitative methods for analyzing FDG PET data can be used to help diagnose parkinsonian patients. These techniques are particularly useful when visual metabolic abnormalities are inconclusive or when experienced neuroradiologists are not accessible. Using single case SPM techniques, several investigators have been able to diagnose individual patients with reasonable accuracy (Juh et al. 2005a; Juh et al. 2005b; Hosaka et al. 2002). The largest series of 135 patients was studied by Eckert et al. (2005), who developed disease-specific statistical map templates from patients clinically diagnosed with IPD, MSA, PSP, and CBD. Individual patients were then prospectively studied by determining a patient-specific map of regional increases or decreases in glucose metabolism, compared to a control group (Figure 1). This patient-specific map was visually compared to the disease-specific templates for each disease to determine the patient diagnosis. Using this technique, they found that non-expert readers correctly categorized 92.4% of scans, compared to the clinical diagnosis after follow-up. While these disease-specific templates are readily available (Eckert et al. 2005; Eckert et al. 2007), there are several drawbacks to this technique. For one, this method requires some degree of technical expertise for image processing of the patient-specific maps. In addition, the final diagnosis is aided by the disease-specific templates but is still ultimately dependent on visual comparison of the patient map to the disease-specific templates. Finally, the disease-specific templates were developed using patients diagnosed after two years of clinical follow-up, but autopsy confirmation of the clinical diagnosis was available in only two patients.

A second quantitative technique available to aid in clinical diagnosis involves the use of disease-specific covariance patterns of individual parkinsonian syndromes. Disease-specific patterns have been developed for IPD, MSA, and PSP by applying a multivariate statistical technique termed principle component analysis to FDG PET images (Eidelberg 2009). There is evidence to suggest that the spatial topography of these patterns is linked to neuronal activity at critical modulatory sites for basal ganglia output (Trost et al. 2006; Lin et al. 2008), and it is therefore likely that each covariance pattern represents the abnormal network organization associated with each disease. For example, the Parkinson's disease-related spatial covariance pattern (PDRP) is characterized by increased pallidothalamic and pontine metabolic activity associated with relative metabolic reductions in the premotor cortex, supplementary motor area (SMA), and parietal association areas (Figure 2) (Eidelberg et al. 1994; Eidelberg et al. 1997; Spetsieris and Eidelberg 2011). The MSA-related pattern (MSARP) is characterized by bilateral metabolic decreases in the putamen and the cerebellum (see Chapter 8) (Eckert et al. 2008). Finally, the PSP-related pattern (PSPRP) is characterized by metabolic decreases predominantly in the upper brainstem and medial prefrontal cortex as well as in the medial thalamus, the caudate nuclei, the anterior cingulate area, the ventrolateral prefrontal cortex, and the frontal eye fields (Eckert et al. 2008). The subject score is the degree to which a single subject expresses one of these patterns and can be calculated prospectively in new patients (Eidelberg 2009). Several studies have shown that patients with IPD, MSA, and PSP have increased expression of their respective disease-related patterns compared to age-matched controls (Figure 3) (Eckert et al. 2008; Ma et al. 2007). These findings suggest that elevated expression of a specific disease-related pattern could potentially be used in individual patients to discriminate between parkinsonian syndromes.

More recent studies have shown that simultaneously applying multiple patterns to the same patient population can be used to accurately differentiate specific syndromes in early symptomatic parkinsonian patients (Spetsieris et al. 2009; Tang et al. 2010). Tang et al. (2010) developed a computer-based automated algorithm to classify 167 undiagnosed parkinsonian patients using multiple disease-related patterns with a logistic regression model. Image-based classification was then compared to the final clinical diagnosis established on average 2.6 years after imaging and autopsy confirmation of the clinical diagnosis was available in nine patients. For the diagnosis of IPD, this technique had 84% sensitivity, 97% specificity, 98% positive predictive value (PPV), and 82% negative predictive value (NPV). Imaging classification was also highly accurate for MSA (85% sensitivity, 96% specificity, 97% PPV, and 83% NPV) and PSP (88% sensitivity, 94% specificity, 91% PPV, and 92% NPV). This approach has several advantages. First, it is fully automated and does not require visual interpretation

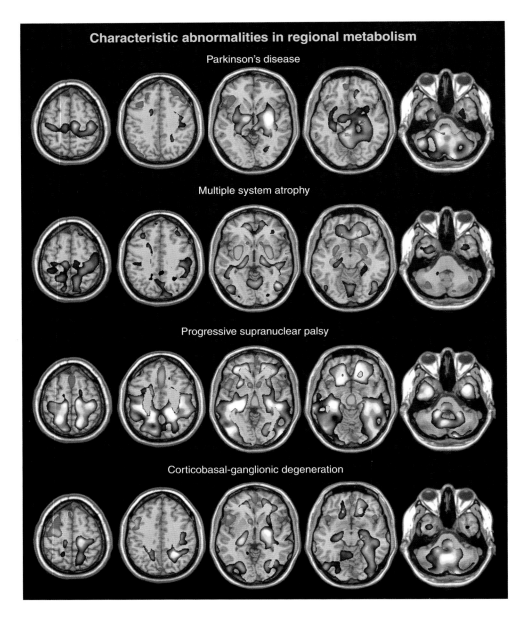

Figure 1 Characteristic patterns of abnormal regional glucose metabolism in Parkinson's disease (IPD), multiple system atrophy (MSA), progressive supranuclear palsy (PSP), and corticobasal degeneration (CBD). The images were obtained using SPM to compare eight patients in each diagnostic category with 10 healthy control subjects. [The red-yellow scale displays relative increases and the blue-green scale displays relative decreases in glucose metabolism for the patient groups relative to controls. Results are overlaid onto a T1 MRI template image.] [Reprinted from Eckert T, Edwards C. The application of network mapping in differential diagnosis of parkinsonian disorders. Clinical Neuroscience Research. 2007;6:359–66. Page 362 Figure 1.]

of the FDG PET data. Second, it was specifically designed to differentiate the three most common final diagnoses in patients presenting with symptoms of nonspecific parkinsonism, namely IPD, MSA, and PSP (Hughes et al. 2002). Third, the initial analysis more broadly distinguishes between IPD and atypical parkinsonian syndrome. This provides the clinician with the most important diagnostic distinction, i.e., IPD versus a non-IPD cause of parkinsonism, before specifically classifying atypical patients as MSA or PSP.

In summary, FDG PET is a readily available imaging modality that can be used by the clinician to help diagnose specific parkinsonian syndromes in individual patients presenting with a bradykinetic rigidity syndrome. Depending on availability, several quantitative techniques have also been developed to further improve the diagnostic

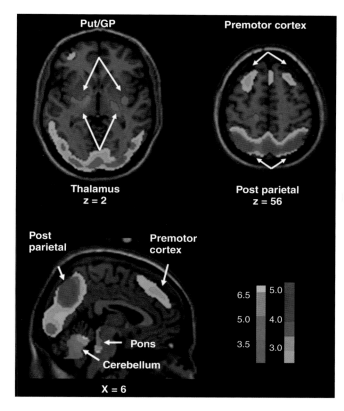

Figure 2 Parkinson's disease-related spatial covariance pattern (PDRP). PD-related motor pattern (PDRP) characterized by pallidothalamic, pontine, and motor cortical hypermetabolism, associated with relative metabolic reductions in the lateral premotor and posterior parietal areas. [The spatial covariance pattern is overlaid on T1-weighted MR-template images. The displays represent regions that contributed significantly to the network and that were demonstrated to be reliable by bootstrap resampling. Relative metabolic increases are color-coded red to yellow; relative metabolic decreases are color-coded blue to purple.] [Reprinted from Ma, Y., C. Tang, P. G. Spetsieris et al. 2007 *J Cereb Blood Flow Metab*: Figure 1A, page 600.]

accuracy of FDG PET, particularly in patients with early symptoms.

PATIENTS WITH TREMOR

Tremor is one of the cardinal features of IPD. However, the differential diagnosis in a patient who presents with isolated tremor is different than that in a patient who presents with a bradykinetic rigidity syndrome. Specifically, drug-induced tremor, ET, and dystonic tremor (DT) are the leading causes of tremor besides IPD (Table 1). Other, less common causes of tremor include orthostatic tremor (OT) and psychogenic tremor. In this section, we will discuss how functional imaging techniques may be used to aid in the

diagnosis of a patient who presents with a primary tremor syndrome.

The only neurodegenerative disorder likely to cause an isolated tremor syndrome is IPD. In patients with other neurodegenerative movement disorders, such as MSA, PSP, and CBD, tremor is usually present only in the setting of more severe bradykinesia, rigidity, or cerebellar symptoms (Williams et al. 2005; Williams and Lees 2009; Geser et al. 2006). In IPD, however, isolated tremor can often be the presenting clinical feature and can precede the onset of bradykinesia and rigidity by several years or decades (Chaudhuri et al. 2005). Tremor in early IPD is classically described as asymmetric and occurring at rest. By contrast, ET tremor is predominantly symmetric and usually occurs with action and posture (Brennan et al. 2002; Poston, Rios, and Louis 2009). In individual patients with atypical tremor, such as asymmetric postural tremor or mixed postural and rest tremor, the clinical distinction between IPD and ET can be challenging (Cohen et al. 2003; Louis et al. 2008). Indeed, clinical studies have suggested that tremor characteristics alone, such as distribution, frequency, and evolution of tremor, are not sufficient for accurate diagnosis (Cohen et al. 2003; Rajput, Robinson, and Rajput 2004; Louis 2005). However, accurate diagnosis in these patients is critical since medication selection, patient counseling, and disease prognosis differ between these syndromes.

Despite the clinical overlap between IPD, ET, and other tremor disorders, the underlying pathophysiology for IPD is unique (Louis et al. 2009; Louis et al. 2005; Braak and Braak 2000). Specifically, neuronal degeneration within the nigrostriatal pathway leads to the primary motor symptoms in IPD, whereas other tremor disorders, such as ET, are associated with preserved neurons and dopamine terminals within this pathway (Louis et al. 2007). Thus, nuclear medicine imaging of the nigrostriatal dopamine terminals can be used to help differentiate IPD from non-degenerative tremor disorders. Indeed, studies using PET and SPECT radioligands to examine the integrity of striatal presynaptic dopamine neurons have reported abnormal radioligand uptake in patients with well-established IPD and in those with early IPD symptoms, when compared with healthy control subjects (Asenbaum et al. 1998; Huang et al. 2001). While some studies suggest that a normal dopamine scan essentially rules out the diagnosis of IPD (Haapaniemi et al. 2001; Schwarz et al. 2000), 5.7% to 14.7% of patients clinically diagnosed with early IPD have normal dopamine imaging and are termed "scans without evidence of dopaminergic deficit" (SWEDDs) (Fahn et al. 2004; Whone et al. 2003; Van Laere et al. 2004a; The Parkinson Study Group 2002). While it is possible that SWEDDs represent

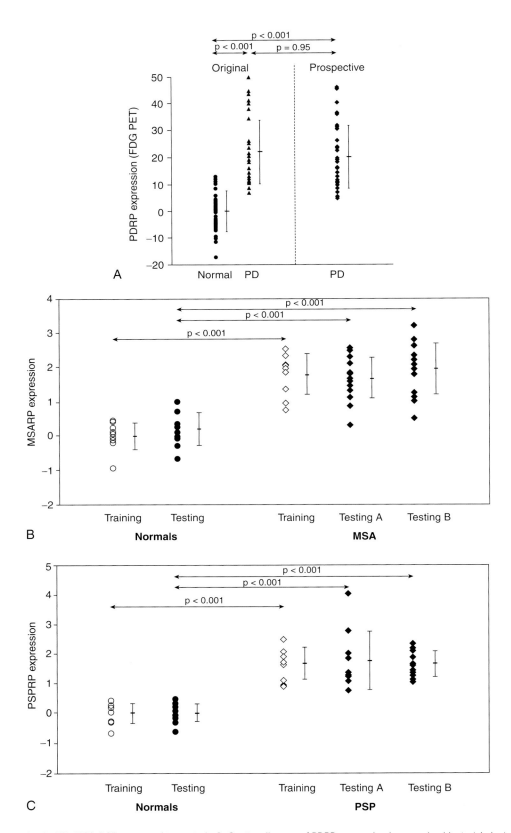

Figure 3 Pattern expression in IPD, MSA, PSP compared to controls **A.** Scatter diagram of PDRP expression in normal subjects (circles) and IPD patients (triangles). PDRP expression (subject scores) was increased in the IPD patients (p < 0.001) relative to the normal subjects. Network expression remained high in a new group of IPD patients (diamonds) (p < 0.001) not included in the identification of the PDRP. Error bars represent standard

(Continued)